Ethics *of* Health Care

A Guide for Clinical Practice
Third Edition

Raymond S. Edge, EdD, RRT
Dean, School of Health Professions (Retired)
Maryville University – Saint Louis
Saint Louis, Missouri

John Randall Groves, PhD
Professor of Humanities
Ferris State University
Big Rapids, Michigan

THOMSON
★
DELMAR LEARNING

Australia   Canada   Mexico   Singapore   Spain   United Kingdom   United States

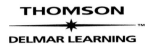

THOMSON

™

DELMAR LEARNING

Ethics of Health Care: A Guide for Clinical Practice, Third Edition

Raymond S. Edge, EdD, RRT and John Randall Groves, PhD

Vice President, Health Care Business Unit:
William Brottmiller

Editorial Director:
Cathy L. Esperti

Acquisitions Editor:
Marah Bellegarde

Editorial Assistant:
Jadin Babin-Kavanaugh

Marketing Director:
Jennifer McAvey

Marketing Coordinator:
Michelle Gleason

Art and Design Specialist:
Alex Vasilakos

Production Coordinator:
Jessica McNavich

Project Editor:
Ruth Fisher

Library of Congress Cataloging-in-Publication Data

Edge, Raymond S.
    Ethics of health care : a guide for clinical practice / Raymond S. Edge, John Randall Groves.—3rd ed.
        p. cm.
    Includes index.
    Includes bibliographical references and index.
    ISBN-13: 978-1-4018-6183-4
    ISBN-10: 1-4018-6183-0
    1. Medical ethics.   I. Groves, John Randall. II. Title.
    RZ24.E27 2005
    174.2—dc22
                            2005048646

Notice to the Reader

This book is dedicated to the practitioners who struggle with these issues on a daily basis. We hope that the students who read this book will join you better prepared to help you shape the future of health care.

Contents

Preface

If only there were evil people somewhere insidiously committing evil deeds and it were necessary only to separate them from the rest of us and destroy them. But the line dividing good and evil cuts through the heart of every human being.

Alexander Solzhenitsyn, *The Gulag Archipelago*

This text is written with allied health practitioners and nurses in mind. These specialties provide over 80 percent of the health care delivery in the United States and are often faced with dilemmas for which they have no previous educational background or experience. Not only must they deal with the ethical problems in regard to their own actions but also they must function as members of a health care team, offering opinions, advice, and leadership. It is for this reason that the text is focused broadly on the vast array of health professionals (rather than a single specialty), whose professionalism and practice require them to assume a greater role in shaping the ethics of health care.

In their books *In Search of Excellence* and *A Passion for Excellence,* Tom Peters and Robert Waterman state that the first step to excellence is caring. While prevention and curing provide the major focus for much of our technical training, the caring aspects of health provision are the major concern of this text. As practitioners, we have a great need for the development and furthering of the value of caring for our patients, our practice, and ourselves. However, just being concerned is not enough; concern must be translated into appropriate language and actions. Much of this book is dedicated to teaching the language of biomedical ethics and the critical thinking skills needed to deal with these issues.

Ethical decision making is a complex task. Practitioners must deal with facts, concepts, basic principles, and people. They must make decisions in an arena of passion, prejudice, and ambiguity. Regardless of the complexities, however, the fact remains that if we as health care professionals are to be listened to as members of the health care team, it will be because we can support our views. Emotion alone, even if intensely felt and forcefully expressed in regard to an ethical problem, will not be enough to persuade others of the cogency of our views. The value attributed to our advice and decision will be based directly on the reasoning that we have invested in the deliberative process.

ORGANIZATION

In this third edition, several chapters have been retitled and new sections added to reflect the current environment of health care practice. The Introduction at the beginning of the text has been strengthened (with objectives, key points, and case studies) to allow it to serve as a separate educational unit. The focus of the material is the need for new clinicians to gain an understanding and mastery of the legal, professional etiquette, and ethical dimensions of practice. As in the previous editions, Chapters 1 through 4 provide the needed background foundation for the study of value development and ethical theories as they relate to health care practice. The reader is expected to gain an understanding of the basic principles involved in health care ethics, as well as to become familiar with the language and decision-making processes with which these issues are examined. These initial chapters review value development, decision-making formats, basic principles, and the nature of rights.

Chapter 5 provides an examination of the principle of confidentiality. Current health care team practice creates a situation in which, on the average, over seventy-five different practitioners have legitimate access to a single patient's health record. Many of these providers have cost-containment and reporting functions rather than patient care as their major concerns. In the modern environment of electronic data, increased need-to-know categories, and loss of general privacy in our lives, confidentiality becomes a difficult principle to uphold. Included in the updated chapter materials is information regarding the federal Health Insurance Portability and Accountability Act of 1996 (HIPAA) and human subject research.

Chapter 6 examines the issues of role fidelity and the requirements of professional practice. How does the nature of our specialties affect the requirements of ethical practice? Issues such as disparagement of colleagues, sexual involvement with patients, scope of practice, whistle-blowing, and self-referral are examined in the light of current practice. Additional materials regarding practices categorized as "gaming the system" have been added to this edition.

Chapter 7 discusses the nature of patient autonomy and how it often conflicts with our desire as health professionals to make decisions for our patients. The chapter provides information regarding the elements of informed consent, standards of disclosure, and competency determination. Additional material regarding the problems associated with patient demand for futile care has been added to this edition.

Chapter 8 examines the principle of justice as it relates to the fair and equitable distribution of health care in our society. Spiraling costs, ineffective efforts toward cost containment, and increasing levels of maldistribution of health care benefits have combined to make the principle of justice perhaps the most critical issue in health delivery today. As health care providers, we are being asked to serve many masters, and it is often difficult to remain true to our patient advocacy and focus while implementing cost containment strategies. The chapter provides a focus on decision making in macro and micro allocation of scarce resources and examines a variety of proposed distribution models.

The focus of Chapter 9 is an examination of the issues involved in withholding and withdrawing life support, and Chapter 10 presents the current status of legislation involving the modern euthanasia movement. Additional materials regarding the critical shortage of organ donations and current legislation regarding physician-assisted suicide have been added to this new edition. These chapters will be of most use to those involved in intensive and emergency care.

Chapter 11, which in earlier editions dealt only with the examination of the debate surrounding abortion, has been retitled and new sections added to cover the issues involved in human reproduction. New sections examine in vitro fertilization and surrogacy.

Chapter 12 retains as its emphasis and title the subject of AIDS and examines the ethical problems associated with this disease. The AIDS focus serves as a historical case study examining professional conduct during this epidemic. However, perhaps more important, the struggle to deal with AIDS also serves as an effective metaphor or cautionary tale as to professional conduct in all epidemics when we must struggle to answer such questions as whether there is a "duty to treat," a "duty to warn," a need for "mandatory screening," and "what is to be done with an infected practitioner." We are living in a rapidly shrinking world in which an outbreak of a new disease in any part of the world could rapidly be transmitted anywhere. Additional materials have also been added to examine the problem of "lifeboat ethics." What is the duty of an advanced and rich nation such as the United States in regard to epidemics in developing parts of the world, where the resources to handle an epidemic effectively appear inadequate?

Chapter 13 examines the issues involved with the advances in genetic science and the potential for biological manipulation. This is a powerful arena of change, and new questions must be answered as we appear to be approaching a historical watershed when humanity will not only be able to determine how we are going to live but even who we are going to be. New materials have been added that address the issues of stem cell research, the genetic causes of behavior, and theories regarding posthumanism. J. Rostand perhaps best described our current situation in his 1939 book *Pensées d'un Biologiste:* "Science has made us Gods, before we are even worthy of being men."

Chapter 14, previously titled "Transcultural Health," has been retitled "Culturally Appropriate Health Care." The emphasis of the chapter, however, remains the same. In our nation of immigrants, health care providers must not only celebrate diversity but seek to understand that in a society such as ours, many times the provider and the patient will have different perspectives regarding the nature of wellness, health, and health care provision. If not recognized and overcome, these differences in perspective can lead to the unwanted results of inadequate patient care. Health care is not a one-size-fits-all business, and no culture or health care tradition possesses the totality of truth. The chapter provides a review of two very strong ancient health care traditions, that of China and India, and examines how practitioners and clients from these cultures might view health care. A new section has been added that examines the Islamic faith and how Western health care providers might be of more assistance to patients with this background.

We acknowledge that any chapter that attempts to deal with the ethical imperatives associated with the provision of culturally appropriate health care must in the end be inadequate, given the vastness of the subject area. In a nation such as ours, all practitioners must come to understand that they will be serving a multicultural clientele with very different perspectives from the majority culture in regard to health, and that failing to understand and accommodate these differences can be detrimental to the process. It is our hope that Chapter 14 will serve to stimulate in the reader a desire to continue this study.

Throughout the text, we provide examples of the questions that practitioners are currently facing. For this edition, case studies have been added throughout the work to enhance understanding of the issues and provide opportunities for decision making. Where necessary, the reader will be provided with a background of the legal aspects of the issues. Ours is a litigious society, and although good law may at times promote reprehensible practice, it is important to understand the current legal positions that have an impact on health care decisions. Americans have a great respect for the law, and when there is disagreement, we often seek legal clarification, even for issues involving individual values.

FEATURES

Objectives and Review Exercises: Each chapter begins with instructional objectives designed to focus the reader. Review questions at the chapter's end encourage the reader to explore the theoretical positions found in the material and to practice decision making.

Key Terms: A list of key terms is provided for each chapter These terms are set in boldface type at first occurrence in the text to help the students focus on important concepts.

Case Studies: These scenarios are found throughout the chapters and are followed by critical thinking questions that encourage synthesizing of information.

Key Concepts: Key concepts have been added at the conclusion of each chapter. This list will allow the reader to gain a quick overview of the important ideas found in the unit.

Glossary: A glossary has been added at the end of the book for easy reference.

ALSO AVAILABLE FOR THE INSTRUCTOR!

Electronic Classroom Manager to Accompany Ethics of Health Care: A Guide for Clinical Practice is a robust, computerized tool for your instructional needs! A must-have for all instructors, this comprehensive and convenient CD-ROM contains:

- An **Instructor Manual** with a sample syllabus, critical thinking study questions, Internet research activities, role-playing exercises, and lecture notes.

- The **ExamView Computerized Test Bank** contains over 550 questions. You can use these questions to create your own review materials or tests. The software allows you to use the questions as is, customize the questions, or add your own.

- The **PowerPoint Presentation,** containing 200 slides, is designed to help you in planning your class presentations.

Acknowledgments

The authors wish to thank all those who have assisted with this text in the areas of reading, critiquing, and arguing for change. Perhaps the greatest assistance in this has been our students. We have refined and shaped the clarification exercises within our classes over the years, and therefore we owe our students a great debt for their tolerance. Marilyn Edge made an important contribution: her grammar sense and attention to detail has made the text eminently more readable. All failure in this regard should be attributed to her husband, who rarely likes to be told he is wrong.

A sincere debt of gratitude is owed to Gary Packingham for his cartoons found in this and previous editions of the text. The concepts behind the cartoons are excellent and unfortunately show how little progress we have made in this critical area, given that they are still as relevant as they were ten years ago, when we included them in the first edition of the text.

A special personal debt is owed to Dr. Robert Francoeur whose own text on the subject was the original model for our book. His years of patient mentoring, friendship, and personal kindness are much appreciated.

No list of those we wish to acknowledge would be complete without the name of Marah Bellegarde, who served as editor for this project. We appreciate your vision, which has made this edition ever so much more than it would have been without you. We also appreciate your voice of calm when deadlines were pressing.

A special thank you to the reviewers of this edition:

Marilyn Bennett, PhD
College of St. Catherine
St. Paul, Minnesota

Patti Biro, M. Ed
Del Mar College
Corpus Christi, Texas

Cindy Farrar, MBA
Del Mar College
Corpus Christi, Texas

Suzanne Tuthill, PhD
Del Tech Community College
Wilmington, Delaware

Robert L. Von Kanel, RN, MSN
Ivy Tech State College
Sellersberg, Indiana

Finally, as with all materials of this nature, many of our ideas for cases and problems have been borrowed and adapted from sources hidden within the mists of long discussions into a thousand evenings. To these sources we must add our thanks in the nature of the immortal words of Blanche DuBois: "Whoever you are—I have always depended upon the kindness of strangers."*

---

*Tennessee Williams, *A Streetcar Named Desire*.

Introduction

GOAL

At the end of this introductory material, the student should understand the need for the health professional to develop both the science and professional conduct aspects of his or her craft.

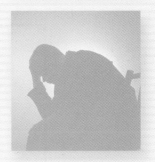

OBJECTIVES

Upon completion of this chapter, the reader should be able to:

1. Explain the dual nature of health care practice and the need to match clinical expertise with appropriate professional behaviors.

2. Explain how an individual's worldview will shape his or her decision making in the arena of morals and values.

3. Compare and contrast the professional conduct areas of ethics, law, and etiquette.

4. Define *nihilism, relativism,* and *hedonism,* and explain why each of these philosophical positions provides an inadequate basis for ethical decision making for the health care provider.

5. Compare and contrast the sanctions associated with inappropriate legal, ethical, and professional etiquette conduct.

6. Evaluate a series of ethical dilemmas using his or her specialty's code of ethical conduct.

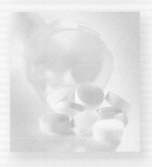

7. Identify a source for his or her profession's code of ethical conduct, and provide an analysis of its strengths and weaknesses.

8. Define *standpoint theory,* and explain why it is useful when considering ethical dilemmas.

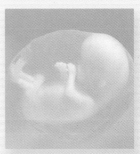

KEY TERMS

Ethical dilemmas	**Legal requirements**	**Standpoint theory**
Ethical, legal,	**Nihilism**	**Value**
professional etiquette	**Professional ethics**	**Worldview**
Hedonism	**Relativism**	

Every man should expend his chief thought and attention on his first principles; are they or are they not rightly laid down? And when he has duly sifted them, all the rest will follow.

Socrates, Greek philosopher (496–399 B.C.)

What Should You Do?

1. When, if ever, is it permissible to take a gift or gratuity from a patient?

2. When it is legitimate and perhaps mandatory to break a patient's confidence?

3. Is it permissible to lie to a client if it is for his or her own good?

4. Can I work in a hospital and refer patients to a durable medical supply company that I have contracted with to provide outpatient equipment orientation services?

5. What should I do if I make a medication error that no one else knows about but it appears harmless to my patient?

6. What obligations do I have to a colleague and fellow practitioner when I suspect that the colleague I am working with is abusing alcohol or appears chemically impaired while on duty?

7. What if I come upon a practice that is legal but appears to me personally to be unethical?

There are many occupations that one may choose, but few will find their choices as rewarding, engaging, exciting, meaningful, frustrating, and overwhelming as those who take up the practice of health care provision. Health care practice is the best of science, the noblest of human arts, and offers careers that never stop growing, challenging, and providing opportunities for personal development.

If one were to examine the health care team prior to the twentieth century, one would find few assigned practitioner roles. The role of the physician, dentist, nurse, and pharmacist was reasonably well established though evolving. During the twentieth century, as a result of technological and therapeutic advances, over 100 specialists were added to the health care team under the umbrella title known as *allied health*. Some of these specialists, such as physical therapists and dietitians, are well known to the public, while others (cytologists, extracorporeal perfusionists, athletic trainers, and music therapists) provide meaningful services but are virtually unknown outside their specialty areas. The growth of the allied health specialties is an important aspect of American health care as they, along with nursing personnel, provide over 80 percent of the direct patient care.

To enter the practice of health care provision is to enter into a social compact not only with the patients you serve but with all other practitioners and the community at large. The honoring of this social compact will require a commitment to excellence in clinical practice and a commitment to a set of appropriate **legal, ethical**, and **professional etiquette** behaviors. For those that meet these obligations, the practice of health care is personally and fiscally rewarding. At a foundational level, this book is designed to assist you in gaining an understanding of the ethical aspects found within this important social compact and to assist you in advancing your career.

Often in clinical practice the appropriate answer is the product of evaluating, understanding, and using scientific information. Many of the clinical questions have been reduced to formulas, and when one plugs in the appropriate stroke volume, tidal volume, rectal temperature, or whatever data you are collecting a reproducible answer comes forward. This is the science of our practice, and advances in health technologies and therapeutics have brought the practice of health care from folk nostrums to magic bullets. And, as it has been said, "the best is yet to come."

Prior to the twentieth century, the patient had less than an even chance of benefiting from an encounter with a physician. Often early health care practitioners had little else to offer than a caring attitude as they sat by the beds of the afflicted and watched disease processes run their course. In the last hundred years, many of the dreaded diseases that plagued humankind for ages have been brought under control. Some have been eradicated. Yet for all the advances of the past century, it appears that even greater wonders lie ahead. Will the puzzle of cancer be solved? Will genetic engineering allow us to live longer and healthier? What are the future implications of the technology of cloning? Will we find the mechanisms for aging and have the longevity of Methuselah? Where will the science of health care take us in this new century?

The wonders of scientific advances are not just interesting questions that exist in a vacuum but rather have implications for our practices, patients, the health of our communities, and the very fabric of our common humanity. The uses of science and technology in health care must always be assessed. We must not only ask where the science of health care will take us but whether we really want to go there.

The practice of health care goes well beyond technical competence: all practitioners must also attend to the legal, ethical, and professional etiquette requirements of their roles.

Practitioners who fail to master these duties will be a continual frustration to those who must work with them and will find themselves facing sanctions for their activities.

We can think of our legal requirements for practice as the need to follow a set of principles and processes by which the people within a society settle disputes and problems without resorting to force or violence. In some sense, law can be considered the minimum standard of expected performance between individuals in a society. To ensure that practitioners abide by this lowest standard, many codes of professional ethics contain rules that require us to stay within the law in our professional conduct. An example is the American Medical Association's (AMA) 1996 Code of Medical Ethics, Current Opinions:

> A physician shall respect the law and also recognize a responsibility to seek changes in those requirements which are contrary to the best interests of the patient.[1]

The AMA's clarification statement regarding the relationship between law and ethics holds that while ethical values and legal principles are usually closely related, ethical obligations typically exceed legal duties. In general, when practitioners believe a law is unjust, they should work within the system to change the law.

The professional etiquette requirements of our roles in health care are usually based on the traditions of good practice and good manners. In our personal lives, social etiquette provides answers to questions such as "How long do I have to write a thank-you note after someone has given me a gift?" or "When I am invited to dinner, must I wait for the host to begin eating before I begin?" Professional etiquette involves issues such as the need to avoid talking badly about another practitioner, especially to patients, or the need to stay within the role boundaries of our specialty. Rules of etiquette help those involved in health care provision maintain order and civility. Often professional development classes discuss these issues, and when you begin practice, more mature practitioners will mentor you in the obligations of professional etiquette. These rules typically are not written or codified, but a practitioner who breaks them can face serious consequences.

Like rules of professional etiquette, health care ethics are also designed to promote order and maintain civility. However, there is a major difference: with ethics, you are not just dealing with something that could be considered bad manners; instead, you are dealing with the rights and welfare of other people. Individuals who do not master the skills of professional courtesy and decorum are considered boorish and rude, and where possible, others will avoid them. When practitioners fail to maintain an appropriate standard of professional ethics, the level of harm is more serious because they have infringed on the rights of others. Table I-1 differentiates the types of sanctions commonly associated with lapses in appropriate legal, ethical, and professional etiquette. Note that a single act could have consequences that involve an individual's ethical, legal, and professional standing.

For most of us, to clone or not to clone is not the question. Our practices will be filled with far more mundane ethical dilemmas. Consider the following case.

CASE STUDY

Mr. Franke and the Dilantin Prescription

Mr. Franke, a school bus driver for the high school, has seen his physician and received a prescription for Dilantin (medication used to control epileptic seizures). After the visit, he stopped at the clinic reception desk to arrange for the next scheduled visit and inadvertently left his prescription as he walked off. As he was leaving the waiting room, the medical assistant noted the prescription and called after him. "Mr. Franke, don't forget your Dilantin prescription." Several other individuals in the waiting room overheard the remark.

1. Does the health care provider have a legal, ethical, or professional etiquette problem?
2. Is it possible to be in a situation where one action causes problems in the three areas of legal, ethical, and etiquette requirements?

TABLE I-1

Sanctions Associated with Lapse in Ethical, Legal, or Professional Etiquette

AREA	JUDGMENT	SANCTION
Ethical conduct	Right or wrong	• Loss of professional reputation • Loss of professional consortium • Personal remorse
Legal Requirements	Legal or illegal	• Loss of professional reputation • Loss of professional consortium • Punishment as prescribed by law
Professional etiquette	Proper or improper	• Loss of professional respect and fellowship

Unlike matters of science and clinical practice, in which the scientific method will often reveal reproducible answers, the answers to questions regarding legal, ethical, and etiquette issues are not subject to comfortable formulas. Often you will come to an answer with which there is little agreement. In this text, we focus on decision making in health care ethics. Health care ethics reside in the realm of human **values,** morals, individual culture, intense personal beliefs, and faith. Often the individual finds the answer not by examining and substantiating the external facts but by checking within her particular **worldview.**

Questions involving ethical positions are often intensely felt by those involved. These discussions reach to the very heart of our perceptions of ourselves as individuals. Practitioners quickly become aware that the value given to their opinions is directly linked to the quality of the reasoning and rationales that they can provide for them. Specialists who know that something is wrong but cannot articulate their reasons or the methods by which they derived their beliefs are at a real disadvantage. They fail to provide appropriate advocacy for their ideas or the patients they serve, and they also inflict stress and discomfort upon themselves and their colleagues.

One of the frustrating aspects of reasoning through these questions is that people you know and respect will often come to different opinions regarding the best answer. Because values are not subject to scientific analysis or deal with areas that are easily quantifiable, value arguments are deeply felt and rarely won. Because of their personal nature, those who disagree with your personal value system are often not only classified as being wrong but are also somehow evil in their wrongness. Consider the two sides currently involved in the abortion debate.

Yet you are entering professions where there is an abundance of value questions that must be dealt with daily. As professionals, even in our opposition our standing up for our position—and, if necessary, our becoming a majority of one—it is important that we remain constructive and appropriate in our actions.

To acknowledge that individuals can have different opinions on ethical issues is not the same as saying that all opinions are equal and have the same worth and credibility. In health care there are decisions that must not be made. Whereas tolerance is generally considered a virtue, there are actions that must not be tolerated.

There are some who subscribe to a philosophy of moral **nihilism**. They believe that there are no moral truths, no moral facts, no moral knowledge or responsibilities. For those who hold this position, nothing can truly be wrong or right in a moral sense. For the moral nihilist, morality, like religion, is a mere illusion. If you followed this reasoning to its conclusion, heinous acts such as the rape and torture of children would not necessarily be wrong. This is, fortunately, a position that most would feel uncomfortable in accepting.

A moderate form of nihilism is ethical **relativism**, which holds that morality is relative to the society in which one is brought up. In this sense, nothing can truly be right or wrong without a consideration of the culture and social context. Ethical relativists go beyond just recognizing differences between cultures, and hold that in questions of morality, rightness or wrongness is always relative to and determined by culture.

Others ground their personal philosophy solely in a **hedonistic** worldview. Their major guideposts for decision making are desire and aversion, and nothing can be right or wrong apart from them. This attitude of self-absorption was captured in the slogan, "He who dies with the most toys wins." Figure I-1 lists the values associated with this worldview. Gross, personal self-interest provides an inadequate framework for ethical decision making in health care. In health care provision, an attitude of "anything goes" is unacceptable.

One useful concept that helps avoid the problems of self-interest in deciding ethical issues is **standpoint theory**. This theory holds that one should always try to adopt or listen to the standpoint of the most marginalized and vulnerable persons involved. This is similar to the "walk a mile in their shoes" advice. While it may be impossible for you to truly understand the position of the addicted woman who takes drugs while pregnant, or the pregnant prostitute who refuses to be tested for AIDS, even when the knowledge would be useful in helping her fetus avoid the infection, it is a useful exercise, especially when you are making judgments about their behaviors.

To involve ourselves in unethical practice harms the patients we serve; by association it harms all fellow practitioners; and in that it lowers the level of trust and esteem in which health care providers are held, it harms the community at large. An analogy is that health care practice can be considered a community commons. All practitioners in the community use the field and are responsible for its continued upkeep. It is unthinkable and unwise to believe that the

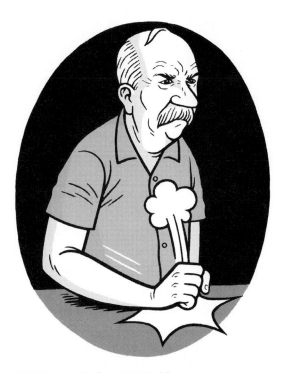

Happiness
Self-aggrandizement
Maneuverability
Pleasure
Power
Self-preservation
Security
Absence of pain

FIGURE I-1   Hedonistic Worldview

maintenance of the health care commons is the responsibility of some other group of practitioners. The obligations to provide ethical care, refine the quality of practice, and provide community service are the obligations not of the few but of the many. It is our privilege to labor in the community commons; it is our obligation to maintain the space so that we can come again, and when we finally leave, leave the commons healthy so that others can replace us in the labor. Nothing damages the health care commons more than unethical practice.

As health care practitioners, we are responsible for our personal ethics and for that of our colleagues. As a member of a professional group, you take on the obligation to be a peer to others on the health care team. Some of these obligations can be considered gatekeeping functions, where you look out for the interests of the profession and others in similar practice.

One of the basic criteria for a profession is that it is self-regulating. A significant part of these processes is our professional codes of ethics, which are an attempt to regulate the conduct of practitioners within a specialty. However, most professional codes are vague and incomplete as to duties and prohibitions. It will be a rare exception when a practitioner involved in a health care ethics dilemma can find the correct answer by just reading the professional code, although it is not a bad place to start.

Health care practice is rapidly evolving. A book that provided the answers to ethical questions would provide the reader with only yesterday's solutions. Part of the evolution of health care is that things are changing so rapidly that even if we knew yesterday's answers, we would find that the questions have changed. This book then cannot be an answer book but is dedicated to asking the right questions.

Questions regarding health care ethics rarely have easy answers; in fact, there are no easy answers. If the answers were easy, these problems would not be called ethical dilemmas. This book will provide you with sufficient background and the right questions to ask when examining these issues.

Figure I-2 lists the important mental attributes needed to reason through ethical dilemmas.[2] Ethical humility is perhaps the most important. At the very minimum, you will need to develop

- **Ethical humility**—awareness of the limits of one's own ethical insights
- **Ethical courage**—willingness to assess fairly ideas, beliefs, and viewpoints differing from our own
- **Ethical empathy**—a willingness to attempt to understand the opinions of others and try to see the issue from their position
- **Ethical fair-mindedness**—to hold one's own beliefs and opinions to the same standard of proof and evidence that we require for the opinions of others

FIGURE I-2   Essential Mental Attributes

enough humility in regard to your own opinions and enough moral imagination to at least leave open the possibility that your initial reaction to issues presented may be wrong.

The first several chapters of this text provide you with the background knowledge and skills needed to examine health care ethics issues and formulate your own solutions. The final chapters examine several major issues under consideration by practitioners for which answers are still being formulated. What is the best method for a just nation to distribute scarce health care resources? Is there a right to health care? What issues are involved in the discussions regarding abortion, right to die, genetics, and experimental research using humans? As health care providers, the answers that we come to regarding these issues will speak volumes about the nature of our professions and us.

CONCLUSION

The value placed on our opinions as allied health and nursing personnel will not be determined by how intensely we feel about an issue or how loud our voice is, but rather by the quality of our reasoning. Ethical decision making is a complex task. Practitioners must deal with facts, concepts, contexts, basic principles, and people. They must make decisions in an arena of passion, prejudice, and ambiguity. Regardless of complexities, however, the fact remains that if we are to be listened to as members of the health care team, it will be because we can support our views. Emotions alone—even if intensely felt and forcefully expressed in regard to an ethical problem—will not persuade others of the cogency of our views. The value attributed to our advice and decisions will be directly based on the reasoning that we have invested in the deliberative process.

If all within the team are to be considered colleagues, then each of us must be part of the decision-making process. Modern health care is a team practice, and the team must involve and get the best from all of its members to be truly successful. Health care ethics issues are challenging, and as health care professionals we need to come to decisions that represent the best interests of our patients, colleagues, and community.

Our view of Reality is like a map with which to negotiate the terrain of life. If the map is true and accurate, we will generally know where we are, and if we have decided on where we want to go, we will generally know how to get there. If the map is false and inaccurate, we generally will get lost.

M. Scott Peck, *The Road Less Traveled*

This book is designed to assist you in gaining an accurate map to negotiate the arena of health care ethics. It will provide you with the tools to reason in this important aspect of health care practice. The text is not intended to provide a definitive source for any of the issues discussed but is a starting place that will stimulate in you a desire to continue the exploration for a professional lifetime. Health care practice is a wonderful adventure, and ethical practice is an important element in a successful career. We wish you good fortune.

KEY CONCEPTS

- To enter the practice of health care provision is to enter into a compact with not only the patients we serve, but will all other practitioners and the community at large.

- To honor the compact requires not only excellence in clinical skills but also appropriate legal, ethical, and professional etiquette behaviors.

- An important criterion for all professions is that they are self-regulating. A significant part of this self-regulation is in the arena of professional ethics.

- Hedonism, relativism, and nihilism are philosophical positions that distort the ability of individuals seeking to make ethical decisions that honor the rights of all parties within an ethical dilemma and respect the traditions of health care practice, where "anything goes" cannot be the answer and where some actions must never be tolerated.

- Standpoint theory holds that one should always adopt or at least listen to the standpoint of the most marginalized persons involved.

- The study of health care ethics requires the development of enough humility and moral imagination to at least imagine that your heart-felt initial reaction to a problem could possibly be wrong.

REVIEW EXERCISES

A. Review the code of ethics for your professional specialty (many are included in the appendix) to see if they have rules that answer the following questions:

1. When, if ever, is it permissible to take a gratuity?

2. When is it legitimate and perhaps mandatory to break a patient's confidence?

3. Is it permissible to lie to a patient if it is for his or her own good?

4. Can I work at a hospital and refer a patient to a durable medical supply company that I have contracted with to provide outpatient services?

5. What must I do if I make a medication error that no one else knows about and it appears harmless to my patient?

6. What obligations do I have as a colleague and fellow practitioner when I suspect that the therapist that I am working with is abusing alcohol or appears chemically impaired?

7. What if I come upon a practice that is legal but appears to me personally to be unethical?

B. In that it is unlikely that the particular code of ethics for your specialty will provide direction to each of the above questions, think about how you personally would go about making a correct decision in regard to an ethical dilemma in a case not covered by your professional code.

C. In many specialty codes there is a rule that forbids practitioners from taking gifts or gratuities from patients. Beyond just stating that it is forbidden by the specialty code of ethics, what is wrong with the practice?

NOTES

1. Council on Ethical and Judicial Affairs. *Code of Medical Ethics: Current Opinions with Annotations*, 1996–97 Edition. Chicago: American Medical Association. 1996.

2. Richard Paul and Linda Elder, *The Miniature Guide to Ethical Reasoning*. Dillon Beach, CA: The Foundation for Critical Thinking. 2003.

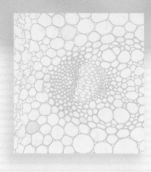

CHAPTER 1

Human Value Development

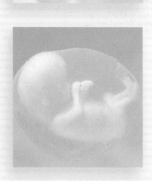

GOAL

To understand the nature of the human value system and relate this to the developmental theories of Lawrence Kohlberg, Jean Piaget, Morris Massey, and Carol Gilligan.

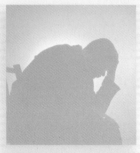

OBJECTIVES

Upon completion of this chapter, the reader should be able to:

1. Differentiate between needs and values.
2. Describe and compare the value development positions of Massey, Kohlberg, Gilligan, and Piaget.
3. Outline the nature of the controversy found in the works of Kohlberg and Gilligan in regard to value development.
4. Describe the three general levels and six stages of value development as outlined by Kohlberg.
5. List the highest value levels as described by Kohlberg and Gilligan, and relate them to gender development.
6. Describe the four value cohorts as outlined by Morris Massey.

KEY TERMS

Altruism   **Egocentric**
Amoral   **Value cohort**

NEEDS AND VALUES

Two things fill my mind with ever increasing wonder and awe: . . . the starry skies above me and the moral law within me.

Immanuel Kant, *Critique of Practical Reason,* 1788

A major preoccupation of sages, philosophers, and social scientists throughout all ages has been a desire to understand the nature of human behavior. Although it is easy to see that human behavior is nonrandom, and designed to produce some end, it is less easy to determine the cause and effect of our actions. One useful model is to look at human behavior as a reflection of our attending to perceived needs or values.

In his classic work, Abraham Maslow listed a "hierarchy of needs" that provide motivation for actions.[1] According to the theory, feelings of isolation stimulate activities such as attending church or joining a bowling team, whereas hunger might stimulate food gathering. Under most situations, our actions are explainable in that we are seen as attempting to satisfy a given set of needs. According to Maslow, as each need level is satisfied, the needs of the next level become the dominant motivators for our actions. If the hierarchy of needs is correct, an observer who could determine which level of need was operational could predict the nature of our next actions (Figure 1-1).

There are times, however, when the individuals appear to move from needs-based motivation to attending to an inner subjective set of feelings, attitudes, beliefs, and opinions that make up their personal value system. In these cases, the individuals seem to ask themselves not what they would do but rather what they should do, and the outcome is less predictable. In some sense, the difference is that found in Hume's law, which holds that there is an unbridgeable gap between fact and value, or as it is classically portrayed between "is" and "ought."[2] The facts of the physical universe can tell us what is, but it is our values that guide us to an understanding of what ought to be as it relates to human behavior. Figure 1-2 lists values that are important to our everyday choices in regard to health care. The list is by no means complete, and each individual's experiences will shape the way these values will be considered in personal decision making. Consider how a patient who placed a high value on personal independence, self-determination, personal privacy, and freedom from disability might react to a spinal injury that left him paralyzed and in need of his bodily functions being cared for by others. It is conceivable that someone might view the loss of these characteristics of the "good life" as being so

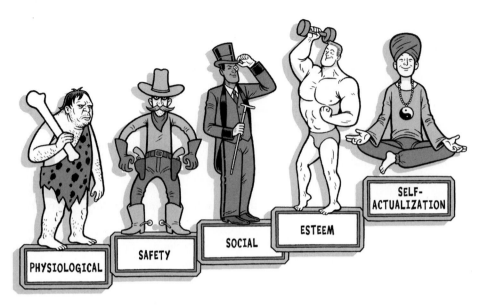

FIGURE 1-1   Hierarchy of Needs

important that the option of no life might be preferable. The same injury to another individual with a differing set of values—perhaps including a view that this life is a mere test for rewards given in an afterlife—might lead that person to cling to life with great tenacity, never considering death as a viable option.

To see how different a value system is from that of a needs system, one need only look at the conduct of the male passengers during the sinking of the Titanic. Obviously their need for sur-

- **Independence**—Freedom from constraint
- **Autonomy**—Self-determination
- **Privacy/confidentiality**—Fear of invasion
- **Self-esteem**—Need to value oneself
- **Well-being**—Freedom from pain and suffering
- **Security**—Control of fear and anxiety
- **Sense of belonging**—Group identification
- **Sexual and spiritual support**—Fulfillment
- **Freedom from disability**—Physical/mental capacity
- **Accomplishment**—Personal fulfillment

FIGURE 1-2   Common Decision-Shaping Values

vival might have motivated a host of actions such as forcing their way onto the lifeboats. However, the predominant value of the time was that men should protect women and children. Therefore, as the ship went down, the bands played and the men stood aside, even at the peril of their lives. Similarly, the health care providers who sacrifice some level of personal safety to work with contagious patients and the mother who takes on the 250-pound bully in the park to protect her children are acting from a position of value and making decisions based on a feeling about what one ought to do. Consider the following value case study to explore the professional implications of personal values.

CASE STUDY

Personal vs. Professional Values

Ray's dad was an alcoholic and abused his family until he died of acute alcoholism at the age of forty-three. As a result of his past experiences, Ray is avidly anti-drinking, and when given a chance, he will explain his views on the matter.

Ray works as a physician assistant in the local hospital's emergency room. One night Mr. Chang is brought in by his family and is in an alcoholic rage. Ray thinks about his own past and begins to lecture Mr. Chang on his drinking and family responsibilities.

1. Is Ray right in lecturing Mr. Chang?
2. How does Ray's role as a physician assistant affect what he can or should say to Mr. Chang?

VALUE DEVELOPMENT

Where then do we receive our values? As humans we are born with a series of undifferentiated potentials. As an example, we have the capability to learn a language, but the particular language is not prescribed by our genetic heritage. In this same sense humans have the innate capacity to acquire ethical beliefs. But the value system that we develop is dependent on the cultural framework in which we live. This capacity to become ethical beings and to conform to some universal principles of mutual cooperation and altruism seems as old as the species itself. One of the earliest found skeletal remains of Neanderthal human was that of an individual, approximately fifty years of age, whose bones indicate that he suffered from a severe, debilitating form of arthritis. His impediment made it unlikely that he could hunt or engage in strenuous activity, and he therefore was dependent on the caring of his group for his survival. While Neanderthal humans may not have had the words to express such concepts as love, altruism, and individual respect, they seemingly exhibited behaviors by which these terms are defined.

In that we are born without a prescribed set of rules for what we should do in any given situation, value development is a product of our interactions with our cultural environment. The foremost theorists in value development are Jean Piaget[3] and Lawrence Kohlberg.[4] Both stress that value development is intimately tied to the individual's cognitive and psychomotor development. In their models, they describe the individual as growing through several stages of value orientation.

In 1935, Piaget's groundbreaking book, *The Moral Development of the Child,* established much of the current thinking regarding value and moral development. Piaget's observations of children at play led him to describe four stages of moral development. The first stage is known as the amoral phase, which occurs up to age two. During this time period the child is totally self-centered. Around age two to seven the child is in the egocentric stage. During this stage children are not particularly interested in or concerned with rules. In a game of marbles, three-year-old children will move marbles to get a clear shot and be unconcerned when their shooting hands cross into the marble ring. The emphasis at this stage is on fun rather than on the observation of rules.

The third stage described by Piaget is known as the heteronomous stage and occurs around the seventh to twelfth year. In this stage children enter a period of behavior described as the morality of constraint. During this period rules are taken very seriously, and children tend to view behavior as right or wrong. They assume everyone views behavior in a similar way, basing their belief on an admiration or fear of adults who appear to be all knowing and powerful. In the latter part of this stage, the child enters a time described as moral relativism and begins developing a morality of cooperation. The perspective of punishment of children at this stage broadens, and they come to understand that differing degrees of wrongdoing require differing levels of punishment. During this phase, intentions become important, and children often wait to consider a person's intentions before making a moral judgement.

Kohlberg's Stage Theory of Moral Reasoning

The Kohlberg model is very similar to that of Piaget except that it ignores the initial amoral phase of the infant and expands on three general levels of development (preconventional, conventional, and postconventional) and further divides each of these levels into two stages. Figure 1-3 shows the three basic stages and the source of the value orientation. In the model, the individual matures through six phases from a value orientation based on punishment and obedience to a final autonomous stage characterized by a universal ethical orientation where one is guided by an internal moral compass. Kohlberg's technique in developing his model was to

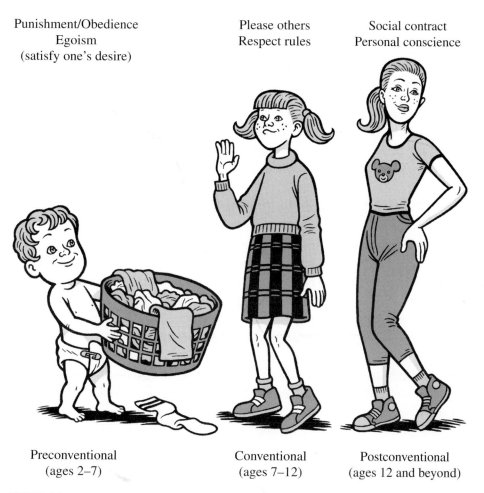

Punishment/Obedience
Egoism
(satisfy one's desire)

Please others
Respect rules

Social contract
Personal conscience

Preconventional
(ages 2–7)

Conventional
(ages 7–12)

Postconventional
(ages 12 and beyond)

FIGURE 1-3   Orientation of Stages

observe and interview children and adults and to pose moral dilemmas, which he would ask them to puzzle out verbally so that he could follow their reasoning. One of his most famous dilemmas concerned a man named Heinz:

> A man named Heinz had a very sick wife who was dying of an unusual cancer. There is only one special drug that the doctors feel might save her. This formula had recently been discovered by a local pharmacist and was available only from the single source. The medicine was expensive to make, and given that he was the only source, the pharmacist was charging ten times what the drug cost him. The daily charge for the medication was $2,000, and Heinz's wife needed at least enough for a two-week trial. Heinz did not have enough money to pay the pharmacist and attempted to borrow and sell whatever he could to get the money. Finally, in desperation, he approached the pharmacist and told him about his dying

wife, asking him to reduce the price, or at least sell it to him on the basis that he would pay what he could now and would pay the remainder later. But the pharmacist said, "No, I discovered the drug, and I'm going to make money from it." So Heinz went away. Later that night, he broke into the man's store to steal the drug for his wife. Should Heinz have done that?

This is both a simple and complex story: there are reasons that can be given for stealing the drug and also reasons for not stealing, and many variations in between. After interviewing and rating hundreds of individuals as they struggled with Heinz's and other similar dilemmas, Kohlberg outlined the following developmental process for moral reasoning.

Level 1: Preconventional Morality (Ages 2–7)

Although infants are essentially amoral, very young children are moral in a rather primitive way, which Kohlberg described by the two preconventional stages.

Stage 1: Reward and Punishment. During this stage, children have no real understanding of values and accept the authority of others. They assume that powerful individuals in their lives have the right to hand down a fixed set of rules, which they must obey. Issues of good or bad depend on the physical consequences. Does the action taken lead to punishment or reward? Many children at this stage will say that Heinz should not steal because he will be caught and punished.

Stage 2: Individualism and Exchange. During this stage, children begin to recognize that other individuals have their own interests, which need to be taken into account. This is the "I'll scratch your back if you scratch mine" phase, a time of simple exchange and reciprocity. Human relations are viewed in the pragmatic terms of the marketplace rather than in considerations of loyalty or justice. In this regard, Heinz should attempt to meet his own self-interests. Some egoist theories hold that this stage, where the individual is focused solely on personal satisfaction, is all there is to morality.

Level 2: Conventional Morality (Ages 7–12)

As they approach elementary school age, children are usually capable of conventional morality, in which they conform to the societal expectations of family or group in order to win the approval of authority figures. Kohlberg called this *conventional morality* because it is where most of us find ourselves, most of the time.

Stage 3: Good Boy/Good Girl. During this period, the child seeks to conform to the expected social conventions. Good behavior pleases or helps others; one earns approval by being nice and having good intentions. Children often adhere to a concrete version of the Golden Rule during this time. In regard to Heinz, they might consider it acceptable for him to steal the drug given that he was trying to save his wife's life.

Stage 4: Law and Order. Here the focus becomes fixed on rules, social order, and respect for authority. Right conduct consists of doing one's duty. The value system exemplified by Boy and Girl Scouts would have real meaning at this level of development. In response to the Heinz dilemma, they might respond that while they could understand that his motive for stealing the drug was good, they could not condone the theft because "if everyone who needed something just stole it, the result would be chaos."

Level 3: Postconventional Morality (Age 12 and above)

The focus of this level is the development of the social contract and autonomous decision making apart from outside authorities. The level allows the individual to rise above morality based on authority to one based on reason.

Stage 5: Social Contract and Individual Rights. During this stage, the individual will explore the idea that the creation of the good society requires a social contract into which people freely enter to work for the benefit for all. A good society protects the rights of its citizens and, where injustices are found, allows changes to be made through the use of democratic processes. In regard to Heinz, someone at this stage might indicate that while he or she could not agree with the decision to steal because that would be breaking the law, the wife also had a right to life, which might take precedence over the druggist's property rights.

Stage 6. Universal Principles. This is the highest level of moral development, a time when the individual makes a personal commitment to the universal principles of equal rights, social justice, and respect for the basic dignity of all people. When there is a conflict between these values and the social contract, the contract takes a back seat to the basic principles. The individual essentially becomes an autonomous agent following the dictates of personal conscience. In the Heinz case, individuals might suggest that each of the players in the conflict (Heinz, the wife, the pharmacist) acts out the situation as if he or she does not know which position in the drama he or she actually holds. The pharmacist, while playing the wife's part, would recognize that her right to life was a higher value than the right to property.

Challenges to Kohlberg

In recent years, the Kohlberg developmental model has come up for criticism, as most of his research data were gathered from the decision-making activities of young males. Using his model, females generally were found not to progress into the final autonomous stage of value orientation (postconventional level), but seemed arrested in the second stage of the conventional level. Instead of becoming essentially morally autonomous, females seemed to reach a plateau in value orientation based on pleasing others rather than being true to their own moral compass.

This difference between males and females is often highlighted by posing the Heinz dilemma to young boys and girls. While young men will often work out a legalistic rationale for stealing the drugs, young women will often want Heinz to return to the pharmacy, believing that if the situation were explained better, the pharmacist would understand and supply the medicine.

Carol Gilligan has challenged the Kohlberg model and the assumption that males and females see value problems in the same light.[5] One interesting aspect of her research was the study of boys and girls at play. Boys tended to play longer and more complicated games than girls, and, during play, often settled disputes by arguing out a set of rules under which the game could go forward. Girls, on the other hand, seemed to play games with fewer rules and ended a game when disputes developed. The rationale given for this difference was that boys were willing to subordinate relationships to rules and principles, while girls were not. Gilligan argues for a separate value development pathway for females that results in a different highest value—personal responsibility for females and legalistic equality for males.

It is interesting to note that the difference observed by Gilligan is somewhat confirmed by the typographical profile created by Isabel Myers and Katherine Briggs, which looks at normal human behavior.[6] Men and women score equally on all the major dimensions of the instrument with the exception of decision making. In this area, men fall predominantly within the "thinking" category for decision making, being more comfortable with following rules, laws, formulas, and the like, and subordinating relationships to principles. Women, on the other hand, are more likely to fall into the "feeling" category, in which decisions are based on relationships and personal outcomes rather than on legalisms and rules. Whether this is truly a difference between men and women, or just a function of what has been fostered by our culture, is yet to be determined and will become clearer as the traditional roles of the sexes are further blurred. Thinking and feeling are just two described methods of making decisions—neither being preferred or useful in all situations. Unfortunately, as a culture we have only recently begun to value the feeling method of decision making. Everyone uses both approaches; however, females predominantly use the feeling pathway and males the thinking pathway. Gilligan's criticism was well taken by Kohlberg. In his writings after 1985, Kohlberg revised his scoring methodology to account for this possible gender bias.

Massey's Value Cohorts

The rather subjective screen of feelings, attitudes, beliefs, and opinions that make out value system and with which we view and judge our world is taught to us by our early environment. According to some value theorists, the critical period of value programming is between birth and teens, with approximately 90 percent of our value system being firmly in place by age ten. Beyond this age, our general values rarely change unless we are affected by some significant emotional event. The value theorist Morris Massey uses the phrase "you are what you are because of where you were when" to emphasize that we are programmed by events that occurred around us as we were growing up.[7] In that certain events happen to us as a group, these shape us as a generational **value cohort**. An excellent example of cohort programming can be seen in the population that was young during the Great Depression of the 1930s. As a group, this is a very security-conscious portion of our population. Whether real or imagined, the ideas of doing without, or "walking five miles through the snow to school," or "a penny saved is a penny earned" are important to them, and yet these notions seem almost mythical to those born after 1940.

In his work, Massey describes four general value cohorts programmed by the events of recent national history. Although some individuals may escape the impact of certain eras (for example a hermit may escape the impact of urbanization, and the idle rich may escape economic downturns), most in the society will be shaped and programmed by the value-molding forces around them. The major current generation clusters identified by Massey are broken down into four broad categories of worldview value differences:

1. Traditionalists

This group received their value programming by the events of the 1930s and 1940s, when family structure was extended, and clearly identified roles were still in place. The war traditionalists fought was generally successful and popular. As a result, this group tends toward patriotism as well as the recognition of authority and legitimate chain of command. Several periods of economic scarcity were included in this time era, leaving the group with a certain level of materialism based on the concept that whatever we do without as we grow up is important to us.

According to Massey, traditionalists have been shaped to believe in a set of prescribed codes of action that determine how a person behaves on the job, at home, and socially. For them, society is best structured with everyone knowing, and being in, his or her appropriate place. In some way, they view life as a team sport in which all the players should support the action and be happy in their assigned roles. Even wildly popular cultural heroes such as Generals Patton and MacArthur could not escape their assigned roles and suffered when they were considered nonteam players.

Several cultural trends, such as the decline of the work ethic, the loss of defined family roles, and the emergence of minority groups, have seriously undermined and challenged traditionalist values. This value cohort seems somewhat dislocated in time. Traditionalists still, however, form much of what we recognize as the "establishment" and are in positions to make decisions that affect all of us.

2. In-Betweeners

The values shared by this cohort were those commonly programmed in the late 1940s and 1950s. This group is caught between the traditional values of the pre-1940s and the highly individual values expressed after the mid-1960s when concepts of structure and set roles were in disarray. They seem caught between the values expressed in the phrases "I am a company man," and "You can take this job and shove it." The dynamics of being between these two polar views have left them uncomfortable with either end of the spectrum. This allows the in-betweeners not only to recognize and accept regulations but also to make calculating assessments in regard to their personal needs. In their work lives, they often appear more like the traditionalist, conforming to standard dress and protocol, while in their private lives they may lead very individualistic and informal lifestyles.

In an attempt to maintain individuality within structure, in-betweeners often shift between conformity and experimentation. This pursuit of a personal place leads this group to be the major consumers of the "How to be _____ books." One of their great values to society is their ability to speak the language of both the pre-1940s and post-1960s, thereby forming a bridge of understanding between two very different value orientation cohorts.

3. Challengers

This cohort shares the basic programming of the early 1960s through mid-1970s. They are the products of a period of wealth and power. Just as scarcity made the traditionalists somewhat materialistic, this group appears to take for granted and to devalue the world of abundance. Challenge to authority and societal values, informal dress, and experimental lifestyles are all hallmarks of this cohort.

Challengers were programmed in a period of permissiveness, when individuality was prized above team play. As a result, they appear to challenge standards unless conformity benefits their own personal requirements. In organizations, they expect and demand participation and personal consideration. It is these demands for consideration of individual needs that have been the impetus for such personnel packages as flextime, employer day care centers, pregnancy leave for men, and similar benefits.

4. Synthesizers

This is the latest of the value cohorts described in Massey's works—the programming period from the 1980s onward. This group has borrowed something from each of the three preceding value cohorts. They are more conservative than challengers, yet more cynical and skeptical than either traditionalists or in-betweeners. The synthesizers perceive a finite and perhaps shrinking world, where the future may well hold less for them in both a qualitative and quantitative sense.

Unlike the challengers before them, the synthesizers see the system as both the problem and the solution. They appear to accept the role of adapting to change and the creation of new systems that both provide and sustain.

Individually, we possess an organized system of thoughts, feelings, opinions, and beliefs (worldview) with which we screen the events occurring around us. It is with this subjective screen, based on our culture and life experiences, that we judge the rightness or wrongness of actions as they pertain to what a person should do in a given situation. Whether individuals feel comfortable taking pens from work, pushing to the front of a line, buying goods beyond their needs, or listening quietly as elders speak is a reflection of their particular worldview and value programming.

CONCLUSION

In his book, *The Closing of the American Mind*, Allan Bloom proposes that students entering the university may come from the left or right in regard to political views but will almost always share the position that truth is relative.[8] This proposition is based on an accommodation to a pluralistic culture. History is viewed as a past in which men thought that they possess the truth, and in the name of this truth justified outrageous persecutions, wars, slavery, xenophobic racism, and even witch burning. The point that these students take from this reading of history is that the "true believer" is a dangerous person, and that only as we are able to avoid thinking that ours is the one right way can we survive. Openness and tolerance have become for these students the only plausible stance in the face of various claims to truth and an appropriate lifestyle. With this belief in relativism, the rational person then would not be concerned with correcting the mistakes from the past but rather would decide that all truth is relative and one view is equal to all other views.

In some sense, Massey subscribes to ethical relativism, a view that holds that there are no universal or absolute principles that bind human beings, and that the standards of right or wrong are always relative to the society or culture. In this light, the rightness or wrongness of customs or traditions that allow the placing of the aged on an ice floe to die, or the obligation of a brother to marry his dead brother's widow, could be examined only in reference to the Arctic Eskimo or African cultures from which they spring. The relativist would hold that there is no basis for saying that a particular act is right or wrong, independent of its cultural framework. Whatever we might believe in regard to relativism and the lack of perfect truth, it would still seem reasonable that if we were in a position to do so, we would stop cannibals from eating missionaries and families from burning widows. Figure 1-4 offers a listing of some acts that most would consider ethically wrong regardless of cultural orientation.

- **Rape**—forcing unwanted intercourse
- **Slavery**—human bondage
- **Genocide**—attempting to eliminate an entire people
- **Torture**—inflicting severe pain in order to gain benefit
- **Sexism**—unequal and harmful treatment based on gender

FIGURE 1-4   Unacceptable Acts

Few health care practitioners would be comfortable in taking a relativistic view of values. The decisions we must make are of such significance that the flip of a coin will not do. Some answers truly are better than others, and some decisions must not be made. To take an amoral position that somehow all answers to moral questions are equal would be unacceptable in health care practice. The philosopher Nietzsche was correct in his declaration that we are valuing animals. However, in regard to our values, humans are not programmed, as is the beast of the forest, to a proscribed set of correct actions but are condemned to lives of freedom and choice. In the practice of health care a position of "anything goes" is unacceptable. John Steinbeck, in his book *Of Mice and Men,* pointed out how bankrupt we had become in regard to moral values when one of his characters commented, "There's nothing wrong anymore."[9]

This book is about the process of choice making in the value-laden area of health care. The purpose is to provide the practitioner with the conceptual framework and language skills needed to examine value issues, and to look at a series of systems that are currently employed in making these difficult decisions. Modern health care is overflowing with value choices that must be made, and the choices we make will determine to a great extent the shape of our careers and the pleasure we derive from the services we perform. There is a tradition of practice whereby health care providers will not conduct themselves in an egoist manner, but will consider the needs of the patients and the profession. Our patients are filled with expectations that we will perform in an ethical manner, even if it is unclear to them and us exactly what that entails.

Value theorists such as Lawrence Kohlberg, Jean Piaget, and Carol Gilligan have investigated the development of these worldviews and have provided models that show maturation and acquisition of value orientation throughout our childhood. The highest level of maturation described by Kohlberg and Piaget seems to be an autonomous decision-making system based on legalistic equality. Gilligan has provided a feminist perspective and argues for separate developmental pathways for men and women, with the highest value for women being personal responsibility.

This text is not an answer book that will provide you with comfortable solutions to these tough issues, for in truth there are no easy answers. This is a book that seeks to provide you with the right questions, so that you are at least comfortable that the issue has been examined appropriately.

KEY CONCEPTS

- Value-based motivation is more subjective and therefore more difficult to understand than motivation based on an individual's needs.
- Humans have an innate capacity to acquire ethical beliefs. The belief system that we develop is dependent on the cultural framework in which we live.

- Jean Piaget and Lawrence Kohlberg are important value theorists who believe that human value development is intimately tied to an individual's cognitive and psychomotor development.

- The Kohlberg model expands on three general levels of development—preconventional, conventional, and postconventional—and subdivides each level into two stages.

- The highest-level value development according to Kohlberg is when the individual makes a personal commitment to the universal principles of equal rights, social justice, and the respect for the basic dignity of all peoples as individuals.

- Carol Gilligan has presented a challenge to the Kohlberg developmental model and argues that it is biased toward males. She argues that young women follow a different value development path than boys do and that for them, the highest level of value development is personal responsibility and caring.

- Morris Massey is a business organization theorist who provides insights into the shaping of generational values based on historical events that tended to shape generational cohorts.

REVIEW EXERCISES

A. Massey holds that certain significant emotional events shape generational cohorts in such a way that they have a unified worldview or shared value patterns. Consider the traditionalists, the group that was value programmed in the 1930s and 1940s. The significant events were the Depression, World War II, extended family structures, and the rise of America as a world power. Describe how you think these events might have created a common value structure toward the following:

1. Patriotism

2. Value of work

3. Family member roles

4. Cooperative action

- Consider that this value cohort participated in a popular and successful war against seemingly evil groups. The end result of this has been a strong feeling toward national pride and priority placed on the need for an adequate defense.

- Select someone you know who was involved in the World War II period and think of how he or she feels about patriotism, work, family roles, and cooperative action. Is the person like or unlike the generalizations you created?

- Imagine a time and place in which children are brought up (programmed) in a situation where these circumstances are common: single-parent families, poverty, no meaningful work, violent streets where people drive by and kill strangers, inadequate school systems where children enter through a metal detector, and popular media that pander to a nightmarish mixture of sexuality, violence, and consumerism. Describe how you think the above might create a common worldview set of values toward the following:

1. Patriotism

2. Family member roles

3. Value of work

4. Cooperative action

B. Recently there have been attempts to update the Massey historical cohorts to include such groups as the baby boomers, Generation X, and Generation Y. Read over the following descriptions. Write a statement as to whether you think this newer formulation of groups captures significant value changes in our society. List at least three significant emotional events from the history of their eras that might have programmed each of the newly described cohorts.

- Traditionalists: This group received their value programming in the 1930s and 1940s. Traditionalist values are influenced by the experiences of their parents, whose values go back to the late 1800s. The significant emotional events that shaped this value cohort are the Great Depression and the patriotism and sacrifice of World War II. As a result, this group is fiscally conservative, tends to be patriotic, and recognizes the need for authority figures and chain of command. Traditionalists tend to value:

  - Privacy

  - Hard work

  - Loyalty and trust

  - Formality

  - Authority and social order

- "Baby boomers" are the largest of the generational cohorts. Baby boomers are the children of the World War II generation, born between 1945 and 1965. This group was value programmed in good economic times. For the most part, they have experienced the good life. Their traditionalist parents wanted them to have the best, and as a result the "Me" generation arrived. The very fact of their numbers has made them the focus of societal change and accommodation. Society has adapted its school systems, clothing fashions, musical tastes, and value norms, all in response to the aging of this group. Even today when we are thinking in terms of changes in the social security system, it is in response to the knowledge that the vanguard of this very large group is about to arrive. Baby boomers tend to value:

- Competition
- Change
- Hard work
- Teamwork
- Skepticism in regard to rules and legal actions
- Inclusion

- Generation X-ers: Coming from a generation that declared itself to be the "brightest and the best" the X-ers were at first an underrated generation. They appear more economically conservative, remembering double-digit inflation and the family stress caused by parents who faced on and off employment. Unlike their predecessors, they do not believe in or rely on institutions for their long-term security. X-ers tend to value:

  - Entrepreneurial spirit, which often seems to others to be disloyalty
  - Independence and creativity
  - Information and feedback, which promotes flexibility

- Generation Y: This group represents people who have grown up during the high-technology revolution. They have never known a world without high-speed video games, speed dial, and ATM machines. They seem to value:

  - Positive reinforcement
  - Autonomy
  - Positive attitudes
  - Diversity
  - Technology
  - Money

C. In the next case, make your decision first using legalistic equality (male pathway) as the highest value, and then using responsibility and relationships (female pathway) as the highest value.

The case involves a man, his wife, his mother, and his son. The family is out in a boat and the man is needed to hold the tiller in order to keep the boat steady. A great wind comes in and the boat begins to founder. It becomes obvious that someone must leave the boat and drown to save the lives of the others. In that the man is needed to hold the tiller or all must perish, which of the others (the mother, son, or wife) should be sacrificed?

Legalistic equality must involve the following of rules or principles, while responsibility must be shown to take into consideration the impact on the lives of the individuals involved.

D. Beginning each statement with "A person should," write a value statement that corresponds to your views in regard to the following areas:

1. Family

2. Work

3. Honesty

4. Abortion

5. Confidentiality

E. In the Kohlberg model there are three basic levels and six stages. Match each of the following six statements to the appropriate level and stage.

1. I do not say bad words because my daddy will be angry with me.

2. I vote not because it is expected of me but because it is the right thing to do.

3. For ice cream, I will pick up my room.

4. I pay taxes because it is the law.

5. I help elderly people across the street because it is one of the Scout laws.

6. I don't run in the hall because my teacher does not like it.

F. One of the applications of Gilligan's work is the writings about a separate Ethic of Caring which is seen as being different and separate from the Ethic of Equality and Justice. Could an ethic of caring exist and function without an ethic of equality and justice?

NOTES

1. Abraham Maslow, *Motivation and Personality,* 2nd ed. (New York: Harper and Row, 1970).

2. David Hume, *A Treatise of Human Nature,* ed. L. A. Selby-Bigge (Oxford: Oxford University Press, 1988).

3. Jean Piaget, *The Moral Judgment of a Child,* trans. M. Gabain (New York: Free Press, 1964).

4. Lawrence Kohlberg, *Philosophy of Moral Development* (San Francisco: Harper and Row, 1981).

5. Carol Gilligan, *In a Different Voice* (Cambridge, MA: Harvard University Press, 1982).

6. Isabel Myers, *Gifts Differing* (Palo Alto, CA: Consulting Psychological Press, 1980).

7. Morris Massey, cited in Michael O'Connor and S. Merwin, Mysteries of Motivation (Carlson Learning Company, 1988).

8. Allan Bloom, *The Closing of the American Mind* (New York: Simon and Schuster, 1987).

9. L. Puenell and B. Paulanka, *Transcultural Health Care* (Philadelphia: F. A. Davis, Co., 1998).

10. John Steinbeck, *Of Mice and Men* (New York: Modern Library, 1937).

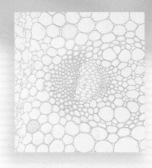

Decision Making in Value Issues

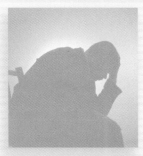

GOAL

To examine the common theories and methods used in making value decisions.

OBJECTIVES

Upon completion of this chapter, the reader should be able to:

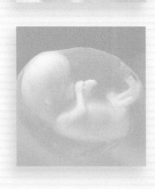

1. List the theorists who are considered the fathers of contemporary duty-oriented, consequence-oriented, and virtue ethics reasoning.

2. Outline the theoretical position known as utilitarianism, and analyze a clinical problem following its framework.

3. Outline the theoretical position of Kant, and analyze a clinical problem following his duty-oriented reasoning.

4. Differentiate between act and rule utilitarianism. State how rule utilitarianism is similar to duty-oriented reasoning.

5. List the major criticisms of duty-oriented and consequence-oriented systems.

6. Outline the theoretical position known as virtue ethics.

7. List the major criticisms of the virtue ethics position.

8. List several sources from which basic principles have been derived by duty-oriented theorists.

9. Define the theoretical position known as divine command ethics and analyze a problem following this line of reasoning.

KEY TERMS

Act utilitarianism	Divine command ethics	Principle of utility
Agape	Duty-oriented system	Rule utilitarianism
Categorical imperative	(deontological perspective)	Teleological
Consequence-oriented system	Equal consideration of interest	Utilitarianism
(teleological perspective)	Euthanasia	
Deontological	Mean	

VALUE CONFRONTATIONS

This is the heyday of the ethicist in medicine. He delineates the rights of patients, of experimental subjects, of fetuses, of mothers, of animals, and even of doctors. (And what a far cry it is from the days when medical "ethics" consisted of condemning economic improprieties such as fee splitting and advertising!) With impeccable logic—once certain basic assumptions are granted—and with graceful prose, the ethicist develops his arguments . . . Yet his precepts are essentially the product of armchair exercise and remain abstract and idealistic until they have been tested in the laboratory of experience.

F. J. Ingelfinger, M.D.

CASE STUDY

Am I Sure It Is My Job to Handle This?

You are a respiratory therapist graduate from a community college program in a rural area. You graduated first in your class, and a large, internationally famous medical center has hired you as a therapist. The atmosphere in this urban area is much different from the small rural hospitals where you did your clinical education, but you work hard and seem to be fitting in with the more experienced team members. Even Peter, the chief therapist, has taken the time to commend you on how well things are going.

Recently you noticed that Peter has been taking longer and longer lunches outside the medical center and seems to be less competent when he returns in the afternoon. When you work closely together in the intensive care unit, you smell alcohol on his breath. This bothers you and given that you have recently reviewed hospital policy, you know that drinking during working hours is forbidden. However, you are new, your coworkers have been around a long time, and no one else seems concerned.

(continues)

Am I Sure It Is My Job to Handle This? (cont.)

You decide to ask another therapist what to do. She does not outright say it, or condone it, but in general she confirms that Peter is drinking during lunch. She advises you not to get involved and just do your job. She then gives you three pieces of advice to think about. First, it is not your business. Second, you do not know the pressure that Peter is under. Third, it is important to remember that often it is the last person hired who is the first person fired!

1. Do you have an obligation in this case?

2. If you do, what is your next move, and why?

As practitioners, we are educated in the science and art of our specialties. Questions in regard to drug preparations, pathologic entities, and appropriate therapeutics often seem to have straightforward and comfortable answers. We know that if we apply the right set of equations or follow the correct procedures, a best answer comes forward. These answers are often reproducible and can be verified, and one need only present the facts in order for everyone to come into agreement. Yet health care is also an arena in which values play a commanding role in what is right and good for patients. Unfortunately for all practitioners, in the arena of values there is often disagreement, and rarely are the answers comfortable.

It is our values that tell us what is right and wrong, good and evil, and that imply a preference in regard to correct human behavior. This rather subjective screen with which we surround ourselves often countenances strong feelings or intense attitudes that are backed by rational justifications. Although we tend to think of value problems in the "big ethics" sense—those problems that are involved in choices dealing with life and death—we are also bedeviled by rather everyday questions that call for judgment based on a perception of right and wrong.

Perhaps the most frustrating aspect of value choices is that honorable individuals often come to very different positions based on reasoning from their particular worldviews. Some will base their opinions on formal philosophical or religious beliefs, while others will try to weigh the potential outcomes—seeking to choose those that provide the greatest good for the greatest number. Still others really don't use a formal system at all to determine the right answer but will rely on current practice or past experiences as their guides.

As professionals, it is necessary, even in our opposition, to attempt to be constructive, not destructive, in the methods we use when we come to disagreements over issues involving personal values. For example, accommodation in regard to the issue of abortion might be more easily attained if each side had not cast the other as "baby killers" or "antiwomen."

To acknowledge that individuals can come to different opinions in regard to value issues is not to say that all opinions have the same worth or credibility, or that one particular answer is better than another. Often we will find ourselves with no "right" answer or several "right" answers that seem to fit the situation. In order to make better value decisions, we must often move beyond our initial thoughts and feelings in regard to these basic issues and to build a framework for examining them. Several theoretical positions have been proposed that allow us to examine value-laden issues.

Although worldviews are individual, certain traits have been described and allow generalizations across individuals and groups. In all cultures there are a variety of common worldviews and ethical systems. One polar dichotomy found is that of the **consequence-oriented** and **duty-oriented** worldviews and theories.

TELEOLOGICAL (CONSEQUENCE-ORIENTED) THEORIES

Consequence-oriented theories judge the rightness or wrongness of decisions based on outcomes or predicted outcomes. Those following a consequence-based theory would decide that what is right also maximizes some good. The right thing to do, then, is the good thing to do. These theorists may argue about what constitutes the good, but once agreed, they would have no problem, theoretically, in deciding on a right course of action. In their works focused on the health care setting, T. L. Beauchamp and L. B. McCullough offer health (prevention, elimination, or control of disease), relief from unnecessary pain and suffering, amelioration of disabling conditions, and the prolongation of life as intrinsic goods.[1] Figure 2-1 lists a variety of consequences that have been claimed as intrinsic goods.

Jeremy Bentham (1748–1832) and John Stuart Mill (1806–1873) are considered the fathers of **utilitarianism,** the most common form of consequence-oriented reasoning.[2] To a utilitarian, the good resides in the promotion of happiness or the greatest net increase of pleasure over pain. To elevate the theory beyond a "pig philosophy," where a satisfied pig enjoying its life would constitute a higher moral state than a dissatisfied Socrates, Mill defined happiness as a set of higher-order pleasures such as intellectual, aesthetic and social enjoyments rather than mere sensual pleasure.

To assist in the process of calculating which of the various options produce the highest degree of utility, Bentham offered seven categories and seven attendant questions as a method for determining the level of utility.[3] When presented with a variety of options, one need only score each possibility to mathematically work out the correct moral option.

1. Intensity—How intense was the pleasure?
2. Duration—How long does the pleasure last?
3. Certainty—How certain are you that the pleasure will occur?
4. Proximity—How soon will the pleasure be experienced?
5. Fecundity—How many more pleasures will happen as a result of this one?

- Life, consciousness, and activity
- Health and strength
- Pleasure and satisfaction of all or certain kinds
- Happiness, beatitude, contentment
- Truth
- Knowledge and true opinion of various kinds, wisdom
- Beauty, harmony, proportion in objects contemplated
- Aesthetic experience
- Morally good dispositions or virtues
- Mutual affection, love, friendship, cooperation
- Just distribution of goods and evils
- Harmony and proportion in one's own life
- Power and experiences of achievement
- Self-expression
- Freedom
- Peace, security
- Adventure and novelty
- Good reputation, honor, esteem

FIGURE 2-1　Proposed Intrinsic Goods

Source: William Frankena, *Ethics* (Englewood Cliffs, NJ: Prentice Hall, 1973), pp. 87–88.

6. Purity—How free from pain is this pleasure?

7. Extent—How many will experience the pleasure?

The purest form of this line of reasoning is **act utilitarianism**, in which the decision is based on listing the possible alternatives for action, weighing each in regard to the amount of pleasure or utility it provides, and selecting the course of action that maximizes pleasure. There is some criticism that this hedonistic form of reasoning might lead to situations in which one group derives pleasure from the pain of others and justifies its actions on the basis of utility. To overcome this objection, some newer consequentialist formulations have required that the principle of **equal consideration of interest** be shown, in which the individual is not allowed to increase his share of happiness at the expense of another. Each person's happiness must be considered equally. The basic formulation for act utilitarianism can be captured in the principle that one

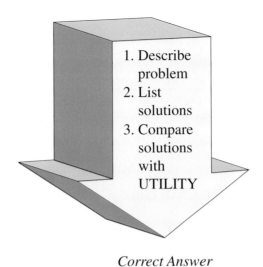

Correct Answer

FIGURE 2-2   Consequence-Oriented Reasoning

ought to act so as to produce the greatest balance of happiness over unhappiness, everyone considered. One of the real problems of act utilitarianism is that the individual must somehow predict and calculate the various levels of happiness promoted by each choice. In the worst-case use of utilitarianism, individuals might be seen to shift from one position to another as they weigh the various levels of happiness and pain avoidance and, in the process, lose their sense of self.

Utilitarian systems are referred to as teleological theory, taken from the Greek word *telos,* which means end. The basic concept is that the right act is that which brings about the best outcome. Often, individuals attempt to use utilitarian theory when they seek to divide scarce resources such as health care. They might justify the denial of a single individual access to a heart transplant if the money could be spent on providing vaccine for thousands. Figure 2-2 is a flowchart model of how decisions are made using a utilitarian system.

Criticisms of Utilitarianism

1. The calculation of all the possible consequences of our actions, or worse yet our inactions, appears impossible.

2. Utilitarianism may be used to sanction unfairness and the violation of rights. In order to maximize one person's or one group's happiness, it may be necessary to infringe on the happiness of another individual or group.

3. Utilitarianism is not sensitive to the agent-relativity of duty. We are inclined to think that parents are obligated to care for their children and that physicians are wrong to harm patients. Both of these examples could be allowed under utilitarianism, if doing so maximized overall utility.

4. Utilitarianism does not seem to give enough respect to persons. Under this theory, the ends justify the means, so it may be moral to use a person merely as a means to our ends.

5. Under utilitarianism, it is justifiable to prevent others from doing what we believe to be harmful acts to themselves. Such a paternalistic view could justify unacceptable governmental intervention into the private lives of individuals.

6. Utilitarianism alone does not provide a basis for our own moral attitudes and presuppositions. If followed, utilitarianism may recommend behaviors that are in conflict with personal fundamental moral beliefs and give rise to a sense of loss of self.

Utilitarian Responses to Criticisms

Those who criticize utilitarian reasoning often do so on the basis that it appears to allow using other people as a means to an end rather than as an end in themselves. In order to show the problem with utilitarianism, they might create a scenario such as the one following, which appears to show high utility in using another person.

Let us imagine that you wanted to get to know a young woman by the name of Judy. In order to do that, you become friends with her roommate Betty, whom you know casually from work. Utilitarians tend to respond to their critics by making three types of defense.

1. Utilitarians could deny that the critic's scenario would play out as claimed. When it is claimed, for example, that utilitarianism will permit using people, utilitarians will say using people always leads to less-than-optimal results. If you use Betty to get to Judy, then you will invariably alienate both and injure your reputation as well.

2. Utilitarians might argue that the supposedly counter-intuitive result should issue in a revision of our intuitions rather than a change in or rejection of the theory. One might say that if Betty doesn't mind or was even happy to facilitate your eventual contact with Judy, and if Judy is also happy with the result, then using Betty was the right thing to do.

3. Utilitarians might move to rule utilitarianism. While one might be able to argue that a particular instance of using someone to maximize utility, one certainly cannot make the claim concerning all cases of using people.

A formulation of utilitarianism that seems to avoid the problem of exact quantification required in act utilitarianism is **rule utilitarianism**. This theory holds that an action can be deemed to be right if it conforms to a rule that has been validated by the **principle of utility**. The principle of utility requires that the rule bring about positive results when generalized to a wide variety of situations. Rules forbidding the abridgment of free speech or the forceful housing of military in private homes might qualify as suitable, even if under certain rare situations they might bring about a decrease in happiness or pleasure.

Consequence-oriented viewpoints are often very persuasive in that they give comfort to modern cynicism in regard to absolute truths, and speak to our better selves with respect to tolerating the views and cultures of others. This is especially true in such formulations of utilitarianism as Joseph Fletcher's situation ethics, in which the good is agape, which can be defined as general goodwill or love for humanity.[4] He holds that human need determines what is or is not ethical. If an act helps people, it is a good act; if it hurts, it is a bad act.

In his writings, Fletcher provides six guidelines for making ethical choices:

1. Compassion for people as human beings

2. Consideration of consequences

3. Proportionate good

4. Priority of actual needs over ideal or potential needs

5. A desire to enlarge choice and reduce chance

6. A courageous acceptance of the need to make decisions and the equally courageous acceptance of the consequences of our decisions

As can be seen, the six guidelines provide for no appeal to an absolute principle, no authority that one can rely on; the only possible test of rival solutions lies in the consequences. This proposal is similar to the clinical model of medicine, in which the best therapeutic regime choice is the one most likely to result in an improvement in patient well-being. The following act utilitarian case study examines the difficulties associated with this position.

CASE STUDY

Act Utilitarianism: Calculating the Pleasures and Pain

Mr. Jimenez is a seventy-eight-year-old chronic pulmonary disease patient (emphysema) who has smoked two packs a day for forty years. He takes great enjoyment and satisfaction in smoking and does not want to quit.

In that his illness is exacerbated by the smoking, his physician is demanding that he quit. Each time he tries to quit smoking, Mr. Jimenez becomes irritable and unhappy. His wife and family hate it when he is not smoking because he becomes difficult to live with.

1. Consider this case from the position of act utilitarianism and create a pleasure-gained and pain-avoided list to see if you can determine whether Mr. Jimenez should continue or quit smoking.

DEONTOLOGICAL (DUTY-ORIENTED) THEORIES

Duty-oriented ethicists feel that the basic rightness or wrongness of an act depends on its intrinsic nature rather than on the situation or the consequences. This position is often described as a **deontological** theory, taken from the Greek word for duty. An act in itself would be either right or wrong; it could not be both. This particular worldview is codified in several major ethical systems and religions. In the classic work *Groundwork of the Metaphysic of Morals,* Immanuel Kant (1724–1804) held that the consequences of an action were essentially irrelevant.[5] Kant based his moral philosophy on the crucial fact that we are rational beings, and a central feature of this rationality was that principles derived from reason are universal. He held that morality is derived from rationality, not from experience, and that obligation is grounded not in the nature of man or in the circumstances of the world but in pure reason. These universal truths applied to all people, for all times, in all situations. Kant held that the human mind works the same way, regardless of who you are, where you are, or when you are. An action could be known to be right when it was in accordance with a rule that satisfied a principle he called a **categorical imperative**. By "categorical" he meant they do not admit exceptions. An "imperative" is a command derived from a principle. These imperatives were formulated by finding a maxim that could be understood as universal law. The imperatives seem to have three elements; (1) universal application (i.e., binding on every individual), (2) unconditionality, and (3) demanding an action. An example might be the unconditional duty of a lifeguard to enter the water to save a drowning swimmer. The mental process for the lifeguard would be a series of questions: "Should all paid lifeguards attempt to rescue drowning individuals?" "Is this duty to rescue unconditional?" and, finally, "Does this particular incident require the actions of a lifeguard?" If the lifeguard answered yes to all three questions, according to Kant, she would have a binding moral duty to act.

One such maxim relevant to health ethics is, "We must always treat others as ends and not as means only." Kant saw people as having an absolute value based on their ability to make rational choices. Accordingly, our dignity was derived from this capacity, and this was violated whenever a person was treated merely as a means to an end (a thing) and not as a person. From this one maxim, you could derive the other principles used in the ethics of health care. An action, then, could be judged right or wrong by determining its relationship to a categorical imperative even without knowledge of the particular circumstances. Figure 2-3 provides a flowchart showing the processes of duty-oriented reasoning.

Not long ago the media told of a family who could not find an acceptable bone marrow transplant donor for their daughter, who suffered from a rare form of cancer. In order to gain acceptable bone marrow, they decided to have an additional child, hoping that the child would provide the match. Kantian theorists would find this action unacceptable, inasmuch as the baby was being used as a means rather than as an end of its own.

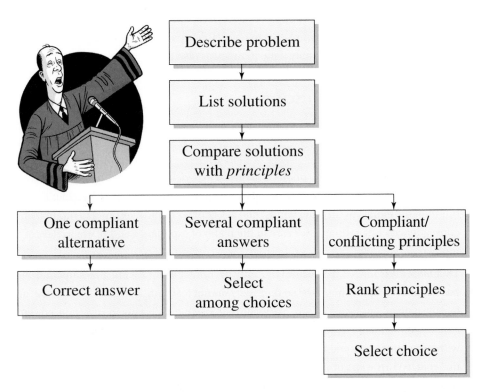

FIGURE 2-3   Duty-Oriented Reasoning

Criticisms of Kant

1. The exceptionless character of Kant's moral philosophy makes it too rigid for real life. Real-life situations are so varied that it is impossible to create rules that can guide us in all circumstances.

2. Morality cannot be derived from pure reason. The fact that we can feel pain and pleasure is central to morality. It is unlikely that we would care about morality if we did not feel pain or pleasure.

3. The disregard of the consequences of our actions can lead to disastrous results. We all have been hurt by well-meaning people who were overly concerned to "obey the law." It is often the spirit of the law, rather than the letter, that provides the arena for rational decisions. The Robert Bland proverb, "We may grasp virtue so hard that it becomes vicious," captures the essence of not considering the consequences of our decisions.

4. Even though nonhuman animals feel pain and pleasure, for Kant they do not have any independent moral standing since they are not rational beings.

5. It is possible to be faced with a conflict between two duties equally supported by an imperative. (The nurse who promises not to reveal that a patient has asked questions about euthanasia is asked by the family if the matter was discussed.)

Kantian Responses to Criticism

In response to the five criticisms, those who follow this philosophical position might respond with the following justifications:

1. To believe that one needs exceptions is to regard experience as central to morality, which is metaphysically incorrect, for exceptions are required only if one is led by experience to question the moral law. In other words, one needs exceptions to respond to nonmaximal consequences. But consequences are in the realm of experience and so are irrelevant to morality.

2. That *morality* is indeed the basis of morality becomes clear if we imagine someone who has her pain receptors impaired so that she does not feel pain. Even though she may not feel the pain of, say, losing an arm, we would still say that such a person was injured since she would be unable to pursue her goals and purposes as effectively. Since interfering with someone's goals and purposes amounts to a lack of respect for that person, any action that led to the loss of an arm, even painlessly, would be immoral. A utilitarian would respond that the reason losing an arm is bad even without the pain would be the unhappiness caused by the inability to use the lost arm. At this point we are down to a disagreement over basic intuitions, a type of disagreement very difficult to resolve.

3. Disregarding consequences does sometimes lead to unhappiness, but the world is full of unhappiness and even death, so the complaint is not really against Kant's morality but against the suffering in the world. We can't stop all pain; what is crucial is that we act with dignity and respect in the face of suffering.

4. Kant has rules against the mistreatment of animals, but the source of our duty to animals is indirect. We refrain from abusing animals because of the effect it will have in reducing our respect for people. Hurting animals owned by others is an injury to the owners of the animals.

5. The Kantian responds in two ways. First, there is often a way out of an apparent dilemma, sometimes by refusing to act either of the two ways that would seem to violate a perfect duty. Second, life may very well be tragic in that we are sometimes obliged to violate the law. In such cases, one would be obliged to choose the less egregious violation of our duties to others or ourselves.

Duty-oriented theorists obviously wish to promote a good result; however, they feel that merely serving the good is not an adequate foundation for ethics. For these theorists, the right action is one based on a correct principle regardless of the results. For instance, if life is sacred, then murder is wrong, regardless of the circumstances leading to the act. Duty-oriented theorists argue among themselves as to how principles are derived, with some claiming the basis to be natural law, while others look to religious dictate, intuition, social contract, pure reason, or common sense.

One influential formulation of duty-oriented reasoning is the contract theory of John Rawls. In this theory Rawls proposes that if a reasoning individual were placed in a social situation requiring a value choice without knowing what role he was playing in the situation (Rawls calls this the original position), the individual would chose the alternative that supported or favored the most disadvantaged person. This, then, becomes a restatement of the "golden rule"—that when actions have an impact upon another, for these actions to be morally defensible, it must be the case that the actor would choose to be the recipient of an identical action by someone else under identical circumstances. The first principle of the social contract is to secure basic liberties for all individuals within the covenant:

> Each person possesses an inviolability founded on justice that even the welfare of the society as a whole cannot override. For this reason justice denies that the loss of freedom for some is made right by a greater good shared by others . . . the rights secured by justice are not subject to political bargaining or to the calculus of social interest.[6]

Following this line of reasoning, the concern of an ethical society would be toward the care and support of its most disadvantaged citizenry, as they are the ones who are least able to speak for themselves. This is a decidedly duty-oriented position in that it establishes the duty of moral equality, which could not be bargained away regardless of social interest or the welfare of the society as a whole.

The individual whose intuitive moral sense leads him or her to believe that abortion is wrong under all circumstances, and the priest who maintains the confidentiality of the confessional even in the case of unreported incest, are both following the dictates of a duty-oriented or absolutist system. It is the exceptionless character of the duty-oriented position that gives most practitioners pause, as we seem always to be in situations of gray rather than black or white. The following duty-oriented case study provides an opportunity to examine principle-oriented reasoning.

Neither theoretical position, consequence or duty oriented, has produced a theory that can be accepted under all circumstances. Both duty and consequence ethics pose grave problems in modern decision making. If we take, as an example, the question of the sanctity of life and an absolutist view prevails, modern medicine and technology might be placed on the side of saving every living individual from death regardless of intolerable costs, suffering of the family, or inability to restore life in a meaningful sense. Conversely, if a utilitarian view prevails, we might see arguments that would allow certain categories of handicapped individuals to be subjected to euthanasia on the basis that their removal served the best interest of society. Today,

---

CASE STUDY

Duty-Oriented Reasoning: A Matter of Principle

Juan and Joe are good friends. They both graduated from the same program and have gone to work in the same radiography department. Part of their duties is to be sure that the standby equipment is ready for service on the wards. Juan and Joe are working the night shift, and while playing around, Juan inadvertently bumps the equipment, tips it over, and breaks the standby instrument.

In that it was an accident, Juan asks you, as a friend, not to tell anyone it was his fault. "Accidents do happen." The two of you switch out the equipment, sending the broken piece down for maintenance, and put a working instrument on standby.

In the morning your boss comes in and notices that the equipment had been sent down to maintenance. He asks what happened, and Juan says, "I dunno. Someone from out of the department must have bumped it or something." The boss looks at you and asks you the same question.

1. Solve this problem using duty-oriented or principled reasoning. Remember that in this form of reasoning, it is not the consequences that are considered but rather the principles involved.

2. What principles are involved in this case?

3. Do any of the principles involved conflict with each other?

4. Do some principles have a higher value than others?

---

biomedical decision making is often based on an uneasy truce between the absolutist and consequentialist views, as practitioners seek a viable middle ground. In practice, rarely do you meet the individual who fails to consider the consequences of the situation, or one who is comfortable with decision making without reference to principles.

VIRTUE ETHICS

The lack of a convincing formulation for a duty-based or consequence-based ethical system that is able to overcome the major criticisms of each has led to an exploration of ethics not understood as a set of rules to guide actions but as an attribute of character or role duty. As an example, let us suppose that a borderline sleazy technologist, after long deliberation, decides not to enter into a conflict-of-interest business deal because he fears being caught and brought up for Medicaid fraud. Is there any difference between his choice and that of another technologist with the same suspect business opportunity who never considers entering into the practice?

Consequence-oriented systems focus on reasoning to an appropriate action. It is the action itself rather than the character of the agent that is the heart of the matter. In this light, the practitioner who is borderline sleazy and the practitioner whose moral disposition never leads her to consider the fraud are equally moral if the action they take is the same in a given situation. There are some who might argue that the borderline sleazy technologist is the more honorable of the two, in that he was first tempted, almost succumbed, and finally resisted the temptation.

In his *Nicomachean Ethics,* the philosopher Aristotle suggests a different solution than the action-centered ethical systems of duty-oriented and consequence-oriented reasoning when he places the focus not on the particular action but rather on the heart of the moral agent:

> We may go so far as to state that the man who does not enjoy performing noble actions is not a good man at all. Nobody would call a man just who does not enjoy acting justly, nor generous who does not enjoy generous actions, and so on.[7]

In posing the problem, Aristotle is following not duty or consequence-oriented traditions but rather a third path known as aretaic ethics (taken from the Greek arete, which can be translated as either excellence or virtue). The primary focus of virtue ethics is the heart of the moral agent making the decision rather than the reasoning to a right action. In this view, it is not the weak person who is mightily tempted and who finally does right things that is to be admired but rather the individual who has the emotional disposition and habits of virtue that manifest their being in actions or nonactions. Virtue ethics places its focus on the sorts of characteristics, traits, or virtues that a good person should have. The belief is that someone who has appropriate moral virtues such as courage, temperance, wisdom, and justice will naturally act in certain ways.

The question then is not, "What shall I do?" but rather, "How should I carry out my life if I am to live well?" The emphasis is taken off individual actions and the quandaries in which we find ourselves and put instead on what we can do to produce the sort of character that instinctively does the right thing. Virtue ethics holds that it is not only important to do the right thing but equally to have the right disposition, motivation, and traits for being good and doing right.

A good virtuous character manifests itself in the display of traits such as courage, magnanimity, honesty, justice, and temperance. Virtue ethics is primarily about personal character and moral habit rather than a particular action.

Over the past several decades philosophers such as Alasdair MacIntyre,[8] Elizabeth Anscombe,[9] Bernard Mayo,[10] and Richard Taylor[11] have argued for a return to virtue-based ethics. They argue that the action-based ethical systems are essentially negative and fail to inspire or motivate to excellent behavior. Without the foundation of individual character to motivate action, the action-based systems seemed more mental gymnastics and hair-splitting than the basis for morality.

The moral virtues, then, are produced in us neither by nature nor against nature. Nature, indeed prepares in us the ground for their reception, but their complete formation is the product of habit.

Aristotle (384–322 B.C.)

In his teachings, Aristotle saw a function or essence for humanity. As examples, doctors were to make the sick well, rulers were to govern wisely, and citizens were to place their individual reason in the pursuit of a good life. This essence or function was considered neither natural nor unnatural, and it was thought to be produced by the practice of virtue. Goodness of character, then, was brought about by the practice of virtues such as courage, honesty, and justice. This practice created the habit of taking pleasure in virtuous acts, which then acted as a sign of a good life. One becomes just and temperate by doing just and temperate things. Aristotle's traits of a virtuous character provided that:

1. Virtuous acts must be chosen for their own sakes.
2. Choice must proceed from a firm and unchangeable character.
3. Virtue is a disposition to choose the mean.

The virtuous person had a disposition of moderation toward the **mean** between two extremes. We have all experienced times when we needed to swing hard against the directions in which our passions were leading us. (Not every passion has a mean; for instance, there is no mean of murder, as murder is itself an extreme in interpersonal conduct.) Better examples can be found in justice, courage, liberality, pride, ambition, good temper, veracity, and shame.

Beyond character or moral virtues, Aristotle also believed in intellectual virtues, such as practical wisdom. This he defined as the power of deliberation about things good for oneself. Whereas intellectual virtues could be directly taught, moral virtues or character virtues must be lived in order to be learned. Arguments and instruction by themselves do not have the power to make the individual good. In this sense, Shakespeare's advice in *Hamlet* was correct: "If one were to have virtue, one must first assume it." Goodness is a matter of character, and character is developed by actions over time. One attempted to live well by practicing right habits. These right habits through practice became intrinsic to the individual and thus became the individual's virtues. Neither intellectual virtues such as practical wisdom nor character virtues could exist independently from each other.

The contemporary philosopher who has expanded Aristotle's work into a modern formulation of ethics is Alasdair MacIntyre. MacIntyre holds that there have been many different conceptions of virtue that revolve around ideal characters associated with a variety of traditions. He isolates and describes several idealized characters such as Homeric (strength/warrior), New Testament (humility/slave), and Early American (industry/capitalist). Beyond these ideals, he believes in a core idea of virtue, of which courage, justice, and honesty are essential components.[8]

In this ethical formulation, practices are the arena in which the virtues are exhibited, and it is only in terms of the particular practice that virtues can be defined. MacIntyre is thinking of social roles that provide standards of excellence and obedience to rules as well as common achievement goals toward some perceived good. To enter into the role of the physician, priest, or teacher is to enter into a practice, as well as to accept the authority of the standards of that role. In the example of the physician, once the individual accepts that practice, duty is determined by the role and the history of medical ethics. Figure 2-4 displays how decisions are made using virtue ethics reasoning.

In that practices have histories, the individual enters into a relationship not only with contemporary practitioners, but also with those who preceded her in the role. This is especially true of those who have come before and have extended the practice to its present point. In this way, we learn from tradition, but tradition also learns from us. Our rapidly changing specialties do pose some problem for virtue ethics in that what may be considered a virtue at one time may be inappropriate later. The best example is perhaps nursing. The good practice in the 1950s and 1960s would have contained ample portions of virtues like submissiveness and respectfulness, whereas today these are being replaced with virtues such as patient advocate and patient teacher. It is quite possible that on the same shift, one could have several groups of nurses with differing views of what the "good nurse" is all about.

If we truly examine our actions as practitioners and look at what goes into our decision-making processes—in calculations of what is right or wrong in regard to professional duties—we would find we often are following the dictates of an idealized role. We are asking ourselves, "What does the good nurse, physical therapist, or radiographer do when faced with this situation?" In this sense we are not calculating our duties from a teleological or deontological

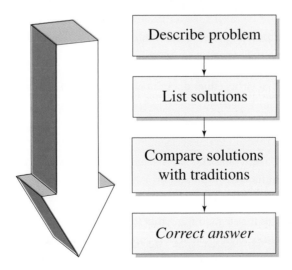

FIGURE 2-4   Virtue-Oriented Reasoning

orientation, but are being guided by the duties imposed by our role and position in the health care team and society. One of the real problems with virtue ethics is that as today's practitioners, we are being confronted by situations for which no role practices have been created, for which tradition provides no answers. An example of this new ground might be the nurse or respiratory therapist in the position of not only disconnecting a ventilator from a patient in a persistent vegetative state, but also removing the feeding tube and IV lines.

Criticisms of Virtue Ethics

1. Virtue ethics generally does not provide specific directions in regard to decision making.

2. In that virtue ethics relies on traditional practices, it does not quickly respond to changes in the practice that require new sorts of moral responses.

3. The derivation of duty from one's social role is likely to lead to or perpetuate classism, sexism, paternalism.

4. A traditional emphasis makes morality depend on past experience rather than on reason. This environment provides little respect or personal autonomy or the use of reason in moral judgments.

5. Practitioners often find themselves attempting to address more than one set of idealized roles, which may come into conflict, (for example, the need to be a team player and the need to be a whistle-blower in a case of negligent action).

6. Virtue ethics often yields results that do not maximize happiness.

Virtue Ethics Responses to Criticism

The advocates for a virtue ethics orientation would respond to the above criticisms with the following justifications for their position.

1. While it is true that virtue ethics does not give specific directions, it does not have to, for virtue ethics is concerned with character, not action. Virtuous people will automatically do the right thing because it is in their character to do so, or because it is an obligation of some social role relevant to the decision at hand. This is not to deny that there are difficult choices to make at times, but this is a problem faced by all ethical theories. And in the case of either Kantianism or utilitarianism, there is just as likely to be a rationalization of a decision made from character as it is that these theories will provide a definitive answer.

2. Virtue ethics takes it as a good thing that it does not change quickly in response to the whims of the masses. We should be very careful to be sure that a proposed change in tradition or social roles is for the better. In fact, rapid change in social norms often leads to what the philosopher Alvin Toffler has called "future shock." People often find themselves adrift when times change faster than they can adjust to them.[12]

3. While virtue ethics does not emphasize the rationality of the individual decision maker, it does rely on a higher reason: the wisdom of the ages. Virtue ethicists regard the reason of individuals as a poor imitation of the accumulation of rationality that embodies tradition. On the autonomy issue, many virtue ethicists believe that many of our contemporary social problems are the result of too much autonomy and too little respect for tradition.

Virtue ethics seems to add an important dimension to ethical discussion but does not supply the full answer. In that virtue ethics instructs us to first become compassionate, honorable, and truthful beings, it reminds us of important considerations often overlooked in action-focused theories. Yet even kind, honorable, compassionate beings often do not know the right thing to do. Perhaps virtue ethics is an important supplement to duty and consequence theories in that it reminds us that in the realm of values, the nature of the individual making the choice is often as important as the ability to reason to a correct answer. The following case study supplies an opportunity to examine the nature of virtue ethics.

CASE STUDY

Virtue Ethics: Saints and Sinners

Maria is the student in your clinical laboratory science class that you as a teacher think is least likely to make a good health care provider. Although very bright, she comes from a rough-and-tumble background, and while she is making satisfactory progress in your class, she is also the one who appears to be cutting the most corners.

On your way out of the office, you leave your office open and the final examination on your desk. Maria works in the building as a work-study student. She knows that you have gone for the day and notices that the door is open. She enters your office and sees the exam.

It would be so easy to copy the exam, she thinks as she moves toward it. However, at the last moment, she stops and thinks to herself that she knows she is prepared for the exam, and she doesn't need the grief if she should ace the exam and someone sees her leave the office.

She backs out of the office, looks to be sure that no one has seen her, and locks the door. She thinks to herself, *If I can't see the exam, I will be sure that no one else will either.*

(continues)

Virtue Ethics: Saints and Sinners (cont.)

Arthur is the model student in your clinical laboratory class. You often daydream of the perfect class, and in every seat the student who is sitting there looks like Arthur.

On your way out of the office, you leave your office open and the final examination on your desk. Arthur works in the building as a work-study student. He knows that you have gone for the day and notices that the door is open. He enters your office and sees the exam.

Once Arthur sees that the exam is on the desk, he backs out of the office and locks it. He thinks, *I will warn the instructor to be more careful with the door*. It really did not occur to him to copy the exam, although he also feels well prepared.

1. In virtue ethics, which of the following is the more noble: the tempted sinner who makes the right choice or the unconcerned saint? Defend your answer.

DIVINE COMMAND ETHICS

Divine command ethics is a fourth type of theory that is often used in ethical debates, so it merits inclusion in this survey of standard ethical theories. The idea is a simple one: there is a divine being who has set down a finite series of rules that adherents claim can provide guidance to most, if not all, moral decisions. An important example is the set of rules known as the Ten Commandments taken from Judeo-Christian traditions. It includes key moral prohibitions common to most cultures, as well as some specific rules set down to exact adherence to a particular religion. For our purposes, the specific moral injunctions are the focus. The Ten Commandments provide rules against stealing, adultery, murder, and so on. These basic rules are taken as guides to behavior in a wide range of cases by extending the reasoning behind each of the rules to related kinds of cases. Hence the rule against murder is claimed by some to imply that euthanasia and abortion are wrong. Of course, almost as many deny that the rules can be extended in such a manner.

A variant of divine command theory is a command theory based on a nondivine but morally exemplary individual such as the Buddha. Buddhism's Four Noble Truths and the related Eight-Fold Path, as well as sets of rules for nuns and monks, follow the same logic as divine command theory, the only difference being their origin is the teachings of a nondivine person. In both cases, the Judeo-Christian religion and the Buddhist religion, the logic of the teachings is the same. There are central moral injunctions that we are supposed to obey upon pain of divine retribution in the Judeo-Christian tradition, or failure to achieve nirvana in the Buddhist tradition.

Criticisms of Divine Mandate Theory

1. Command theories assume belief in either divine beings or exemplary individuals. To the extent that these beliefs can be questioned, so can the theory.

2. Command theories cannot cover all possible cases of moral decision. This problem often leads to either a fundamentalism, which merely states that the extensions of the basic rules to other cases are unproblematic, or it leads to differences in interpretation of the basic rules and therefore differences in people's moral views.

3. Command theories generally have a "no exceptions" clause, either explicit or implicit. This is a problem for people living in morally complicated times.

4. Command theory has what may be called the "Euthyphro Problem," from the Platonic dialogue from which it originated. The question arises, Is an action morally unacceptable because the divinity or exemplary individual (arbitrarily) says so? Or is it a case that the divine being or exemplary individual is basing the rule on some justifying reason? Is an action good because God loves it, or does God love it because it is good? If it is the former, it is hard to imagine why we would feel compelled to obey a rule so arbitrarily chosen. If the latter, then we can eliminate the middleman and refer directly to the justifying reason. In either case, one could question assenting to rules provided by command theory.

Divine Command Responses to Criticism

Followers of divine mandate ethics might answer the criticisms with the following justifications:

1. While there is no convincing response to the first criticism when dealing with unbelievers, the supposition of a divine being or exemplary being is unproblematic when dealing with believers. For the true believer, it is simply a matter of seeing the light.

2. The response here is simply to argue that the questions of interpretations are not insurmountable. With enough study and faith, one can come to generally acceptable interpretations that extend the reasoning behind the basic rules to fit all current situations. It is simply a matter of likening the text and admonitions to ourselves.

3. It is believed that the very need for exceptions to revealed truth is a sign of a decadent time, and perhaps a greater adherence to the rules will lead to a more morally sound society.

4. A command theorist could argue that there are reasons behind a religion's moral injunctions but that we are unable to completely fathom the justification due to our personal limitations. Hence, we are asked to obey on faith in the superior wisdom of the divine being or the exemplary individual.

It is clear that divine command ethics often provides a meaningful system for decision making for those who believe. Yet this is a world of believers and nonbelievers, a world of complex problems never before faced by previous generations. It is difficult to imagine that the ancient texts will resolve with a high level of certainty issues such as cloning, or whether it is appropriate to collect and freeze the sperm from a dead spouse so that artificial insemination can take place at a later time. The complexity and context of the questions associated with modern health care will stretch any absolutist theory such as divine command ethics seemingly to their limits. Yet when one examines the decisions regarding organ donation by a variety of religions, it is clear that divine mandate reasoning can be remarkably adaptive.

While divine command ethics seem suitable for personal decision making, it appears somewhat problematic when one is required to reason together with those of a different belief system and come to a decision acceptable to all. Individuals who perceive that they have revealed truth may find it difficult to see the value of other opinions, or of exploring the myriad options that surround problems. This is understandable when one considers that unlike the other ethical systems that seek the correct or right answer, the answer provided by divine mandate ethics is not only right but good, which places the opposite view as not only wrong but perhaps bad.

CONCLUSION

Over the course of our lives, each of us develops a coherent set of attitudes, feelings, and opinions with which we judge the world of actions around us in terms of good and bad, right or wrong, positive or negative. This value system or worldview is culturally shaped by the events of our lives and the traditions of our people.

Several ethical systems have been proposed to assist and bring order to value-laden decision making. Clearly the settling of these issues by the flipping of a coin is unacceptable, as it would lead to an ethical pluralism, where any choice is as good as another. To allow a morally neutral society is not in keeping with social order and progress. Currently, the ethical systems with the highest level of acceptability are duty orientation, consequence orientation, divine mandate, and virtue ethics. Each of these allows the examination of ethical problems and provides a framework for decision making. Each of these general systems with which we look at ethical problems has contemporary theorists with varying models, which can be classed as being duty, consequence, divine mandate, or virtue ethics oriented.

Each of the general ethical systems has been subjected to legitimate criticisms that they fail to overcome, and none at this point seems to have universal acceptance. When we examine our own personal value systems, we can be found to be duty oriented in some decisions and consequentialistic in others. An individual could be very duty oriented in regard to an issue such as abortion, and yet approach the withdrawal or removal of life support from a consequence orientation. It has been noted that just as in the foxhole there are no atheists, in the practice of health care, there is little comfort in decision making without a situational framework or the reliance on principle. Van Rensselaer Potter, who is credited with coining the word *bioethics,* explained that this new discipline had as its focus the traditional task of medical ethics: aiding the individual practitioner to make decisions and to live with them.[13] Ethics, then, is a generic title that we give to systems that seek to bring sensitivity and method to the human task of decision making in the arena of moral values.

Whatever ethical framework one chooses in order to solve problems, usually the method will contain the same basic steps.

Step 1—Identify the characteristics of the problem. Describe the problem, and identify the principles involved. Who are the concerned parties? Who is charged with making the decision?

Step 2—Gather the facts of the case. What is fact? What is opinion? What are the legal ramifications? Has this issue been decided by the courts before? What documentation exists that outlines the problem?

Step 3—Examine the options with initial credibility. The more options you can think of, the more likely you are to find one you can support.

Step 4—Weigh and evaluate the potential options. What happens to the individuals involved, given each option? Has everyone been considered equally? What principles are favored and which are sacrificed? What ethical system are you going to use to make the choice: utilitarianism, duty oriented, or virtue ethics?

Step 5—Make your decision, and act on it.

Step 6—Assess and evaluate the results.

The next several chapters deal with health care issues and the methods used in coming to decisions. Within the clarification exercises, a variety of methods will be examined, but most deal with the six basic steps as outlined.

KEY CONCEPTS

- Several theoretical systems for solving ethical dilemmas have been developed. Perhaps the most commonly used are utilitarianism proposed by Jeremy Bentham and John Stuart Mill, Kantian ethics proposed by Immanuel Kant, virtue ethics first proposed by Aristotle with a modern formulation by Alasdair MacIntyre, and divine command ethics, which has many proponents and founders.

- Act utilitarianism is the purest form of utilitarianism. One judges the utility of an act by listing the possible options and then calculating the amount of pleasure each provides and selects the course of action that maximizes pleasure.

- Rule utilitarianism is a form of utilitarianism that seeks to avoid the hedonic calculus of act utilitarianism in which each option must by measured by the principle of utility. Rule utilitarianism holds that an action can be right if it conforms to a rule that has been previously validated by the principle of utility. An example of such a rule might be that unless there is a fire, one should not yell "*Fire*" in a dark theater.

- When using utilitarian ethics, it is important to give equal consideration of interest. Everyone involved must be taken into account. Some theorists claim that it is necessary to adopt or at least listen to the standpoint of the most marginalized individuals in the situation.

- Kant proposed that consequences were essentially irrelevant, that morality is derived from rationality, not from experience. Kant held that through reason, one could find universal truths that created obligations of action binding on all people, for all times, in all situations. An important example of such a rule would be, "We must always treat others as ends and not as means only."

- The primary focus for virtue ethics is the heart of the moral agent making the decision rather than reasoning to a right action. According to the theory, an individual by living well and practicing virtues could develop the habit of being virtuous. Such an individual, when confronted by an ethical dilemma, would act according to his heart and choose well.

- Knowing and practicing professional virtues makes professional decision making easier and often better. However, it is important to remember that even in virtue, the ancient Greeks urged moderation and the golden mean.

- The basic idea of divine command ethics is that there is a divine or exemplary being that has set down a finite series of rules that can provide guidance for most, if not all, moral decisions. An example of such a set of rules is the Ten Commandments.

- In a world of believers and nonbelievers, an appeal solely to faith for an ethical answer is often not beneficial in gaining understanding and agreement.

- Over time, theorists have developed several methods by which to evaluate health care issues involving values. None of these has clearly carried the day, and often you will find yourself combining them in your decisions.

REVIEW EXERCISES

A. For this case, first justify your decision using duty-oriented reasoning and then follow using consequence-oriented reasoning.

As the local pharmacist, you have known the Smith family for years and consider them friends as well as customers and clients. Missy Smith has always been a favorite of yours and you have watched her grow into a very pretty thirteen year old. One day when no other customers are present, Missy asks you for a kit to test for pregnancy and pleads with you not to tell her family that she is sexually active.

B. Using the labels (cultural relativism, hedonism, consequence oriented, virtue ethics, divine command, and duty oriented), identify the following statements:

1. "If it feels good, do it."_____

2. "Don't criticize until you walk a mile in their shoes."_____

3. "The cost of maintaining the elderly on ventilators is beyond the cost the society can bear. After the age of eighty-five, the elderly should not be placed on a ventilator or should be taken off." _____

4. "At the moment of conception a human comes into being, with all the rights and privileges of all other humans. In that life is sacred, nothing should be done that would sacrifice the fetus regardless of the situation." _____

5. "As practitioners of the healing arts, we are to take care of the sick, even if they have conditions that threaten our personal health." _____

C. Early utilitarians offered a system by which to quantify utility. This method consisted of seven categories and seven attendant questions. When presented with several potential choices of action, one need only score the possibilities to scientifically calculate the correct moral action.

Intensity: How intense is the pleasure?

Duration: How long will the pleasure last?

Certainty: How certain am I that the pleasure will occur?

Proximity: How soon will I experience the pleasure?

Fecundity: How many more pleasures will happen because of this one?

Extent: How many will experience the pleasure?

Assume a scoring system of 1 to 5 with 5 being the highest utility and 1 the least. Work out the utility for the following problem. Should I take a gratuity from a patient, ($50 in an envelope) even though I know that the hospital policy manual forbids it.

Score for yes _____ Score for no _____

Would you feel comfortable using this as a system for determining utility?

D. Virtue ethics depends on an identifiable set of good practices. List some value-oriented acts that you are expected to assume as a practitioner of your specialty.

E. The following questions involve value judgments. Answer each with a yes or no decision, and identify whether you arrived at your decision by duty-oriented, consequence-oriented, divine mandate, or virtue ethics reasoning.

1. Should I take a gift from a patient?

2. Is it acceptable to own a portion of a diagnostic clinic to which you refer patients?

3. Should a pharmacist criticize a physician if the doctor will not change a drug order that is clearly not in the best interest of the patient?

4. What is the nurse's duty when another nurse makes an error?

5. Should you tell a patient who asks about the quality of specific medical care that in your opinion the physician is a jerk?

6. As a radiographer you did a portable chest X-ray on the wrong patient in Room 407. In that the patient is not coherent and was not hurt by the process, do you have to report the error?

7. As a physical therapist, if the patient could not afford the care but needed to continue therapy, would it be acceptable to falsify insurance papers in order to provide the appropriate care for your patient?

8. As a respiratory therapist would it be acceptable to accept a finder's fee from a home health equipment company to which you referred your hospital patients?

9. Would a surgical nurse with strong pro-life values be correct in refusing to take part in a therapeutic abortion?

NOTES

1. Tom Beauchamp and Laurence McCullough, *Medical Ethics: The Moral Responsibilities of Physicians* (Englewood Cliffs, NJ: Prentice Hall, 1984), p. 37.

2. John Stuart Mill, *Utilitarianism, On Liberty,* and *Essay on Bentham,* ed. with intro, by Mary Warnock (New York: New American Library, 1974).

3. David Ingram and Jennifer Parks, *Understanding Ethics* (Indianapolis, IN: Alpha Books, 2002).

4. Joseph Fletcher, *Situation Ethics* (Philadelphia: Westminster Press, 1966).

5. Immanuel Kant, *Groundwork of the Metaphysic of Morals,* trans. J. J. Paton (New York: Harper and Row, 1964).

6. John Rawls, *A Theory of Justice* (Cambridge, MA: Harvard University Press, 1999).

7. Aristotle, *Nicomachean Ethics,* trans. T. Irwin (Indianapolis, IN: Hackett Publishing Company, 1985).

8. Alasdair MacIntyre, *After Virtue* (Notre Dame, IN: University of Indiana Press, 1984).

9. Luke Gormally, ed., *Moral Truth and Tradition: Essays in Honor of Peter Geach and Elizabeth Anscombe* (Dublin: Corners Press, 1994).

10. Bernard Mayo, *The Philosophy of Right and Wrong* (New York: Routledge, 1986).

11. Richard Taylor, *Ethics, Faith, and Reason* (Upper Saddle River, NJ: Prentice Hall, 1985).

12. Alvin Toffler, *Future Shock* (New York: Bantam Books, 1971).

13. Van Rensselaer Potter, *Bioethics: Bridge to the Future* (Englewood Cliffs, NJ: Prentice Hall, 1973).

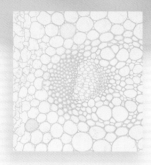

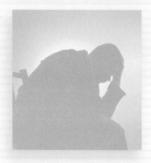

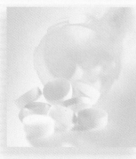

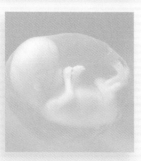

CHAPTER 3

Basic Principles of Health Care Ethics

GOAL

To introduce the reader to the basic principles used in the analysis of moral dilemmas and to show how these principles function in health care delivery.

OBJECTIVES

Upon completion of this chapter, the reader should be able to:

1. Differentiate between morals and ethics.

2. Identify the basic principles involved in medical ethics, and show their application in our ethical codes.

3. Define the basic principles found in health care ethics.

4. Define paternalism and show how in the best sense it is a conflict between the principles of autonomy and beneficence.

5. Outline the nature of the special fiduciary relationship between the practitioner and the patient.

6. Differentiate among compensatory, retributive, procedural, and distributive justice.

7. Outline the ethical problem associated with side effects and the duty of nonmaleficence, and show how the principle of double effect is an attempt to resolve the issue.

8. Explain how the principle of informed consent is derived from the basic principle of autonomy.

9. Explain the types of cases in which benevolent deception might be justified.

KEY TERMS

Autonomy	Informed consent	Principle of double effect
Beneficence	Justice	Professional Codes of Ethics
Benevolent deception	Morality	Role fidelity
Confidentiality	Nonmaleficence	Therapeutic privilege
Ethics	Paternalism	Veracity
Fiduciary relationship	Placebos	

APPLIED ETHICS

It appears to me that in Ethics, as in all other philosophical studies, the difficulties and disadvantages, of which history is full, are mainly due to a very simple cause: namely to the attempt to answer questions, without first discovering precisely what questions it is to which you desire an answer.

G. E. Moore, *Principia Ethica,* 1903

CASE STUDY

Tuskegee Study

Syphilis is a chronic, contagious bacterial disease that is most often sexually transmitted but is sometimes congenital. Since about 1946, the disease has been successfully treated with antibiotics. Prior to 1946, individuals with the disease had an inevitable progress through its sequelae, from the primary lesion and chancre to rash, fever, and swollen lymph nodes to the final stage of nervous system and circulatory problems, and finally death. The progress of the disease is often thirty to forty years.

Around 1929 there were several counties in the South with a high incidence of syphilis. The U.S. Public Health Service (USPHS) began a demonstration project to treat those afflicted with the disease in Macon County, Alabama, home of the famous Tuskegee Institute. With the Great Depression, funding for the project decreased and finally the demonstration project to treat the men became an opportunity for a study in nature. A *study in nature* means that the researchers were not to treat the patients but rather were to observe the natural progression of the disease. To conduct this study in nature, the USPHS selected 399 African American men who had never received treatment.

(continues)

Tuskegee Study (cont.)

The research group was told essentially that they had "bad blood," and they had been selected for special free treatment. Except for an African American nurse, Eunice Rivers, there was very little continuity with staffing of the experiment, as the federal doctors would come every few years to check on the progress of the disease. To induce the participants, they were promised free transportation, free hot lunches, free medicine (for everything but syphilis), and free burials. An interesting although somewhat dramatized version of the study can be seen in the film *Ms. Ever's Boys* (1997).

Although antibiotics were available in adequate supply by 1946, the study subjects were never treated. In fact, the local draft board was provided their names so that they could not enter the army, where they would have been treated as a matter of course. The local members of the County Medical Society were also provided their names and were asked not to provide them with antibiotics.

In July 1972, Peter Buxtun of the USPHS, who had been criticizing the study since 1966, told the story to an Associated Press reporter, and the research became headlines across the nation. In 1997, President Clinton officially apologized to the remaining study participants on behalf of the United States government.[2]

It is from our general worldviews that we have developed our societal morals and legal rights. These are in a continual state of evolution: As an illustration, society at one point in history will embrace slavery and then reject it, oppress women and disregard the disabled and then struggle to create a legitimate space for all. These societal swings may come as reactions to such vague concepts as to "do good and avoid evil," or the "inherent dignity of the individual."

These concepts become part of the foundational fabric of our morals and ethics, and they undergo constant reinterpretation for every age and time. An excellent example of how certain values seem to capture the day and then fade to be replaced by others is the mid-nineteenth-century slogan, "Twin Relics of Barbarism: Slavery and Polygamy." Today this has little emotive impact, and yet in its time it justified the movement of armies. Likewise, the societal impact of pro-choice and pro-life arguments will eventually also run their course and seem to future generations as quaint as the twin relics.

To gain a clearer picture of the differences between morals and ethics, we might examine the distinction offered by the ethicist Joseph Fletcher, who stated that "**morality** is what people believe to be right and good . . . , while ethics is the critical reflections about morality and the rational analysis of it."[1] **Ethics,** then, is nothing more than a generic term for the study of how we make judgments in regard to right and wrong. Ethics offer a way of examining moral life.

Professional ethics, such as those found in medicine and law, are applied ethics designed to bring about the ethical conduct of the profession. In health care delivery, the major purpose might be the pursuit of health, with the prevention of death and the alleviation of suffering as secondary goals. The basic ethical principles that have been developed to allow health professionals to determine right and wrong in regard to value issues involving these goals are **autonomy**, **veracity**, **confidentiality**, **beneficence**, **nonmaleficence**, **justice**, and **role fidelity**. Figure 3-1 illustrates a general hierarchy of thinking in regard to biomedical ethics, as we proceed from a general worldview, to universal principles, to rules as found in our ethical codes, and finally to decisions. The universal principles have application for other areas of human endeavor such as politics, business, and the conduct of war.

The end good or major purpose of these various other pursuits will shift the focus from that given when the goal is health. This shifted focus can be seen in an incident taken from the World War II Battle for North Africa. The allies were faced with the dilemma of having two groups of soldiers needing antibiotics and only enough medication for one group. One group contained the traditional heroes, wounded in battle against the tank forces of the enemy, while the other group—perhaps equally traditional but less heroic—had received their wounds in the local brothels, having contracted venereal disease. Who should receive the limited antibiotics? If the choice had been purely medical, the decision might have been to treat the heroes wounded in battle, based on the severity of the wounds, or even by lottery to assure equality of access. However, inasmuch as the major factor became who could be made well quickly and returned to the battle line (a nonmedical focus), the easy decision was to treat those wounded in the brothels.

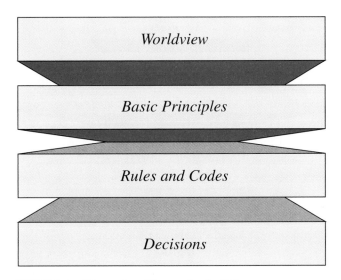

FIGURE 3-1   Hierarchy of Reasoning by Values

UNIVERSAL PRINCIPLES OF BIOMEDICAL ETHICS

In the cases and problems that follow in later chapters, we will examine the focus that health care gives to the universal principles (Figure 3-2). It is from these principles that we derive the rules found in our professional codes of ethics. Although the principles are listed in a set order, it is not intended that they should be considered in any hierarchy of importance.

Autonomy

The word comes from the Greek *autos* (self) and *nomos* (governance). In health care, it has come to mean a form of personal liberty, where the individual is free to choose and implement her own decisions, free from deceit, duress, constraint, or coercion. Three basic elements seem to be involved in the process: *the ability to decide*—for without adequate information, and intellectual competence, autonomy seems hollow; *the power to act on your decisions*—it is obvious that those in the death camps of World War II could have made all the decisions they might have wished but lacked power to implement them; and finally *a respect for the individual autonomy of others*—it is the provision of a general respect for personal autonomy for both practitioner and patient alike that ennobles and professionalizes the process. The term *self-determination* is often used synonymously with *autonomy*.

From the basic principle of autonomy, we have derived the rules involved in **informed consent**, which generally contain the elements of disclosure, understanding, voluntariness,

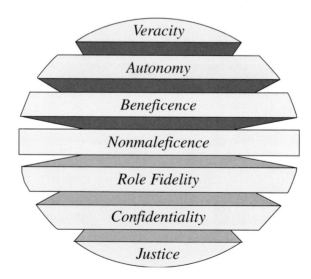

FIGURE 3-2   Universal Principles

competence, and permission giving. It is obvious that the patient is not free to select an appropriate path if not given adequate information, stated in a manner that allows understanding. The information must be provided at a time when the patient is able to sort options rationally and is in a position to grant or refuse consent. Legal exceptions to the rules of informed consent under **therapeutic privilege** have been made in cases of emergency, incompetence, waiver, and when there is implied consent. A problematic area of therapeutic privilege is that of **benevolent deception**, in which the practitioner is allowed to intentionally withhold information based on his sound medical judgment that to divulge the information might potentially harm a depressed and unstable patient.

One of the great areas of struggle in health care ethics is that of autonomy versus paternalism. **Paternalism** is the intentional limitation of the autonomy of one person by another, in which the person who limits autonomy appeals exclusively to grounds of benefit to the other person. Health care professionals have a special **fiduciary relationship** with patients based on the confidence placed in us and the inequality of our positions with regard to information. This relationship places an affirmative duty on practitioners to seek the best for patients. What, then, is to be done when the patient, acting on the impulse of personal autonomy, chooses a path away from health? Does the patient have the right to be wrong?

The American Hospital Association's *The Patient Care Partnership: Understanding Expectations, Rights and Responsibilities* provides the following statement with regard to autonomy and right to refuse treatment.

> **Discussing your treatment plan.** When you enter the hospital you sign a general consent to treatment. In some cases, such as surgery or experimental treatment, you may be asked to confirm in writing that you understand what is planned and agree to it. This process protects your right to consent to or refuse a treatment. Your doctor will explain the medical consequences of refusing recommended treatment. It also protects your right to decide if you want to participate in a research study.[3]

This right to refuse treatment in no way speaks to the quality of the decisions, only to the patient's right to make them. As practitioners, we are fortunate to serve in professions that generally are viewed by our patients and clients as positions of confidence and trust. This allows most health care questions to be solved through a process of negotiation based on fidelity, respect, and shared values.

Complicating the process of autonomy are the cases in which it becomes necessary to limit autonomy because the patient could not be expected to comprehend sufficiently to make an authentic decision. For example, should a patient in severe pain be allowed to make a decision to refuse treatment based on the current pain, when the treatment will be lifesaving and restore normal function?

As our population continues to age, we have an ever-increasing number of individuals who are physically frail or suffer from dementia. Even if we must, in the end, suspend some portion of their autonomy, who decides how much? The issue of autonomy and competency will be further discussed in Chapter 7.

Veracity

Veracity binds both the health practitioner and the patient in an association of truth. The patient must tell the truth in order that appropriate care can be provided. The practitioner needs to disclose factual information so that the patient can exercise personal autonomy.

The special fiduciary relationship that exists between patients and their health care practitioners is such that patients have the right to expect a higher level of truthfulness from us than others with whom they deal. If you were to buy a used car, you would hope that the dealer would tell you the truth. If asked a direct question about a specific problem and the dealer lies, he is committing fraud, but in most jurisdictions he is not required to volunteer the information. The practitioner, however, is bound within the limitation imposed by her role to disclose all relevant information. The limitation imposed by role fidelity will be discussed in Chapter 6.

Even under the guise of benevolent deception, the idea of not telling the truth to patients is rather suspect. The suggestion is that the individual is not strong enough to tolerate the truth, or more time is needed to prepare the patient for an unpleasant fact. Unfortunately, this lack of truth telling leads to a slippery slope, for while it gives comfort to the one individual, it teaches all others involved—for example, family members, friends, housekeeping staff, and hospital volunteers—that health care practitioners lie to their patients. When these others become sick themselves, they remember the previous deception and feel they cannot rely on the word of the professionals. It would be a rare case that truly justified lying to a patient. Modern health care is based on a complex set of covenants between the practitioner and patients, which work best under conditions of trust, veracity, and fidelity.

In *The Death of Ivan Ilych,* Leo Tolstoy beautifully explains how benevolent deception forces the patient into the madness of playing a role unsuited to the circumstances:

> What tormented Ivan Ilych most was the deception, the lie, which for some reason they all accepted he was not dying but was simply ill . . . what tormented Ivan Ilych was that no one pitied him as he wished to be pitied. At certain moments after prolonged suffering, he wished most of all (although he would have been ashamed to confess it) for someone to pity him as a sick child is pitied. He longed to be petted and comforted.[4]

Medicine's attitude toward truth telling has always been in somewhat of an ambiguous place because of the way in which it can clash with the desire to do the best for the patient. The use of substances known as **placebos,** which the practitioner knows to be biomedically inert but which the patient feels are therapeutic, is a good example. Fundamental to the use of placebos is that the practitioner must engage in nondisclosure and deception in order for the practice to work. The defense offered is that the deception is used only for the welfare of the patient. This is a triumph of doing good (beneficence) over patient autonomy, which virtually forms the definition of paternalism. Figure 3-3 lists suggested rules to be considered and questions to be asked prior to participating in placebo therapy.[5]

Whereas it is conceivable that lying to the patient might become necessary to avoid some greater harm, it cannot be entered into lightly as it interferes directly with the person's autonomy. Tolerance for lying damages the system of health care delivery. Patients believe lies only because truthfulness is expected from health care providers. Once the patients begin to look for deceit, an essential element of good health care delivery will be lost.

In *The Justification of Paternalism,* Gert and Culver developed the following criteria to determine whether a paternalistic lie is justified:[6]

1. The lie benefits the person lied to; that is, the lie prevents more evil than it causes for that particular person.

2. It must be possible to describe the greater good that occurs.

3. The individual should want to be lied to. If the evil avoided by the lie is greater than the evil caused by it, a person would be irrational not to want to be lied to.

4. Assuming equal circumstances, we would always be willing to allow the violation of veracity.

Allied health and nursing specialists should be committed to the truth. When faced with situations in which lying seems a rational solution, other alternatives must be sought. The harm

---

RULES

- Placebos with active agents that may have harmful side effects are not acceptable.
- Placebos should not be given to patients without their consent.

QUESTIONS

- What is the condition being treated?
- What are the motives for the therapy?
- What is the placebo supposed to do?
- Are there alternatives that are less misleading?
- What is the patient-staff relationship?

FIGURE 3-3   Placebo Therapy Rules and Questions

to patient autonomy and the potential loss of practitioner credibility makes lying to patients a practice that in almost all cases should be avoided.

Beneficence

The common English usage of the term *beneficence* suggests acts of mercy and charity, although it certainly may be expanded to include any action that benefits another. Most health care professions have statements that echo the Hippocratic Oath (Figure 3-4), which states that the physician will "apply measures for the benefit of the sick." The obligation to help imposes on

---

HIPPOCRATIC OATH

I swear by Apollo Physician and Asclepius and Hygieia and Panaceia and all the gods and goddesses, making them my witnesses, that I will fulfill according to my ability and judgment this oath and this covenant:

I will apply dietetic measures for the benefit of the sick according to my ability and judgment; I will keep them from harm and injustice.

I will neither give a deadly drug to anybody if asked for it, nor will I make a suggestion to this effect. Similarly I will not give to a woman an abortive remedy. In purity and holiness I will guard my life and my art.

I will not use the knife, not even on sufferers from stone, but will withdraw in favor of such men as are engaged in this work.

Whatever houses I may visit, I will come for the benefit of the sick, remaining free of all intentional injustices, of all mischief and in particular of sexual relations with both female and male persons, be they free or slaves.

What I may see or hear in the course of the treatment or even outside of the treatment in regard to the life of men, which on no account one must noise abroad, I will keep to myself holding such things shameful to be spoken about.

If I fulfill this oath and do not violate it, may it be granted to me to enjoy life and art, being honored with fame among all men for all time to come; if I transgress it and swear falsely, may the opposite of all this be my lot.

FIGURE 3-4   Hippocratic Oath

health care practitioners the duty to promote the health and welfare of the patient above other considerations, while attending and honoring the patient's personal autonomy. In the pledge of the American Nurses' Association, this is clearly stated: "The nurse's primary commitment is to the health, welfare, and safety of the client." Patients' assumption that health care providers are working on their behalf is of great importance to their morale, especially for those who are summoning all their strength to fight illness.

In an earlier age, when medical science had less to offer, the duty of beneficence was rather straightforward. Prior to the twentieth century, even after exhausting all efforts to help, health care providers were often only able to sit by the bed dispensing good psychological support, unable to arrest the disease process. However, with advanced life-support techniques, it is possible and common today to arrest the process of death, but at the same time fail in the restoration of life in a human sense, the life captured in events, life in a biographical sense. Life without awareness, without relationships, is perhaps not a beneficence but an additional form of injury.

Questions arise: Is the restoration of life that appears to have no value to the individual, beneficence? Are the staggering fiscal and emotional costs justifiable? When does the effort cease to be beneficent? With modern medicine, in which technology often overwhelms resources, it has become necessary to use cost-benefit ratio analysis to determine where beneficence ends and maleficence (doing harm) begins. In an earlier time, prior to antibiotics, pneumonia was known as "an old man's friend," as it was commonly the illness that ended a life filled with pain and suffering. In Chapters 9 and 10 we will discuss the issues of withholding and withdrawing life support as well as the current controversy involving active euthanasia.

Nonmaleficence

Most health care professional pledges or codes of care echo the principle paraphrased from the Hippocratic Oath statement: "I will never use treatment to injure or wrong the sick." In some way, this seems very similar to the duty of beneficence, in which the practitioner works to maximize the good for the patient and minimize harm. T. Beauchamp and J. Childress distinguish the principles in the following way:[7]

Nonmaleficence

1. One ought not to inflict evil or harm

Beneficence

2. One ought to prevent evil or harm
3. One ought to remove evil or harm
4. One ought to do or promote good

All the statements of beneficence involved positive action toward preventing, or removing harm, and promoting the good. In the nonmaleficence statement, the admonition is stated in the negative, to refrain from inflicting harm.

The technology of modern health care and therapeutics has made this a difficult principle to follow, because much of what we do has unfortunate secondary or side effects. For example, when steroids are administered to the asthmatic patient to relax the smooth muscles of the airway, often the side effect of Cushing's syndrome occurs. Some of the newer antibiotics given to fight infections have ototoxicity and nephrotoxicity as side effects. Analgesics such as morphine given for pain may lead to a suppression of respiration. In attempting to maintain the ethical position of nonmaleficence in these cases, some practitioners have explained their actions through the **principle of double effect**. With this concept the secondary effects may be foreseen, but can never be the intended outcomes. The practitioner could, when necessary, ethically prescribe or administer morphine for pain, while understanding that the analgesic suppresses respiration—so long as the intended effect is the former and never the latter and the good intentions equal or outweigh harmful effects. The elements contained within the principle of double effect are outlined in Figure 3-5. Although intuitively persuasive and described and defended in many duty-oriented works, the principle of double effect has detractors who feel that unwanted effects of actions that are foreseen and still allowed within the course of treatment become intended effects. Even if the principle of double effect is finally put to rest and found not to be a useful formulation for practice, it still asks the right question: Under what circumstances can one be said to act morally when some of the manifold foreseeable effects of that action are harmful? Figure 3-6 points out how the basic principles are considered almost common sense and intuitively correct.

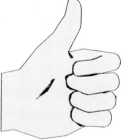

- The course chosen must be good or at least morally neutral.
- The good must not follow as a consequence of the secondary harmful effects.
- The harm must never be intended but merely tolerated as causally connected with the good intended.
- The good must outweigh the harm.

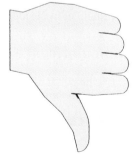

FIGURE 3-5   Principle of Double Effect (Guiding Elements)

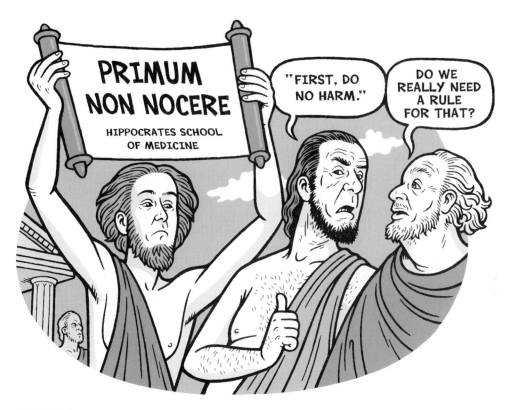

FIGURE 3-6

Confidentiality

The American Hospital Association's *The Patient Care Partnership: Understanding Expectations, Rights and Responsibilities* provides an outline of the current state of practice with regard to the individual's right to privacy in health care:

> We respect the confidentiality of your relationship with your doctor and other caregivers, and the sensitive information about your health and health care that are part of that relationship. State and Federal laws and hospital operating policies protect the privacy of your medical information. You will receive a **Notice of Privacy Practices** that describes the ways that we use, disclose, and safeguard patient information and that explains how you can obtain a copy of information from our records about your care.

Confidentiality is an important aspect of the trust that patients place in health care professionals. If the patient felt that information in regard to his body or condition was the subject of public conversation used to brighten the coffee break in the cafeteria or was subject to release to publications, a great barrier between practitioner and patient would exist. This fear of disclosure has, in the past, led minors with sexually transmitted diseases to suffer without care rather than to seek aid, knowing that the system required the health care system to notify their parents.

With sophisticated information systems, personal confidentiality is beset in all aspects of our lives. This is especially true with medical information systems in which patient information can be brought up on a CRT screen in a variety of areas throughout the hospital, making this information available to all who are on the system.

In a survey that looked at the expectations of patients, medical students, and house staff in regard to the issue of confidentiality, it was found that patients expected a more rigorous standard of confidentiality than that in current practice.[8] In the study, house staff and medical students indicated that they frequently discussed patients with spouses and informally with each other at parties. While current practice may require that cases be discussed in professional settings to gather other opinions, great care must be taken to warrant the confidence of patients. The breaching of confidentiality has serious implications. It threatens to harm patients, professions, and society in general, which depends on the services we provide.

Justice

The maintenance of this ethical principle is seemingly very simple in the abstract and complex in application, as it looks at the concepts of fairness, just deserts, and entitlements. What is due to an individual? In a just society, we require procedural justice or due process in cases of disputes between individuals. In health care, we deal with *distributive justice* as we struggle with the distribution of scarce resources. Perhaps the most famous formulation is that stated by Aristotle that "equals must be treated equally and un-equals must be treated unequally."

In our society we use several methods for the distribution of goods and services, attempting in some measure to provide a system in which individuals receive their due share:[9]

1. To each, an equal share (e.g., elementary and secondary education)
2. To each, according to need (e.g., aid to needy and programs such as food stamps)
3. To each, according to effort (e.g., unemployment benefits)
4. To each, according to contribution (e.g., retirement systems)
5. To each, according to merit (e.g., jobs and promotions)
6. To each, according to ability to pay (e.g., free market exchange)

In health care we are confronted by distribution problems that seem to provide better care to the rich than to the poor, the urban dweller over the rural, the middle-aged over the child or the elderly. Calls for a national health system much like that found in Canada, or the Oregon plan to ration care, can be seen as an attempt to better apply the principle of justice. The problem of providing for fair and equal distribution of health care would be difficult even if we assumed a world of unlimited resources. Once we factor in problems of scarcity, practitioner self-determination, maldistribution of resources, and costs, it becomes overwhelming.

A further discussion of the principle of justice will follow in Chapter 8. Complicating the issue of just distribution is a lack of agreement on what constitutes health. Certain groups, such as the World Health Organization (WHO), define it in the broadest terms: "a state of complete physical, mental, and social well-being, and not merely the absence of infirmity."[10] In that this definition somewhat guarantees everything for everybody, it becomes hard to imagine the distribution system that could accommodate such promises.

Another interesting aspect is the area of compensatory justice, in which individuals seek compensation for a wrong that has been done. This has become a far more important aspect of medicine in the light of the cases such as those where harm was caused by asbestos and other materials placed in our bodies and environment. Recent cases where cigarette smokers have received compensation from tobacco companies for their lung cancer or emphysema suggest how large an issue this may become.

Similar to compensatory justice is the ancient call for retributive justice or "an eye for an eye and a tooth for a tooth." Unlike compensatory justice, in which fines and compensation for injury are requested, retributive justice calls for equal suffering. Given the power of the argument (usually heard first from our mothers) that "two wrongs never make a right," retribution may have very little to do with any form of behavior suitable for the health care arena.

Role Fidelity

Modern health care is the practice of a team, as no single individual can maintain the data bank of information needed to provide rational care. Contained within the designation of allied health are over 100 individual professions, which in combination with nursing provide over 80 percent of our national health care. The nature of these specialties shapes the way in which the individual practitioner will respond to basic questions of biomedical ethics. An example might be the duty of the respiratory care practitioner not to tell a patient's family how critical the situation is, while the attending physician might have an obligation to relate the information. Whatever the assigned role, the ethics of health care require that the practitioner practice faithfully within the constraints of the role. Most often the areas of acceptable practice are contained and prescribed by the scope of practice of the state legislation that enables that profession's practice.

CONCLUSION

In general, morality is concerned with what people believe to be right and good conduct. It is transmitted from generation to generation, evolving and being reinterpreted for each age. This broad understanding of what is right and wrong in human conduct is taught to us by our families, religion, national culture, and legal structure.

Ethics is that part of philosophy that deals with systematic approaches to questions of morality. It provides the intellectual framework that allows us to analyze and make decisions in regard to moral choices. In no area of our lives are we more pressed by value-laden decisions than that of health care. The enormous power gained by our scientific successes raises questions that have never previously been posed, such as:

Should the elderly be provided the same level of health care as that provided for children?

Should patients with "Do Not Resuscitate" orders be treated in intensive care?

Must a health care provider who is HIV positive inform patients?

Who should live when not all can live?

Is there a morality to mercy killing?

Can health care practitioners work for the patient and be socially responsible for cost containment at the same time?

What constitutes life? What is a person?

Is there a right to health care? If there is a right, what is the limit of that right?

Is there a moral difference between removing a ventilator from a patient and removing IV tubes and a nasal gastric tube?

What is the meaning of confidentiality when, on the average, over seventy-five different individuals have access to information from our medical records?

Who shall be denied lifesaving treatment when there is not enough for all?

The increased usage of high technology, breakthroughs in scientific research, team medicine, and easy access to data have brought major changes to the delivery of health care and created a host of new moral dilemmas for which there are no easy solutions. However, answers must be found, because the very concept of value-free medicine is unworkable and because health care practitioners are forced into the process of making choices with which individuals and a society can live.

All forms of professional ethics draw from the same well of basic principles that shape our concepts of right and wrong in all aspects of our lives. The nature of our profession, however, and its basic purposes and goals will give these basic principles a unique focus. Therefore decision-making analysis from a legal, military, or health care perspective will often bring out decidedly different views of what is right in a given situation. Even within the different specialties of health care, the requirements of role duty will shape the analysis of ethical problems. In recent times, many questions involving health care ethics have been litigated in the courts for final decisions. The nature of these decisions does not always flow from ethically correct precepts. Something can be truly socially correct, medically possible, and legally permissible—and yet be morally reprehensible for the individuals involved.

In general, the basic principles involved in health care ethics are autonomy, veracity, beneficence, nonmaleficence, justice, confidentiality, and role fidelity. Often decision making in health care takes the form of an appeal for justification, based on an attempt to be true to one of these basic principles.

Professional codes of ethics can be seen as rules derived from the universal principles to bring about the goals of the profession. Although drawing from the same universal principles, they are shaped by the needs of the specific profession. An example is the clinical laboratory science focus on the need for detail and exactness. Respiratory care practitioners might find a focus in being directed by physicians and staying within the scope of practice. The code of ethics for medical record personnel stresses the duty of confidentiality.

KEY CONCEPTS

- Morality is what people believe to be right and good.
- Ethics is the critical reflection of morality and the rational analysis of it.
- Health care ethics is the application of moral philosophy to the health care arena.
- The seven basic principles of health care ethics are autonomy, veracity, beneficence, justice, confidentiality, role fidelity, and nonmaleficence. These principles will assist you in organizing your thinking when dealing with ethical dilemmas.
- There is no hierarchy for the principles. Although some have received more emphasis, none should be considered to be first or last.
- Paternalism is the intentional limitation of the autonomy of one person by another, in which the person who limits the autonomy appeals exclusively to grounds of benefit to the person whose autonomy is being limited. It is a situation in which I attempt to do you good, even if you desire not to have the "good" done. In its best sense, it is a contest between autonomy and beneficence.

- Although the principle of double effect has many detractors, it is often useful in sorting out issues such as secondary harmful side effects associated with treatment modalities.

- Ethical dilemmas are difficult to solve because they often create the need to choose among competing principles. It is important to take the time to analyze these problems.

REVIEW EXERCISES

A. The chapter begins with a very frustrating case concerning the now-infamous Tuskegee Study. Review the case and answer the following:

1. Consider each of the individual basic principles: autonomy, veracity, beneficence, non-maleficence, justice, role fidelity, and confidentiality. Which of these principles were sacrificed in the Tuskegee Study? Explain your answer.

2. To what extent should blame for the lack of ethical conduct be placed on the shoulders of Nurse Eunice Rivers? It should be noted that during the study, physicians came and went, but Nurse Rivers was the consistent figure throughout the study.

B. For the following code of ethics, identify the universal principle that is being addressed with each rule. For example, a rule that requires a nurse not to disclose personal information would be addressing the universal principle of confidentiality.

ANA Code for Nurses

1. The nurse provides services with respect for human dignity and the uniqueness of the client unrestricted by considerations of social or economic status, personal attributes, or the nature of health problems.

   Principle(s) involved _____

2. The nurse safeguards the client's right to privacy by judiciously protecting information of a confidential nature.

   Principle(s) involved _____

3. The nurse acts to safeguard the client and the public when health care and safety are affected by the incompetent, unethical, or illegal practice of any person.

   Principle(s) involved _____

4. The nurse assumes responsibility and accountability for individual nursing judgments and actions.

   Principle(s) involved _____

5. The nurse maintains competence in nursing.

   Principle(s) involved _____

6. The nurse exercises informed judgment and uses individual competence and qualifications as criteria in seeking consultation, accepting responsibilities, and delegating nursing activities to others.

   Principle(s) involved _____

7. The nurse participates in activities that contribute to the ongoing development of the profession's body of knowledge.

   Principle(s) involved _____

8. The nurse participates in the profession's efforts to implement and improve standards of nursing.

   Principle(s) involved _____

9. The nurse participates in the profession's efforts to protect the public from misinformation and misrepresentation and to maintain the integrity of nursing.

   Principle(s) involved _____

10. The nurse participates in the profession's efforts to establish and maintain conditions of employment conducive to high-quality nursing care.

    Principle(s) involved _____

11. The nurse collaborates with members of the health professions and other citizens in promoting community and national efforts to meet the health needs of the public.

    Principle(s) involved _____

C. Review the code of ethics for your specialty to determine what basic principle is being addressed with each rule. (The codes of ethics for the following specialties are found in the appendix: American Dental Association, Dental Hygienists, Occupational Therapy, Physical Therapy, Physicians, Physician Assistants, Respiratory Care, Nursing, Clinical Laboratory Professionals, Radiologic Technologists, Medical Assistants, and Pharmacists.)

D. Does the code of ethics for your specialty have a rule that addresses each of the basic principles (autonomy, veracity, beneficence, nonmaleficence, justice, confidentiality and role fidelity)?

E. Compare your code to the one for the American Medical Association. In what way does yours differ? In what way does your code reflect the nature of your specialty?

F. In the following cases, identify the principle(s) involved, and state a rule from your specialty code of ethics that might be used to address the issue.

1. In a voluntary outpatient psychiatric clinic in California, a young man disclosed to his psychologist that he intended to kill a young woman. From previous conversations, the psychologist knew the identity of the woman and became very concerned. After the young man had left his office, the psychologist consulted with his superior and they decided to have the man stopped by the security person at the gate.

   When security stopped the man as he was leaving the clinic, they became concerned about his legal rights in that he appeared to them to be rational and to threaten no danger to himself or others. They related this information to the psychiatrist on duty, who then decided to allow the man to leave and ordered the records of the event destroyed.

   The young man then proceeded to carry out his intentions and shortly after took the life of the young woman. The parents of the woman, upon finding out about what had occurred, sued the clinic.

   The clinic staff defended their actions on the basis that (1) many individuals fantasize about doing harm to others without carrying out the threat, and (2) to repeat the information gathered during therapy would bring them into an ethical problem of breaching confidentiality. They held that if the patients did not have faith that what they said during therapy was going to be held in confidence, in actual fact they would not continue to reveal anything of significance.

   Principle(s) involved _____

   In your specialty code of ethics, which rule might have application?

   What is your own personal decision concerning the lawsuit in this case?

2. You and Joseph Bradshaw have been friends and colleagues for some time. You are graduates from the same physical therapy program and now work at the same rehabilitation center. This has been a hard year for Joseph, as he has just come through a very difficult divorce, and you have attempted to befriend him. Recently you have noticed that he has been acting a bit strange, laughing at inappropriate times and having mood swings—between being very quiet to talking a mile a minute. You suspect that your friend has begun to abuse drugs.

   Your suspicions are confirmed one day in a conversation, in which he reveals to you that he has had a hard time sleeping and is taking pills to help him sleep and then other pills to keep him going through the day. Joseph asks you to keep his problem a secret, as he is sure that this is just something that he will need to work out as he gets over his divorce.

   The next day during morning review of the patients, Joseph seems to be falling asleep during report. Later your department head, who knows of your friendship with

Joseph, approaches you and asks, "What is the matter with Joe?" You wonder what to say.

Principle(s) involved _____

What rule in your specialty code of ethics might have application in this case?

Before you come to a personal decision, first list all the options that have some credibility. After you have developed your options list, then estimate how each of the parties involved will fare under each of the options.

G. In Greek literature there are several models for health care practice. Two with significance for our time are the cult of Aesculapius and the cult of Hygeia.

The cult of Aesculapius is strictly a patient-health care practitioner affair aimed at getting the particular individual physically well. In this light, care would be aggressively patient centered, and the practitioner would not mix social, political, or economic considerations with the care of the patient.

The cult of Hygeia (daughter of Aesculapius) uses the broader social or public health model of prevention as well as therapy as the context for care. The term *hygiene* means "good for health." This approach is based on the prevention of disease rather than treatment. *Hygeia* is the public health or public interest way of looking at health care delivery.

Examine the American health care delivery system, and indicate which of the models better fits what we are currently doing in our culture.

Examine the practice of your specialty. Which of the Greek models is it more closely aligned with: Aesculapius, or Hygeia?

H. Are there basic ethical principles missing from your professional code of ethics? If so, write rules that should be added to your code to address these areas.

I. A case often cited that looks at the principle of veracity is that of the husband and wife who are both in a nursing home. The husband has a heart attack and the wife is brought from another floor. Before she can get to the room, the man dies, but to spare the woman pain, the staff allows her to think that he is still alive when she gets to the room. In that she is frail and feeble, with poor eyesight, she does not know that he is dead. The woman is then told that her husband's respiration is growing weaker and that he appeared to have been waiting for her before he died. As she leaves the room, she tells the staff that she is so glad that he waited for her so that she could see him alive one more time.

Using the Gert and Culver criteria listed in the chapter under the principle of veracity, does the above case justify the lying? Explain your answer.

NOTES

1. Joseph Fletcher, *The Ethics of Genetic Control* (Garden City, NY: Anchor Books, 1974), p. xiii.

2. Susan Reverby, ed., *Tuskegee Truths* (Chapel Hill, NC: University of North Carolina, 2000).

3. American Hospital Association, *The Patient Care Partnership: Understanding Expectations, Rights, and Responsibilities.* Washington, DC. 2003.

4. Leo Tolstoy, *The Death of Ivan Ilych and Other Stories* (New York: New American Library, 1960).

5. Marilyn Desmarasis, "The Nurse's Ethical Guide to Placebo Giving," *California Nurse* (May 1988).

6. Bernard Gert and Charles Culver, "The Justification of Paternalism," in *Medical Responsibility,* ed. W. Robinson, and M. Pritchard (Clifton, NJ: Humana Press, 1979), pp. 1–9.

7. Tom Beauchamp and James Childress, *Principles of Biomedical Ethics* (New York: Oxford University Press, 1989), p. 119.

8. Barry Weiss, "Confidentiality Expectations of Patients, Physicians, and Medical Students," *Journal of the American Medical Association* 247 (1982): pp. 2695–2697.

9. Gene Outka, "Social Justice and Equal Access to Health Care," in *Ethics and Health Policy,* ed. R. M. Veatch and R. Branson (Cambridge: Ballinger Publishing Co., 1976).

10. Preamble to the Constitution of the World Health Organization, adopted 1946.

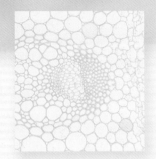

CHAPTER 4

The Nature of Rights in Ethical Discourse

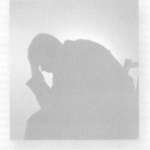

GOAL

To explore the language of rights and the nature of the obligations that are attendant to these rights.

OBJECTIVES

Upon completion of this chapter, the reader should be able to:

1. Define what is meant by a claim to a moral right.

2. Explain how rights and their attendant correlative obligations are grounded in the same overarching principles and rules.

3. Define and differentiate between the following types of rights:

   moral rights

   legal rights

   positive rights

   negative rights

   perfect obligations

   imperfect obligations

4. List three examples each of positive and negative rights.

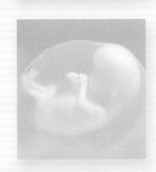

5. Explain how operating from the original position would naturally lead to choices that are founded on the principle of justice and collective choice.

6. Contrast the development of rights from a natural right, consequential, and contractarian position.

7. Explain why the modern tendency to justify all claims on the basis of rights has a negative effect on the value of rights as a concept used in ethical discussion.

8. List four correlative obligations that could be rightfully claimed from us by our patients as a result of our being health professionals.

9. List four examples of natural rights that have found their way into our society as legal rights.

10. Outline the rights problem associated with the U.S. Supreme Court's creation of a negative right in regard to abortion.

KEY TERMS

Contractarian theory	**Legal rights**	**Perfect obligation**
Correlative obligations	**Natural rights**	**Recipient rights**
Imperfect obligation	**Original position**	**Rights**

We hold these truths to be self evident, that all men are created equal; that they are endowed by their Creator with certain unalienable rights; that among these are life, liberty and the pursuit of happiness.

Declaration of Independence

In the case of intrinsic or fundamental, unacquired rights . . . what grip we had on rights has, I think been lost. Rather we are at sea in a tide of theoretical claims and counterclaims, with no fixed point by which to steer.

Raymond Frey

> ## CASE STUDY
>
> ## Poor Piggy Case
>
> In William Golding's classic novel, *Lord of the Flies,* a situation occurs where a small chubby child with the nickname Piggy has lost his glasses to a bully.* Piggy asserts his claim to the glasses in the language of rights, arguing that he has a right to them. In the story, the bully rolls a rock down on Piggy, killing him.
>
> 1. Did Piggy have a right to his glasses?
>
> 2. If not his glasses, did Piggy have a right to his life?
>
> 3. From where might such rights come?
>
> 4. Did Piggy's weakness with respect to enforcing his rights decrease his legitimate claim?
>
> _____
>
> *William Golding, *The Lord of the Flies* (New York: Coward-McCann, 1962).

THE NATURE OF RIGHTS

Although there is often disagreement as to the exact nature of rights, regardless of how they are defined, they appear to be something that is desirable and beneficial. Rights have been described variously as entitlements, interests, powers, claims, and needs.[1] If one is a possessor of a right, one apparently need not feel gratitude to others for its possession. Somehow, the right is ours, something that we own, or is our due and not dependent on the goodwill of others. Rights are not claims to a privilege, which is dependent upon the free will, kindness, or pleasure of another person. When we say that someone has a right to something, we are not indicating that it would be nice or charitable if they received it, but rather that they must be provided with the object or service in question. To quote Ronald Dworkin,

> "a right is something of which no one may be deprived without a grave affront to justice."[2] And, according to Dworkin, "Rights can be thought of as 'trumps' which take precedence over mere expediency or social benefit."[3]

Rights in moral philosophy and political theory are thought of as justified claims. In this sense, if you have a moral or legal right to personal property, then others have an obligation to respect your claim to that property. Rights can be justified by moral or legal principles and rules or in some cases a claim to both moral and legal justification. In the language of rights, we often find the following formulation to explain the obligations and limits of rights: "If John has a right to X, then others have no justification in interfering with John's pursuit or possession of X, so long as John's exercise of his right to X does not infringe on the rights of others." This is significantly different from a privilege, which depends on the goodwill or kindness of others for fulfillment. As an example, if an individual purchases a book, then he has a right to personal property, which includes the book, and others have a moral obligation to respect the ownership of the book. As a rule, we need not thank others for honoring private ownership. However, if you go to the library and receive a book on loan, it is not generally thought that you have a moral or legal right to receive loans of books. In this case, you are exercising a library privilege, and an expression of appreciation might be warranted. Also, there are limits placed on what you can do with the book.

When we consider rights as justified claims, then built within the claim is the correlative thesis of rights and obligations. In this sense, a right creates an obligation in others to behave in a certain way—to provide goods or services or refrain from interference. As an example, the patient's right to informed consent obligates the health care provider to provide appropriate information. If it is possible to examine the obligation of the health care provider regarding providing information to the patient, we could ascertain the patient's right to informed consent, or vice versa. If we could examine the patient's right to informed consent, then we could reason ourselves to the obligation of the health care provider. The correlative thesis implies that both the obligation and the right are being justified by the same overarching principles or rules.[4]

Although we often think of rights as being absolutes, they must compete in the social context with other competing claims. In general, a right to life creates an obligation in others not to kill. However, even the right to life, which seems rather foundational, must compete with the right to life of others who have an equal claim to their lives and with social considerations and moral judgment in regard to self-defense and killing in the time of war. There are cases in which generally accepted rights, such as a right to informed consent, privacy, and personal autonomy in regard to health care choice, are overridden when they come into competition with other rights in a social context. In deathbed situations, often the family will wish for the health care providers to do everything for their loved one. In a sense, they have a right to expect that everything will indeed be done, and the providers have an obligation within a reasonable context to see that everything is provided. Yet one's death is uniquely one's own. If the patient chooses to exercise the autonomy of choice and asks that all heroics be avoided, then the family's right to call for heroics can be interfered with and infringed on.

One primary usage of rights language that is separate from justified claims and duties is the symbolic language of covenants, charters, manifestos, and conventions, which we use to lay out expressions of hope for the future of humanity. These documents usually speak to our better selves and a better future for humanity but are usually not meant to outline a reality that is grounded in law or claims that can be enforced. Examples of this symbolic usage of rights language can be seen in declarations such as the 1948 United Nations Universal Declaration of Human Rights.[5] Article 6 of the declaration states that "everyone has the right to recognition as a person everywhere before the law." It is difficult to imagine the enforcement or ability to honor the *everyone* and *everywhere* portions of these documents. As expressions of hope, these covenants have great symbolic value, but it is very difficult to explicate the status of the rights claimed in them in the sense of correlative obligations.

HISTORICAL BACKGROUND OF RIGHTS REASONING

Historically, the language of rights and their concepts came into general political and moral discourse in the Middle Ages. Natural rights were generally equated to the law of God and found their most succinct expressions in forms such as the Golden Rule. As seen in Figure 4-1, the Golden Rule appears to have almost universal application and understanding. With the age of reformation, both local jurisprudence and international law came to be discussed in the light of natural rights. In the writings of men such as Grotius and Locke, the legitimacy of nation-states could be determined by the respect they paid to the inherent natural human rights.[6] We can see some reflections of this today in the shifting American policy of attaching favored-nation status to human rights improvement in countries such as the People's Republic of China.

Natural liberties are universal moral rights and are thought to exist prior to and independent of the guarantees of a social contract or institutionalized government. The concept writ large into our culture that all men are "endowed by their Creator with certain unalienable rights; that among these are life, liberty, and the pursuit of happiness"[7] is an expression of the universality of natural liberties and moral rights. These are often called *negative rights* in that they obligate others from interference. The right to liberty is really a statement of a personal right to be free from interference of the exercise of that right, such as enslavement. The expression of human rights seems to have been used first by the American firebrand patriot Thomas Paine in his translation of the Revolutionary French document. In his writings, Paine seems to use *human rights* and *natural rights* as synonymous terms.

Human rights, when differentiated from natural rights, seem to flow from a recognition that all humans (*Homo sapiens*) are equally separated from the beasts of the field and are unique unto themselves. As we grow and mature, we come to recognize our common human origins and the needs that are required for our development. If I am without food, I feel hunger, and if this continues long enough, I die. Not only do I know this of myself, I know this for all human beings. There are basic needs that we all share and have come to recognize and respect as a person's just due if he is to remain human. It is clear that animals and humans share a set of common needs, yet most do not grant rights to animals based on a recognition of their shared needs.

ISLAM

No one of you is a believer until he desires for his brother that which he desires for himself. (Sunnah)

JUDAISM

What is hateful to you, do not to your fellow man. (Talmud)

BUDDHISM

Hurt not others that which you would find hurtful. (Udana-Varga)

BRAHMANISM

Do naught unto others which would cause you pain if done to you. (Mahabharata)

CONFUCIANISM

Do not unto others that which you would not have them do unto you. (Analects)

TAOISM

Regard your neighbor's gain as your gain, and your neighbor's loss as your own loss. (T'ai Shang Xan Ying P'ien)

CHRISTIANITY

All things whatsoever ye would that men should do to you, do ye even to them. (The Bible)

FIGURE 4-1   Golden Rules

These claims to goods or services are often termed *positive rights*. These fundamental shared needs form the basis for our concepts of universal human rights. This agreement in regard to universal human rights is a recognition that as humans, we are interdependent, and the welfare of one is the responsibility of all.

Not every human right can be satisfied in all situations. If, for instance, I thirst for water and no water is available, I continue to thirst. Having a right without a means to exercise it does not negate the right; it continues to exist. Other humans know that as they need water, so do I if I am to remain alive and human. I can justly demand water from them if it is available beyond their needs. If they have only enough for themselves, my right to their water becomes inoperative, in effect, canceled out by their needs. I still have a human right to have my needs fulfilled, yet I may not demand what others require to remain alive without violating their fundamental human rights.

It is felt that natural rights and human rights are so basic and universal that people might know of their existence and truth by reason alone. Thomas Aquinas (1225–1274) states in the *Treatise on Law:*

> To the natural law belong those things to which a man is inclined naturally; and among these it is proper to man to be inclined to act according to reason. . . . Hence this is the first precept of law, that good is to be done and promoted; and evil is to be avoided. All other precepts of the natural law are based upon this; so that all the things which the practical reason naturally apprehends as man's good belong to the precepts of the natural law under the form of things to be done or avoided.[8]

The point that Aquinas is making is that some moral principles do not depend on feeling, observation, or demonstration, but are stable, eternal, irresistible, and certain to those who are wise enough to understand their terms. If understood, they would be as unarguable as the statement that all calico cats are cats. Natural rights then are basic truths that can be understood and known by human reason alone and are not dependent on outside dictates.

The ideas of Thomas Aquinas are somewhat echoed in the works of John Locke, who wrote of self-evident principles whose veracity the "mind can not doubt, as soon as it understands the words." According to Locke, the law of nature "teaches all mankind that, being all equal and independent, no one ought to harm another in his life, health, liberty, or possessions."[9] To Locke, these were not matters of truths that one could accept without demonstration or experiment but rather became known and self-evident by these processes.

The concepts of natural and human rights seem based on humans being the measure of all things. The following are the key concepts drawn from the historical traditions of natural law:

- Humans possess a rational nature as a gift from God.
- Natural laws are not dependent on social contract.
- Natural laws are unchangeable and universal.
- Inability to effect natural rights does not distinguish them.
- Natural laws can be discovered even without a knowledge of God.

CONTRACTARIAN AND CONSEQUENTIALIST RIGHTS THEORY

There are other philosophers for whom the whole concept of natural or human rights is patent nonsense. Jeremy Bentham was an implacable foe of the concept of natural rights, holding that they were "*absurd in logic and pernicious to morals.*"[10] So if the concept of rights could not be thought of as stemming from basic human reason or as a preexistent endowment of a kind creator, on what other rational foundation might rights be justified? In his work *Utilitarianism,* John Stuart Mill sets out the following in regard to right and wrong, which might lead us to a source for rights from a utilitarian view.

> We do not call anything wrong unless we mean to imply that a person ought to be punished in some way or another for doing it; if not by law, by the opinion of his fellow creatures, if not by opinion then by the reproaches of his own conscience. This seems to be the real turning point in the distinction between morality and simple expediency. It is part of the notion of Duty in every one of its forms, that a person might rightfully be compelled to fulfill it. Duty is a thing that may be exacted from a person as one exacts a debt. Unless we think that it can be extracted from him we do not call it his duty. Reasons of prudence, or the interest of other people, may militate against actually extracting it; but the person himself, it is clearly understood, would not be entitled to complain. There are other things, on the contrary which we wish that people should do, which we like or admire them for doing, perhaps dislike or despise them for not doing, but yet admit that they are not bound to do, it is not a case of moral obligation; we do not blame them, that is we do not think that they are proper objects of punishment.[11]

What Mill describes as being the distinction between morality and simple expediency is better stated as the distinction between that which is morally required and morally valuable. For Mill, duties were subdivided into two sets: duties of **perfect obligation**, which have inherent within them assigned correlative rights, and duties of **imperfect obligation**, which do not give birth to any right. The basis of perfect obligations was the realm of required duty, while imperfect obligations were those in which the act was obligatory but the particular occasions of performing them are left to our choice. Examples of imperfect obligations can be found in areas of charity and beneficence, which we are called on to practice but not toward any particular person or any prescribed time.[12] The difference, then, is the specified requirement of a duty as opposed to what one might expect on the basis of generosity or beneficence.

Rights from this viewpoint are claims that can be justified on the principle of collective agreement. For Mill, what others were calling moral rights were those that were backed up by the force of law or public opinion. "To have a right, then, is, I conceive, to have something which society ought to defend me in the possession of. If the objector goes on to ask why it ought? I can give him not other reason than general utility."[13] One could imagine a society accepting and enforcing a great number of claims to rights validated by the principle of utility, if by doing so they tended to promote general happiness and their omission produced the reverse of happiness.

This still begs the question as to whether there are distinct moral rights that are separate from rights supported by social sanction. It seems that what Mill is saying is that if a moral justification is worthy of social protection, i.e., an enforceable sanction, then it is a moral right. Yet for some, the fact that there is an antecedent moral right is what has led us to create the social sanction that protects it.

For contractarians, the development of rights principles always comes from practical rationality and collective choice. In **contractarian theory**, the driving force or mechanism for the selection of correct principles is the agreement or bargain reached by the initial agents. Within the tradition, moral agents come to an initial situation and bargain to a choice. This initial situation can be moralized if it places moral constraints on the participants, or nonmoralized if it does not.

Perhaps the most famous of the nonmoralized initial situations is the state of nature described by Thomas Hobbes (1588–1679). According to Hobbes, life in the state of nature prior to the formation of government was "solitary, poor, nasty, brutish and short." Rather than an era of peace and tranquility populated with noble savages, Hobbes envisioned a nightmare of violence where each individual decided only for himself and against all others. In this version of a state of nature, there could be no industry, no crops grown, no security or peace found, and certainly no rights whose claims were equally understood and honored.

> To this war of every man against every man, this also is consequent; that nothing can be unjust. The notion of right and wrong, justice and injustice, have there no place. Where there is no common power; there is no law, no injustice. Force and fraud are in war the two cardinal virtues. Justice or injustice are faculties neither of the body nor the mind. If they were they might be in a man alone in the world, as well as in his senses and passions. They are qualities that relate to men in society, not in solitude.[14]

In the Hobbesian model, the initial agents do not come to the table necessarily as equals. The impetus that brings them to the agreement is a dissatisfaction with the current circumstances. The state of nature fails to serve either the weak or the strong. For Hobbes, nature did not teach lessons of innate human rights, but rather that human nature itself created the need for a leviathan, something so large that it could crush individual will and bring about acceptable behavior from the chaos. In this era, only the law of self-preservation existed. Because precontractual differences existed with this model, it could be predicted that postcontractual inequality in property and human rights would necessarily result. For Hobbes, the leviathan, which needed to be larger than the individual, was a justification for the monarchy but would later be reduced by others to ideas including a social contract or government.

The Hobbesian model does not solve the question of human rights, as it posits a world where the strong and the ruthless armed with force and fraud are the only ones who are allowed to come to the bargaining table. It is difficult to see how the principle of justice that would allow equal protection for all could come from such a gathering.

Perhaps a more useful contractarian model for the development of justified claims for individual rights is the moralized initial situation as described by John Rawls.[15] Rawls offers a kinder and gentler arrangement as the context for the social contract and envisions an initial situation known as the **original position** that is designed to promote rational choice and fairness. In the original position, all individuals are free and equal. There is a veil of ignorance, which denies each of the agents' knowledge of who is to receive the rights to goods and services. When the decision is made, it would need to be made so that the most disadvantaged individual would be willing to accept that position. This formulation of social justice can be seen in the fair opportunity rule.[16]

FAIR OPPORTUNITY RULE

No person should receive goods and services on the basis of undeserved advantage nor be denied goods and services on the basis of an undeserved disadvantage.[17]

In this light, let us consider two agents attempting to determine whether slavery would be a good thing. Neither knows of the other's natural assets or social position. Neither knows who is to be the slave in the new society, if that is the choice. It is clear that in this original position, neither would choose to have slaves. If the choices were made from this original position, the principle of justice would prevail, as Rawls has removed the opportunity for either of the individuals to exploit the determination to their advantage.

Contractarians believe that individual rights are grounded in the principle of justice and collective choice, and it is this collective choice that forms the basis of morality. Yet there are those who state that Rawls in his setting up of the original position has already posited the concept of a moral right to equal concern and respect. If this were true, then it would seem that these rights would need to have existed prior to the collective choice procedure.

LEGAL RIGHTS

Whatever one feels to be the original source of rights, whether from the laws of nature, a generous creator, or social contract, it is more likely that they will be accorded their just due if backed by the sanction of law. Some rights have been seen as being of such importance that they have become **legal rights**. These are rights not only asserted as moral prerogatives but afforded governmental guarantees. Legal rights are created through constitutional guarantees, legislative statutes, judicial review, and governmental agencies. They are ubiquitous, and each of us lives in a literal sea of legal claims that shape our behaviors. These claims can be as comprehensive as a constitutional guarantee, or as small as whether you must separate your garbage into recyclables and nonrecyclables. Table 4-1 lists examples of a few common positive and negative rights that have been afforded the sanction of law.

In general, we have found it easier to put into place laws that protect negative rights, which require others to refrain from interfering with our just claims, than in framing laws that provide

TABLE 4-1	
Positive and Negative Legal Rights	
POSITIVE RIGHTS	NEGATIVE RIGHTS
American veterans' right to health care	Equal opportunity in employment
Right to a public education	Freedom of religion
Indigent right to health care (Medicaid)	Right to bear arms
Licensed drivers' right to use of public roads	Right to personal property
Citizens of Ballwin, Michigan, to garbage collection	No taxation without representation
Right to an abortion

positive or welfare rights, which call for provision of goods and services. This can be seen in the current controversy regarding a right to abortion. In the 1973 case of *Roe* v. *Wade*, the U.S. Supreme Court ruled that the woman's negative right to privacy, that is, a right to noninterference, provided a right to abort her fetus within certain limits. This negative right is justified by considerations of the principle of autonomy and personal privacy. This right to noninterference has even been found to abrogate a husband's veto of his wife's and her physician's decision to terminate the pregnancy.[18]

What is not included in the negative right to noninterference in the decision is the positive right to a claim to the resources and services required for an abortion. The current controversy in regard to denying poor women public funding for legal abortions is based on this difference between negative and positive rights. Arguing that poverty ought not to exclude some women from exercising the negative right to noninterference in regard to abortions, individuals are seeking to create a positive right justified under the principle of distributive justice.

Notice that positive rights are **recipient rights**, which are rights to receive goods and services from another person, organization, or government. Only legal persons can receive legal rights. The characteristics that are commonly attributed to a legal person include that:[19]

- Persons can be injured
- Persons can be thought to have interests
- Persons can be benefited

We should also note that legal rights may or may not be based on established moral claims. The fact that citizens of Ballwin, Michigan, have a claim to garbage collection is a matter of consensus in regard to quality-of-life issues rather than basic moral convictions. Legal rights obviously differ by jurisdiction and nation. They are the product of human action and can be made and unmade. An excellent example of this shifting with time can be seen in U.S. civil rights legislation. In our earliest time, humans with black skins were considered property that could be bought and sold. At a later time, they could not be legally enslaved, but could be denied the rights of other citizens to the vote. Under current law, African Americans must be treated equal to all and if past discrimination can be proved must be given recompense by affirmative action policy.

While it is clear that legal rights are often used to reaffirm moral rights, they do not necessarily coincide. Many legal rights, such as the right to drive and the right to garbage collection in your neighborhood, are not born in deep moral principle. Likewise, there are many moral rights not sanctioned by law.

The enforcement of legal rights is a rather clear process with a designated set of factors (fines, punishments, and constraints) that tend to coerce others to honor an individual's claims. On the other hand, moral rights depend on a more informal set of processes, which include contempt, blame, and social ostracism that are designed to induce appropriate behavior.

Discussions in the health professions regarding rights often involve patients' rights. If these rights are things that the patients possess and are not dependent on the charity or the goodwill of others, where do they come from? It should be clear that discussing and listing of a patient's rights by health care providers cannot itself bring the rights into existence. If the patient already has the rights, any discussion is nothing more than reaffirming our knowledge about them and our acceptance of the responsibilities associated with them. The source of the patient's claim is beyond the listing, and found either in sanctions of law, good practice, or moral duty.

English is a language rich in the symbols, traditions, and terminology of rights. In health care, we will argue our obligations and duties regarding each other in the language of rights. As a group, we will in the near future need to come to an agreement as to whether a basic right to health care exists for all citizens. Along with this issue, we will argue out a right to life for the unborn, a right to die for adults, animal rights, and a host of others. Although it is comforting to base our legal rights to goods and services on natural rights, it is not a necessary condition; many legal rights will be based on an assessment of available resources and the need to guarantee a certain quality of life for all citizens. There are many elements of human existence (such as garbage collection) that we will decide are useful and good and yet need not be described as a moral or legal right.

CASE STUDY

Is Fetal Endangerment a Mother's Right?

Jane is pregnant, twenty-three years old, unmarried, and the mother of four children by three different fathers. She has been an insulin-dependent diabetic since the age of twelve but had no complications from the disease during the earlier pregnancies.

During clinic visits, Jane has been advised of the risks of uncontrolled diabetes for her unborn child, (increased risk for congenital deformities, premature birth, and being stillborn) but does not seem to take the advice seriously. When questioned about how she is monitoring her blood sugar, she complains that she is too poor to buy the test strips, and even when she has the supplies, she often forgets.

At fifteen weeks' gestation, following an office visit, she is admitted to the hospital as an inpatient to treat her diabetes. The next day, against her physician's advice, she checks herself out of the hospital even though the diabetes has not been fully brought under control. Once at home, she again fails to monitor her blood sugar adequately.

At twenty-two weeks' gestation, Jane is again admitted to the hospital as her diabetes is again out of control. The next morning, she again announces that she wishes to check out. The physician and unit staff advise her that her actions are clearly not in the best interest of the fetus. Jane responds negatively to the advice and becomes belligerent, demanding to be released.

1. In this case, who has rights? Whose rights should prevail? Jane's? The fetus's? The hospital staff's?

2. Should the physician attempt to get a court order to keep Jane hospitalized?

MORAL AND LEGAL RIGHTS

Moral or natural rights have several different aspects that are not necessarily shared by legal rights. First, they are universal, and if an individual has this right, then all relevantly alike individuals also have the same rights regardless of historical time or laws of the nation. Second, moral rights provide equality among humans. If a single individual has a moral right, then all individuals of that class have the same right and possess it equally. Men cannot have more moral rights than women, whites over blacks, Christians over Muslims. When it comes to moral rights, we are all born equal. Third, moral rights are believed not to be the product of human creativity, but are inherent to our species. They cannot be brought into existence by democratic vote or taken away by despotic action. These rights continue to exist, even if the means of effecting them are denied.

Some would question the value of a moral right if in fact it were ignored under law. One might argue that each individual has the moral right to personal autonomy in the area of reproduction and that the government has no right to tell individuals how many or how few children they should have. Yet in the People's Republic of China, there is a stringently enforced one child per family policy. What is the value of the moral right if it can be ignored by those in power?

In order to provide greater protection of moral rights, many people feel that they should be converted to legal rights and provided the sanction of law. In the case of the efforts to create an equal rights amendment for women, proponents would argue that this should come into the law based on the moral claims for equality. Obviously, those who claim a right for the unborn, special rights for children, animal rights, and others are also seeking to base these in our foundational claims to universal moral rights.

It is not always an easy process to gain legal protection of needed rights, even when there is general societal agreement that these should be given the status of law. It is said that one should never watch sausage or politics being made. This is perhaps never a truer admonition than the current attempt to move a patient's bill of rights into federal law. While there seems to be general agreement that a set of rights that would protect patients from some of the more problematic practices of managed care should be guaranteed and justified by law, details, such as whether the patient can sue and for how much (trial lawyers in general support Democratic legislators, while Republicans support tort reform to decrease the high judgments against physicians and hospitals), are standing in the way.

THE PROBLEM OF RIGHTS

One of the interesting but perhaps peculiar aspects of humanity and our society in particular is the multiplication of claims to personal rights. People advocate a right to die, a right to health care, a right to smoke hemp products, nonsmokers' rights, smokers' rights, animals' rights, women's rights, abortion rights, a right to die, a right to know, a right not to know, and even a right to a guaranteed annual income with periodic paid holidays. In Fuji, a group of miners claimed a personal right to a sex break during work hours.[20] It is almost as if we have lost the ability to provide arguments for something without appealing in the language of rights. We are either living in an age of sudden awareness where we have evolved and are now aware of a whole new set of rights, or we are confusing what we want with what is somehow our due. The gross multiplication of rights threatens to make the very issue of rights associated with real claims almost meaningless. It appears too easy to move from "I want X" to "I have a right to X."

In order to discriminate between wants and rights, there must first be an understanding and agreement as to the nature of what we are talking about. Prior to some common agreements regarding definitions, it is unclear how we are to judge between the competing claims. Without these agreements, who is to say that the Fuji miners are not correct in claiming a right to a sex break? However, it is clear that human imagination and creativity can create more claims to rights than we could possibly honor.

CONCLUSION

Because of the proliferation of rights language for rather marginal gains, such as the right to eat in a smoke-free environment, some have argued for a moratorium on the use of rights language in moral discourse. What is lost if the right to eat in a smoke-free environment becomes "smoke-free environments for eating are highly valued?"

Aren't there some things so fundamental to our being a just society that merely stating that they have value misses something important? When we claim these things as rights (right to life, free speech, a jury trial), we create immense obligations in others that cannot be denied by mere inconvenience or expense. The English language is rich in rights language, and nothing seems to confer power on these basic claims to the same extent as framing them as rights.

Just as inflation erodes the value of currency by decreasing its purchasing power, so too does the inflation of rights language erode the value of these concepts as justified claims. Regardless of whether you have come to believe that rights are innate or formed as a result of a social contract, they remain an important and vital aspect of the legal and ethical health practice. In the foreseeable future, all patient care providers will be discussing the issue of rights as they relate to the patients served. The parent who wishes to decline lifesaving care for a child, the child who wishes a prescription for contraceptives without parental consent, and the physical therapist who is forced to charge less than what the market will bear for her services due to a governmentally imposed cap are all involved in aspects of the rights controversy.

The concept of human rights, with its attendant creation of obligations, must be limited only to fundamental human needs. Three basic considerations that should be examined prior to declaring new human rights are:[21]

1. Not all human wants can or should be converted to the status of human rights.
2. Human creativity allows us to imagine more rights than we can fulfill.
3. The dilution of human rights by adding new ones threatens established claims.

The most important of these is dilution, in which our creativity as humans causes us to claim rights well beyond limits that can be honored and thereby reduces the meaning of rights as a concept. Soren Kierkegaard, (1813–1855), the father of Christian existentialism, was correct in asserting that ethics should not become merely a statistical exercise.[22] Human rights cannot be created or lost by opinion polls. The daily will of the people is a fickle foundation. It must be remembered that in early Nazi Germany, prior to the atrocities of the holocaust death camps, the popular will of the people first reduced the rights of the mentally ill. It is clear that in this beginning, they came to forget that the most basic of our human rights is the right to be recognized and respected as equal human beings.

In our daily practice as health care providers, more good will be done by honoring the basic human rights that we already have come to know by experience and reason than in imagining a whole host of new ones. Our professions place on us special obligations and additional duties to protect the rights of those we serve. These rights form part of the traditions and conditions of practice and bind us not only to our patients with whom we have entered into a voluntary contractual agreement but to society as a whole. For society and our patient's rights to be operative, we must as practitioners assume the correlative obligations that give them meaning.

Each of us needs to develop a framework for thinking about these issues and the claims they represent. Obviously, when rights claims are deployed on all sides of a single issue, they become diluted and their meaning in regard to understandable obligations is lost. Our failure to form a certain base for the development of human rights does not negate their importance. They are in some way fundamentally important, as they are the essence that we share with all humanity. The respect of human rights is the independent standard by which we judge the merit of nations and the actions of individuals. Most practitioners would feel very uncomfortable in a world where the rights we have intuitively come to accept, regardless of their source, were to be removed from our moral scales.

KEY CONCEPTS

- Rights are thought to be justified claims that others have an obligation to respect.
- Rights often have moral or legal or both moral and legal justification. As an example, most agree that a moral right to life exists, which has found its way into the law against murder.
- Western culture has a rich heritage of rights philosophy and language. These ideas are writ large in documents such as the Declaration of Independence.
- Positive rights can be thought of as recipient or welfare rights as they require that goods or services be provided.
- Negative rights are rights that require that others refrain from interfering with a person's right to something.
- Some have based rights on the development of a social contract. In one moralized formulation, the process is known as the original position. In this formulation, everyone is sitting at the table to decide what type of society will be set up. The formulation requires

that no one at the table knows what position she will hold in the upcoming society, and therefore it is assumed that no one would choose to have individuals in the society be required to do things they themselves would be unwilling to perform.

■ Care must be taken so that new rights for marginal gains do not threaten established claims.

REVIEW EXERCISES

1. In our culture we often talk of special rights for those whom we consider innocent, such as babies and children. How might such rights have evolved and become justified?

2. We often talk of recipient rights, such as the rights that American veterans have to health care. Could one create recipient obligations in regard to this right? As an example, could we predicate this right to health care on the obligation that the veteran would refrain from smoking and drinking to excess? Would this be a good idea? If a right is something for which one need not feel grateful to others, how could others create legitimate obligations in regard to the right?

3. In the chapter discussion regarding abortion, we found that the negative right to abortion only created an obligation to noninterference. In this light, do we currently have a negative right to health care?

4. In theory, once one understood the right, one should be able to reason out the correlative obligations. List at least two obligations associated with informed consent.

5. It is clear that not all wants can or should be converted into rights, yet it seems as if we are being inundated by demands from various groups expressed in the language of rights. If a right can be defined as a justified claim, provide the justification under some ethically acceptable principle for the following claims to rights:

   - nonsmokers' rights
   - smokers' rights
   - gay rights
   - marijuana smokers' rights
   - animal rights
   - women's rights

6. The philosopher John Rawls states that the basic social arrangement is an agreed-on contract to advance the goodwill of all who are in the society. In this communal effort, all would work toward equal distribution of goods and services unless an unequal distribution would serve to everyone's advantage. Others have argued that when this view of an enlightened collective social protection is added to the fair opportunity rule, you can begin to see an actual right to health care. What is your opinion in regard to a right to health care?

7. In some rights discussions, individuals speak of option rights. These are loosely defined as your sphere of autonomy, where you have the right to freedom of action without interference from others. Can you identify in your practice rights that could be considered option rights (where one is free to do or not do what one has a right to do)?

8. It appears that philosophers who hold a contracterian view feel that rights stem from a collective social decision and that these rights gain their power by the fact that they are important enough to be protected by law or social sanction. Theorists like Thomas Aquinas feel that rights exist before society and come from sources such as a consequence of God's creation. These are two very different orientations to rights. Which do you feel provides the strongest protection for the weakest among us, such as the elderly, the disabled, and the premature infant? Explain your answer.

NOTES

1. Bertram Bandman and Elsie Bandman, *Nursing Ethics* (Norwalk, CT: Appleton and Lange, 1995).

2. Maurice Cranston, "Human Rights, Real and Supposed," in *Political Theory and Rights of Man,* ed. D. D. Raphael (Bloomington: Indiana University Press, 1967.)

3. Ronald Dworkin, *Taking Rights Seriously* (Cambridge, MA: Harvard University Press, 1978).

4. Tom Beauchamp and James Childress, *Principles of Biomedical Ethics* (New York: Oxford University Press, 1994).

5. United Nations Universal Declaration of Human Rights, Article 6 (1948).

6. M. P. Golding, "The Concept of Rights: A Historical Sketch," in *Bioethics and Human Rights,* eds. B. Bandman and E. Bandman (Boston: Little, Brown, 1978), pp. 44–50.

7. Thomas Jefferson, *The Declaration of Independence* (1776).

8. Thomas Aquinas, *Summa Theologica,* as quoted in *Social Thought in America* (Boston: Beacon Press, 1966), p. 265.

9. John Locke, *Essay on Human Understanding* (New York: Dover Press, 1959).

10. H. L. A. Hart, *Essays on Bentham: Studies in Jurisprudence and Political Theory* (Oxford: Clarendon Press, 1982).

11. J. S. Mill, "Utilitarianism," in *Great Books of the Western World,* ed. Robert M. Hutchins (Chicago: Encyclopedia Britannica, 1952).

12. L. W. Sumner, *The Moral Foundation of Rights* (Oxford: Clarendon Press, 1989).

13. Mill, "Utilitarianism."

14. Thomas Hobbes, *Leviathan: Parts I and II* (New York: Bobbs-Merrill, 1958).

15. John Rawls, *A Theory of Justice* (Cambridge, England: Clarendon Press, 1971).

16. Raymond Edge and Randall Groves, *The Ethics of Health Care* (Albany, NY: Delmar Publishers, 1999).

17. Beauchamp and Childress. *Principals of Biomedical Ethics.*

18. *Danforth* v. *Planned Parenthood of Central Missouri,* 428 U.S. 52, 49 L. Ed. 2d 788 96 S. Ct. 2831 (1976).

19. W. Gilmer ed., *Cochran's Law Lexicon* (Cincinnati, OH: W. H. Anderson Company, 1973).

20. M. D. Bassom, Introduction to the Fourth Conference on Rights, *Rights and Responsibilities in Modern Medicine,* ed. M. Bassom (n.p.).

21. Raymond Edge and John Krieger, *Legal and Ethical Perspectives in Health Care* (Albany, NY: Delmar Publishers, 1997).

22. Soren Kierkegaard, "Attack on Christendom," in *A Kierkegaard Anthology,* ed. Robert Bretall (New York: Modern Library, 1946), p. 446.

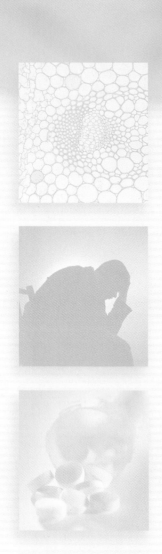

Confidentiality and the Management of Health Care Information

GOAL

To gain an understanding of the current problems associated with the principle of confidentiality as it is applied in modern health care.

OBJECTIVES

Upon completion of this chapter, the reader should be able to:

1. Write a defense for the principle of confidentiality within health care from a utilitarian, duty-oriented, and virtue ethics point of view.

2. Explain the rationale for "the Harm principle" as it relates to the Tarasoff case.

3. List the two basic principles in conflict in the Tarasoff case.

4. Give five instances in which the practitioner would have a legal requirement to report confidential matters that relate to health care.

5. Explain how vulnerability guides the decision-making process when confidentiality is overridden by the duty to warn.

6. List five groups not involved in direct patient care that have a legitimate interest in the medical record.

7. List six safeguards that should be considered in regard to allowing access to confidential patient information.

8. Explain why confidentiality is considered a principle with qualifications.

9. Identify the major purposes of the Health Insurance Portability and Accountability Act (HIPAA) of 1996.

10. List three patient rights in regard to control over patient information that has been provided for or strengthened by the HIPAA legislation.

11. List two measures that are not required of health providers in regard to providing security for health care information.

12. List the basic ethical principles that are foundational to the conduct of research using human subjects.

KEY TERMS

Harm principle	**Institutional review**	**Third-party payers**
Health Insurance Portability and	**boards**	**Utilization review**
Accountability Act (HIPAA)	**Right to privacy**	

CONFIDENTIALITY: A PRINCIPLE WITH QUALIFICATIONS

What I may see or hear in the course of the treatment or even outside of the treatment in regard to the life of men, which on no account one must spread abroad, I will keep to myself, holding such things shameful to be spoken about.

Hippocratic Oath

In this chapter we begin a serious discussion of health care confidentiality and privacy by examining a rather silly item that anonymously came across my desk in an e-mail titled "Pizza 2010" (Figure 5-1).

Operator: Thank you for calling City Pizza. May I have your . . .

Customer: Hi, I'd like to order.

Operator: May I have your NIDN first, sir?

Customer: My National ID Number, yeah, hold on, eh, it's 61020499-45-6332.

Operator: Thank you, Mr. Jones. I see you live at 1742 Block Lane, and your phone number is 494-6332. Your office number is 494-2302, ext. 201. Which number are you calling from, sir?

Customer: Huh? I'm at home. Where d'ya get all this information?

(continues)

Operator: We're wired into the system, sir.

Customer (sighs): Oh, well, I'd like to order a couple of your all-meat specials.

Operator: I don't think that's a good idea, sir.

Customer: Whaddya mean?

Operator: Sir, your medical records indicate that you've got very high blood pressure and extremely high cholesterol. Your national health care provider won't allow such an unhealthy choice.

Customer: What do you recommend then?

Operator: You might try our low-fat soybean yogurt pizza. I'm sure you'll like it.

Customer: What makes you think I'd like something like that?

Operator: Well, you checked out *Gourmet Soybean Recipes* from the library last week, sir. That's why I made the suggestion.

Customer: All right, all right. Give me two family-sized ones.

Operator: Will there be anything else, sir?

Customer: No, nothing. Oh, yeah, don't forget the two free liters of Coke your ad says I get with the pizzas.

Operator: I'm sorry, sir, but our ad's exclusionary clause prevents us from offering free soda to diabetics.

FIGURE 5-1 Ordering a Pizza in the Year 2010

If the ordering pizza story seems funny to you and perhaps only a little bit over the top, it is because at some level, it rings true. Modern communication has made the need for increased emphasis on confidentiality and personal privacy a critical issue in all aspects of our lives and especially in health care. For evidence supporting the need for increased awareness and effort in this area, consider the following stories in articles collected by the Health Privacy Project of Georgetown University.

- Although she had received a positive review and raise, Terri Seargent, a North Carolina resident, was fired from her job after being diagnosed with a genetic disorder that required expensive treatment.[1]

- The medical records of a Maryland school board member were sent to school officials as part of a campaign criticizing performance.[2]

- An Atlanta truck driver lost his job in early 1998 after his employer learned from his insurance company that he had sought treatment for a drinking problem.[3]

- The thirteen-year-old daughter of a hospital employee took a list of patients' names and phone numbers from the hospital while visiting her mother. As a joke, she contacted the patients and told them they had been diagnosed with HIV.[4]

- A banker who served on his county's health board cross-referenced customer accounts with patient information and called due mortgages of anyone with cancer.[5]

- A hacker downloaded medical records, health information, and social security numbers of more than 5,000 patients at the University of Washington Medical Center.[6]

- A doctor's laptop was stolen at a medical conference. The computer contained the names and medical histories of his patients.[7]

- Documents referring to over 125 psychiatric patients of Rapid City Regional Hospital were found in a convenience store trash can. A fourth-year medical student had taken the papers from the hospital and dumped them in the trash.[8]

- An Orlando woman had some routine medical tests. She received a letter weeks later from a drug company touting a treatment for her high cholesterol.[9]

- The chain drugstores CVS and Giant Food admitted to making patient prescription records available for use by direct mail and pharmaceutical companies. Their stated intent was to track customers who do not refill prescriptions and send them letters of encouragement.[10]

These articles are in no way an exhaustive listing of the problems we face providing due care for patient confidentiality and privacy. To get some idea of how big the problem is, consider the more common problems of inadvertent talking in the elevator, at a party after a couple of drinks, or cafeteria gossip that most of us have been guilty of. Our ability to store and share data has opened up an almost unlimited opportunity for health information to be misused. Almost all of us have personal information that we prefer to remain confidential.

A patient's basic right to expect the information he gives a health care practitioner to be held in confidence can be arrived at and defended using any of the four systematic approaches to ethical decision making outlined in Chapter 2. Whether the reasoning is from a utilitarian, duty-oriented, virtue ethics, or divine command standpoint, confidentiality seems to be a settled issue.

From a utilitarian point of view, the long-term consequences of making public any personal information gained as a result of the practitioner-patient relationship would have a chilling effect on the truth telling in that relationship. Since health care practice is normally conducted under a tacit agreement of confidentiality, practitioners who breach this trust are in violation of an agreed-on expectation. This is especially critical in psychotherapy, in which the patient is encouraged to take the risks involved in personal disclosure. If the patient has lost confidence in the process and fails to discuss personal issues with the practitioner, the quality of care that can be provided will be severely limited.

From a duty-oriented perspective, personal privacy is a basic right, with its foundations firmly based not only in long-standing codes of professional practice but also in common law. The unwarranted disclosure of a patient's private affairs, the unauthorized use of a person's photograph, or exploitation of a person's name have traditionally been considered acts that might give rise to legal action on the grounds of invasion of an individual's right to privacy. The legal standard for judging a breach of confidence is clear: you may be found liable for any unauthorized breach of confidentiality that "offends the sensibilities of an ordinary person."[11] The medical duty to protect the confidentiality of patients could be argued on the basis of our general rights as citizens to be free from invasion of privacy. Individuals in our society have the autonomous right to the control of personal information and the protection of personal privacy. In some sense, privacy can be viewed as a person's right, while confidentiality is the professional's duty.

From the vantage point of virtue ethics, the practice of patient confidentiality has been a mainstay of health care practice and forms one of the virtues that one would expect from the "good practitioner."

Confidentiality is a critical principle, and, regardless of the specialty, the good practitioner cannot be viewed as cavalier in regard to protecting patients' confidences and privacy. While it is obvious that confidential information must be shared among practitioners in order to provide the best care for the patient or to extend the body of knowledge within health care, it is equally obvious that this does not take the form of conversations in elevators, in cafeterias, or with friends at a party.

The real question, then, is not whether confidentiality is a good—regardless of what reasoning you use—but whether it is a moral absolute, or might be overridden by other considerations. In the classic *Tarasoff* case, a young man by the name of Prosenjit Poddar confided to his clinical psychologist that he intended to kill a young woman he readily identified as Tatiana. The psychologist, understanding that his patient presented a real danger to the young woman, decided that Prosenjit should be committed for seventy-two hours to allow further evaluation, and he notified security to assist in securing the patient's confinement. The patient, however, convinced the security officers that he was rational, and he was released following his promise to stay away from the young woman. The health care providers rescinded the orders to place Prosenjit in confinement for evaluation, and no efforts were made to warn Tatiana or her family of potential danger. Within weeks of these events, Prosenjit murdered the young woman.[12]

The health care practitioners later defended their decision to maintain patient confidentiality on the basis that they had a duty only to their patient, and in the absence of duty they were not required to protect the life and safety of others. To whom did the caregivers owe duty: to their real patient or to the potential victim? They had chosen to serve the one and ignore the other. Arguments used in their defense were that effective treatment required the patient's full disclosure of his innermost thoughts and that, without the promise of confidentiality, patients needing treatment would fail to seek care.

In its decision, the court recognized the difficulty that a practitioner might have in attempting to predict whether statements made by a patient would actually be carried out. However, the court ruled that the specialist would be held to the standard of reasonable practice, and where that standard indicated a foreseeable danger to another, a duty to warn was created. The protective privilege of confidentiality is limited where the health and safety of others is involved. This breaching of the trust of confidentiality is recognized and allowed by the Code of Medical Ethics: Current Opinions of the American Medical Association, which states that

> the obligation to safeguard patient confidences is subject to certain exceptions, which are ethically and legally justified because of overriding social considerations. Where a patient threatens to inflict bodily harm to another person or to himself or herself and there is a reasonable probability that the patient may carry out the threat, the physician should take reasonable precautions for the protection of the intended victim, including notification of law enforcement.[13]

In her book *Secrets: On the Ethics of Concealment and Revelation,* Sissela Bok cites several instances in which confidentiality is overridden by more compelling obligations.[14] Many of these have found their way into legal statutes, and practitioners are generally required to report cases involving child abuse, contagious diseases, sexually transmitted diseases, wounds caused by guns or knives, and other cases in which identifiable third parties would be placed at risk by failure to disclose the information. Bok feels that the personal protective privilege of confidentiality is limited by the **harm principle**. This principle requires that health care providers refrain from acts or omissions that would foreseeably result in harm to others, especially in cases in which the individuals are particularly vulnerable to the risk.

The harm principle is modified by the level of vulnerability. Consider the case of a married man who tests HIV positive. In that the risk to the community at large is rather minimal, whereas the risk to the man in regard to discrimination, deprivation of rights, and occupational and social harm are great, the practitioner would have an obligation to be very discrete in regard to confidentiality, and to do little more than that which is legally required in reporting the test results. However, in the case of the wife, who is far more vulnerable than the community at large, the practitioner must either be assured that the situation is modified in order to lessen the woman's vulnerability or disclose the information to the woman. It would seem, then, that the practitioner's observance of the principle of confidentiality must always be balanced by the need to protect others from foreseeable harm, especially if the other individual is particularly vulnerable to that harm.

LEGITIMATE INTEREST

The medical record goes far beyond just medical information and contains personal data of a financial and social nature. In general, it is the property of the hospital or clinic, but the patient has a legal interest and right to the information. It is generally considered that the record is confidential and that access to it should be limited to the patient, authorized representatives of the patient, the attending physician, and hospital staff members who have a legitimate interest.

The exact specification of who has a legitimate interest is a great concern to health care practitioners, but some general guidelines are accepted where the need is for patient care, professional education, administrative functions, auditing functions, research, public health reporting, and criminal law requirements. In regard to patient care, any information may be shared among health care providers who are responsible for the patient within the treating facility. Modern medicine is a team practice, and adequate exchange of information is necessary for patient care.

The need for professional education usually permits information in regard to in-house patients to be exchanged for these purposes. This generally includes medicine, nursing, allied health, psychology, social services, or any other professional group involved in patient care. If the information is to be disseminated outside the treating facility (as in a patient case study), this may not be done without prior patient consent or unless the information is in a form that precludes all possible patient identification.

Limited amounts of information as needed for the administrative functions of appointments, admissions, discharges, billing, compiling census data, and the like are necessarily shared among clerical and administrative staff.

Duly appointed quality-of-care auditors, governmental third-party payers, and professional review organizations have a legitimate access to the patient record. The Peer Review Organization (PRO) program, which replaced the Professional Standards Review Organization (PSRO) program in 1982, requires that the PROs disclose review information according to guidelines set forth by the U.S. Department of Health and Human Services. This information is reported to (1) state and federal fraud and abuse agencies, (2) agencies responsible for identification of public health problems, and (3) state licenser and certification agencies.

Data in regard to the conducting of research can generally be shared with all the researchers involved, provided that the patient is not identified directly or indirectly in the process or subsequently in any other report or presentation. Hospitals that permit their staff to engage in research generally have research committees set up to screen the protocols. These **institutional review boards** (IRBs) attempt to balance the potential risk to the patient against the potential benefits of the research. In the absence of more stringent standards, the research committees should require the following as minimum standards.[15]

1. The research results should be presented in such a fashion as to protect the anonymity of the patients.

2. Only those involved in the study will have access to the raw data.

3. Safeguards to protect the patient's privacy will be part of the research protocol.

4. The same level of obligation to maintain patient confidentiality in the practice of health care is expected in the conduct of medical research.

Health care providers often record far more than is needed for documentation or to convey the necessary information required for patient care. It generally is not necessary for confidences to be recorded in explicit detail. A note in the record that a young patient "has a close relationship" with her boyfriend would generally be adequate to jog the practitioner's memory in regard to the need for counseling of a sexually active teenager. The less confidential information written explicitly into the record, the fewer opportunities there are for harmful disclosures involving patient privacy. Only material necessary for documentation and therapeutic care should be recorded; for example, in the case of a stab wound, the practitioner would not necessarily confide to the record other privileged information in regard to the attack on prior crimes or involvement in gang warfare.

It is essential that hospitals establish effective procedures to protect the content of medical records, not only from the standpoint of patient confidentiality, but also against the possibility of intentional falsification or alteration of the record. Unfortunately, records have been doctored by patients and practitioners alike who wished to improve their chances in pending legal actions. To protect the security of medical records the following minimal guidelines are suggested:

- Competent medical records or risk management personnel should review a record before it is examined by the patient or the patient's representative.

- An original medical record should not be permitted to be taken from the hospital's premises except pursuant to legal process or a defined hospital procedure, such as allowing an accompanied patient to transport records to another facility for testing purposes.

- Neither the patient nor the patient's authorized representative is to be allowed to examine the medical records alone.

CASE STUDY

Confidentiality vs. A Right to Know

In 1984, James Gusella discovered the marker for Huntington's disease. This discovery made possible a genetic test for the disease, which became available in 1994. Although the test is now available to indicate whether an individual will contract the disease, there are no successful treatments for those carrying the gene. One hundred percent of the individuals with the gene will have symptoms before the age of sixty-five.

1. Suppose that a parent tests positive for the gene and refuses to tell his children. Should the genetics counselor who performed the test break the parent's confidentiality?

MODERN HEALTH CARE AND CONFIDENTIALITY

In the early 1900s, maintaining confidentiality was a much easier task, as 85 percent of the direct medical care services were delivered by physicians. Access to medical records and the obligation to maintain confidentiality in regard to them was limited to the physician and a very small direct staff. Today over 80 percent of direct patient care is provided by allied health and nursing professionals. In the hospital, only about a third of the patient record is maintained by physicians, with the rest being recorded by other members of the health care team.[16]

The patient record is not only accessible to the attending physicians but also is readily available to a host of technical and administrative staff who generate and handle patient data. Following the complaint of one patient in regard to confidentiality, a survey revealed that at least seventy-five individuals had legitimate access to the patient's record by virtue of the fact that they were involved in providing either direct care or support services.

Moreover, the problem of access to patient information has been exacerbated by the growing use of computerized information systems. The large scale on which information can be stored and the ease of access to these data have made distribution of the information outside the arena of the patient–health care practitioner interface a daily routine, as patient data are used for administration, payment, **utilization review**, teaching, and research. In addition to the health care providers, patient files may be available to the following: insurance companies, (because they pay the bills); public health agencies (to assist in monitoring and investigating disease outbreak patterns); employers (to assess job-related injuries); federal, state, and local government (to develop health care plans and allocate resources); attorneys and law enforcement agencies (as evidence to settle civil or criminal matters); media (to report health hazards and help report medical research development); and accreditation, licensing, and certification agencies (to assess compliance with various criteria and standards).[17]

The concerns of these **third-party payers** with access to medical information may or may not coincide with the patient's best interests, inasmuch as confidentiality and privacy are not necessarily a high priority for groups such as governmental regulators, third-party payers, insurers, or utilization reviewers. Given the tasks they perform, they may favor safety, truth, and knowledge far more than they value the personal privacy of a single patient. The computerized accumulation, analysis, and storage of unlimited quantities of medical information have overwhelmed the medical record professionals who are entrusted with protecting patient privacy and confidentiality. Mark Siegler, director of the Center for Clinical Medical Ethics at the University of Chicago, argues that in hospital medicine, the existence of third-party interests and the development of the team medicine have made confidentiality a "decrepit concept."[18]

LEGAL PERSPECTIVE TO MEDICAL RECORD ACCESS

Many state statutes and a few federal regulations require the reporting of certain types of information, from the medical record, to appropriate agencies with or without the patient's authorization. Common legal reporting requirements found in most American jurisdictions include:

- Child abuse

- Drug abuse

- Communicable disease

- Injuries with guns or knives

- Blood transfusion reactions

- Poison and industrial accidents

- Misadministration of radioactive materials

Often these reporting requirements deal with issues vital to community health and welfare, such as child abuse, poison and industrial accidents, communicable diseases, misadministration of radioactive materials, blood transfusion reactions, injuries with guns or knives, and narcotic use.[19] The child abuse statutes in most states require that hospitals and practitioners report incidents of suspected abuse. In these cases, the practitioners are protected from liability if they are making the report in good faith even if the reported abuse proves to be false. Failure to make a report in regard to child abuse by those required to do so can leave them legally liable for any additional injuries the child may suffer upon return to the hostile home environment. An Illinois statute is illustrative:

> Any physician, hospital administrator and personnel engaged in examination, care and treatments of persons, . . . having reasonable cause to believe a child known to them in their professional or official capacity may be an abused child or a neglected child shall immediately report or cause a report to be made . . . The privileged quality of communication between any professional person required to report and his patient or client shall not apply to situations involving abused or neglected children and shall not constitute grounds for failure to report as required by this Act.[20]

Some states maintain a registry of the names and addresses of all patients who obtain drugs that are subject to abuse. These reporting regulations have been upheld as a reasonable exercise of an individual state's broad police powers. In the absence of a legal regulation to provide patient information, a police agency has no authority to examine a medical record without the patient's authorization.

HIPAA LEGISLATION

By the early 1990s it was clear that the use of computers and complex database retrieval systems was making confidentiality of patient information difficult to maintain. Periodic stories involving computers put up for sale as surplus from medical schools or other agencies that were later found to contain confidential files providing case details of thousands of patients, or marketing companies that advertised databases with literally millions of names and addresses of people with conditions such as bladder cancer, allergies, and clinical depression, underscored the scope of the problem. It was obvious that the patchwork of state laws governing the area left gaps in the protection of patients' privacy and confidentiality.

Recognizing the growing problem, Congress enacted the **Health Insurance Portability and Accountability Act (HIPAA)** in 1996 to encourage the use of electronic transmission of health information (to assist in cost containment) and provide new safeguards to protect the security and confidentiality of the information. The law gave Congress three years to enact comprehensive legislation regarding health care privacy and authorized the U.S. Department of Health and Human Services (HHS) to craft protections by regulation should the Congress fail to act within the time limit. In 1999, HHS proposed regulations guaranteeing new patients' rights and added protections against the misuse or disclosure of health care information. Rather than require immediate implementation, HHS provided an extended period for public review and comment. The final rule took effect on April 14, 2001, and as required by law, most covered entities were given two years, until April 14, 2003, to comply with the final rules provisions.

Entities covered under the law are health care plans, health care clearinghouses, and health care providers that conduct certain financial and administrative transactions (electronic billings and fund transfers) electronically. All medical records and other electronically identifiable health information used or disclosed in any form are protected.

Highlights of the legislation include the following:

- Consumer control over health information
    - Each patient must be given an opportunity during registration at a health care facility to restrict what information can be given out and to whom.
    - Providers and health plans will be required to give patients a clear, written explanation of the conditions of use and disclosure of health information.
    - Patients will be able to see and get copies of their records and request amendments.
    - Health care providers who see patients will be required to obtain patient consent before sharing information for treatment, payment, and health care operations.
    - Individuals will have the right to file a formal complaint about violations of the rule's provision.

- Rules regarding medical record release and use
  - Health information generally may not be used for purposes not related to health, such as disclosures to employers to make personnel decisions or to financial institutions without explicit authorization from the patient.
  - In general, disclosure of information will be limited to the minimum necessary for the purpose of the disclosure.
  - Psychotherapy notes are held to a higher standard of protection as they are not part of the medical record and are never intended to be shared.
  - Emergency circumstances, identification of the deceased, identification of cause of death, public health needs, judicial and administrative proceedings, limited law enforcement activities, and national security needs are areas in which the HIPAA rules permit, but do not require, covered entities to continue disclosures of health information without individual authorization.

- Increased security of personal health information
  - Health care entities must adopt written privacy procedures, including steps to ensure that their business associates protect the privacy of health information.
  - Some health entities will be required to encrypt computer data containing health information.
  - Health care entities will need to train their employees in privacy protections and must designate an individual to be responsible for ensuring the procedures are followed.

- Accountability for medical record use and release
  - Congress provides both civil and criminal penalties for knowingly violating patient privacy.

- Balancing public responsibilities and privacy protections
  - The final rule is considered a foundation law for the protection of privacy. In cases in which more stringent state laws exist, health care organizations must follow the most restrictive law on the books.
  - The provisions of the rules apply equally to both private sector and public sector entities.

Although the new rules are welcomed by privacy and consumer advocates and many health care providers, the nation's health care institutions have struggled to understand and implement them. It is estimated that implementation costs will exceed $17 billion over the first ten years. It is anticipated that the savings from standardizing the computer codes and other efficiencies gained in the legislation will offset the cost of upgrading patient privacy, although these savings may not be realized for years.[21]

> ## CASE STUDY
>
> ## A Question of Priorities
>
> It is clear that the HIPAA legislation regarding patient privacy is attempting to deal with a real problem. However, it is equally clear that the costs of health care are spiraling out of control, and we now have over 45 million Americans without health care insurance.
>
> According to the American Hospital Association, hospitals nationwide expect to spend between $4 billion and $22 billion to comply with the legislation. U.S. Representative Michael Burgess, whose background includes practice as an obstetrician/gynecologist, has argued that implementation should be delayed, saying, "HIPAA is just one more thing layered on that is not delivering one dollar of value to patient care and not increasing our revenue stream at all. This is just money going out of the practice. In effect, it's an overhead increase."[22]
>
> 1. Which of the two arguments, maintaining patient privacy or holding down costs, is more important?
>
> 2. If you were going to convince someone of the value of your argument either for or against the implementation of HIPAA, what would you say?
>
> 3. Prepare a cost-benefit (pro-con) list for each side of the issue.

HUMAN SUBJECT RESEARCH

One of the more interesting and rewarding aspects of health care education and practice is the opportunity for clinicians and students to participate in research. Research projects generally are described in a protocol that sets forth the explicit objectives and formal procedures designed to reach these objectives. The objectives themselves may involve everything from gaining an understanding of normal and abnormal physiological, psychological, and sociological phenomena, to evaluating the efficacy of diagnostic, therapeutic, or preventive interventions and variations in service or practice. To reach these objectives, researchers may conduct both invasive and noninvasive procedures, the collection of body tissues and fluids, the administration of chemical substances, randomization of subjects, modification of diet or daily routine, orchestration of strenuous physical exercise, alteration of environment, administration of questionnaires, reviews of records, and a host of other activities.[23]

The basic ethical principles that need to be considered in planning a research protocol involving human subjects are autonomy, beneficence, nonmaleficence, confidentiality, and justice. Autonomy in these cases flows from two important considerations. The first is that subjects are individual autonomous agents and have the right to expect that the researcher will support their opinions and choices while refraining from obstructing their actions unless they are clearly detrimental to others. One basic application of this principle is informed consent. The researcher has an obligation to ensure that the individual has adequate information on which to base an autonomous choice. The second consideration deals with the fact that not all individuals are capable of self-determination. For individuals who have either not gained the capacity for self-determination or have lost this capacity due to illness, mental disability, or circumstances that severely restrict liberty, special considerations need to be put in place to ensure their protection, even if this means excluding them from participation in the research.

Patient benefit and risk calculations should always be considered in human research under the principles of beneficence and nonmaleficence. Every effort should be made to secure for all participants their well-being. Two general rules that have been formulated to extend to these activities are (1) do no harm, and (2) maximize possible benefits and minimize possible harm. Obviously the process of learning what will in fact provide benefit may involve exposing research subjects to some risk. In all cases of human subject research, this cost-benefit analysis must be done to decide when it is justifiable to seek benefits despite risks and when the benefits should be forgone because of the risks.

The principle of justice involves questions such as who benefits from the research and who bears the burden. Often in the nineteenth and early twentieth centuries, the burdens of serving as research subjects fell disproportionately on groups such as the poor ward patients, and the benefits of improved medical care flowed primarily to private patients.

History is unfortunately replete with the exploitation of unwilling prisoners as research subjects, such as in the Japanese and Nazi concentration camps, and in the exploitation of disadvantaged groups such as in the Tuskegee syphilis study. It is against this historical background of abuse that the consideration of justice within human research takes place. It is critically important that the selection of research subjects be scrutinized to ensure that vulnerable groups (e.g., welfare patients, racial and ethnic minorities, or persons confined in institutions) are not being selected simply because of their easy availability, their compromised position, or their manipulability, but rather for reasons directly related to the purpose of the study.

Finally, a consideration of justice requires that research supported by public funds that leads to improvement of technologies or therapies should benefit more than those who can afford them and that the research should not depend unduly on populations unlikely to be among the beneficiaries of the applications of research findings.[24]

Whenever human subjects are part of the research protocol, great care must be used to ensure professional and ethical standards are followed. Generally the use of human subjects requires that the following are satisfied:

1. Risks to subjects are minimized by using procedures consistent with sound research design that do not unnecessarily expose subjects to risk. Whenever appropriate, the research will use procedures already being performed on the subjects for diagnostic or treatment purposes.

2. Risks to subjects are reasonable in relation to anticipated benefits, if any, to them, and the importance of the knowledge that may reasonably be expected to result. Researchers should consider only risks and benefits that may result from the research (as distinguished from risks and benefits of therapies subjects would receive if they were not participating in the research). Researchers should not consider the long-range effects of applying knowledge gained in the research (e.g., the possible effects of the research on public policy) as among those research risks that fall within the purview of their responsibilities.

3. Selection of subjects is equitable. In making this assessment, the researcher should take into account the purposes of the research and the setting in which the research will be conducted. The researcher also should be particularly cognizant of the special problems of research involving vulnerable populations, such as children, prisoners, pregnant women, mentally disabled persons, or economically or educationally disadvantaged persons.

4. Informed consent will be sought and appropriately documented from the subject or the subject's legal representative, in accordance with the requirements of law and ethical practice.

5. There will be appropriate provision for monitoring the data collected to ensure the safety of subjects.

6. There will be adequate provision for the protection of privacy and the maintenance of confidentiality of collected data.[25]

INSTITUTIONAL REVIEW BOARDS

To ensure satisfactory compliance with appropriate research standards, institutions create institutional review boards to review the research protocols prior to implementation. One of the many important activities gathered under the aegis of role duty is service on an IRB. These boards are established to protect the rights and welfare of human subjects recruited to participate in research activities under the auspices of the institution with which a board is affiliated.

For the purpose of this discussion regarding the activities of an IRB, *research* is defined as a systematic investigation, including research development, testing, and evaluation, designed to develop or contribute to generalizable knowledge. *Human subjects* are defined as living individuals about whom an investigator (whether professional or student) conducting research obtains (1) data through intervention or interaction with the individual or (2) identifiable private information.

Since the end of World War II and the general knowledge of the horrors associated with the concentration camp practices regarding human experimentation, several documents and codes dealing with the proper and reasonable conduct of research using human subjects have been developed. Included in these codes and documents are the Nuremberg Code of 1947, the Helsinki Declaration of 1964 (with later revisions), the Belmont Report of 1979, U.S. Department of Health and Human Services Title 45 of 2001, and the American Psychological Association Code for the conduct of social and behavioral research. Students and clinicians considering participating in research involving human subjects or on an IRB will find these documents a valuable starting place.

CASE STUDY

Tainted Data

Your secretary is a person of Jewish descent who recently read a book about medical experiments conducted in the Nazi concentration camps. In that you teach bioethics as part of your course work, she asks you whether you think it is appropriate for scientists to use the data collected from these experiments. In the conversation, you learn that a recent scientific paper references the material. It also becomes clear that your secretary feels that it is an outrage for the information gained in these experiments to be used.

1. Is she correct? Is the information gathered in the experiments tainted beyond use by the process?

2. Is the information gathered morally neutral?

3. If this information was to be used, should it be referenced differently from other data?

CONCLUSION

Personal privacy appears to be under siege in all aspects of our lives. The use of computers has greatly increased this concern, as it is common knowledge that all of us have dossiers in several major data banks. These governmental and commercial data sources provide information to others in regard to credit ratings, marital status, and even hobbies and interests. It seems at times that one need only provide a small donation to a favorite charity (perhaps to save the woodlands) before being inundated by an avalanche of offers for the type of person who might want to save woodlands, or at least look woodsy.

The general patient population still places a great deal of faith in the manner in which health care providers maintain the principle of confidentiality. Confidentiality seems to serve two basic purposes. First, the principle acknowledges a respect for the individual's **right to privacy** as guaranteed by our legal system and enshrined in our cultural values. Second, and perhaps more important to the health of the patient, the promise of confidentiality provides a bond between the practitioner and patient that allows for a full and honest disclosure of information. In those rare cases in which disclosure is necessary to protect a community interest, confidentiality must be balanced by a duty to warn, especially with vulnerable third parties.

Although the establishment of hospital team medicine and bureaucratic interventions has eroded the principle of confidentiality, it is imperative that, to the fullest possible extent, health care providers take meticulous care to guarantee that patients' medical and personal information be kept confidential. To the degree that health care providers must breach confidentiality to third parties, it would seem that the patient should be notified of the nature and ramifications of these disclosures. If patients understand what will happen to the information, they then would be in a better position to decide which of their personal matters they would choose to relate and what they would prefer to keep private.

Policies must be designed to balance the right to legitimate personal privacy while not offsetting the institutional need to make necessary information quickly and easily available to those who have a legitimate claim to it. It would seem that, at a minimum, these privacy safeguards should (1) define circumstances under which medical information is disclosed to other parties; (2) provide procedures by which patients may gain access to their records; (3) allow access to records to others only on a need-to-know basis; (4) ensure anonymity in aggregating data for research or statistical purposes; (5) carefully balance society's long-term goals and the legitimate need of organizations to have access to medical records with the patient's short-term desire for and right to privacy; and (6) inform the patient of what is meant by confidentiality in the context of current practice.

3. J. Appleby, "File Safe?" *USA Today,* March 23, 2000, p. A1.

4. "Hospital Clerk's Child Allegedly Told Patients That They Had AIDS," *Washington Post,* March 1, 1995, p. A17.

5. M. Lavello, "Health Care Plan Debate Turning to Privacy," *National Law Journal,* May 30, 1994, p. A1.

6. R. O'Harrow, "Hacker Accesses Patients' Records," *Washington Post,* December 9, 2000, p. E1.

7. A. Santana, "Thieves Take More Than Laptops," *Washington Post,* November 5, 2002.

8. C. Brokaw, "S. Dakota Investigates Psych Records," Associated Press, May 26, 2001.

9. "Many Can Hear What You Tell Your Doctor," *Orlando Sentinel,* November 1997, p. A1.

10. R. O'Harrow, "Prescription Fear, Privacy Sales," *Washington Post,* February 15, 1998.

11. *Housh* v. *Peth,* 165 Ohio St 35, 133 N.E.2d 340 (1956).

12. California Supreme Court; July 1, 1976, California Reporter 14.

13. American Medical Association, *Code of Medical Ethics; Current Opinions with Annotations.* (Chicago: Council on Ethical and Judicial Affairs, 1996).

14. Sissela Bok, *Secrets: On the Ethics of Concealment and Revelation* (New York: Vintage Books, 1983).

15. William Roach, *Medical Records and the Law* (Rockville, MD: Aspen Publications, 1994).

16. Marc D. Hiller, "Computers, Medical Records, and the Right to Privacy," *Journal of Health Politics, Policy and Law* 6, no. 3 (Fall 1981): pp. 463–487.

17. William Hafferty, "Whose Files Are They Anyway?" *Modern Maturity* (April–May 1991): p. 70.

18. Mark Siegler, "Confidentiality in Medicine—A Decrepit Concept," *New England Journal of Medicine* 307 (1982): pp. 1518–1521.

19. George Pozgar, *Legal Aspects of Health Care Administration* (Gaithersburg, MD: Aspen Publications, 1993).

20. Ill. Ann. Stat. ch. 23 2054 (Smith-Hurd Supp. 1983–1984).

21. U.S. Department of Health and Human Services, *Fact Sheet: Protecting the Privacy of Patient's Health Information,* May 9, 2001.

22. Mitch Mitchell, "Medical Privacy Laws Stir Controversy," *Fort Worth Star,* Feb. 25, 2003.

23. Saint Louis University, "Guidelines for Investigators in Preparation of Human Research Protocols for IRB Review," Institutional Review Board MPA-119-01-NR, 2000.

24. National Commission for the Protection of Human Subjects of Biomedical and Behavioral Research, "Ethical Principles and Guidelines for the Protection of Human Subjects of Research [Belmont Report]." April 18, 1979.

25. Code of Federal Regulations, Title 45 Public Welfare, Department of Health and Human Services. National Institutes of Health Office for Protection from Research Risks. Part 46. Protection of Human Subjects. Revised November 13, 2001.

26. Raymond Pfeiffer and Ralph Fosberg, *Ethics on the Job* (Belmont, CA: Wadsworth, 1993).

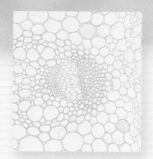

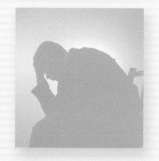

CHAPTER 6

Professional Gatekeeping as a Function of Role Fidelity

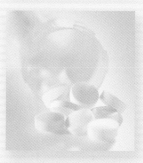

GOAL

To understand how the requirements of professionalism lead to a whole series of gatekeeping tasks under the principle of role fidelity.

OBJECTIVES

Upon completion of this chapter, the reader should be able to:

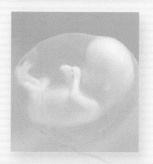

1. List the rationale for a profession's creating a code of ethics.

2. State an ethically based rationale for forbidding sexual relations between patients and health care providers.

3. State an ethically based rationale for discouraging conflicts of interest in our practices.

4. Outline the importance of a scope of practice as it relates to practitioner activities.

5. Define *disparagement,* and state why it is a problem that is to be avoided in health care practice.

6. Outline the ethical obligation that we have toward impaired colleagues.

7. Define what is meant by the term *gaming the system* and provide three examples of the harm this practice has to the health care provider.

KEY TERMS

Disparaging	**Joint-venturing**	**Safe harbor rules**
Gaming the system	**Patient advocate**	**Scope of practice**
Gatekeeping	**Role fidelity**	**Self-referral**

Our responsibility is not discharged by the announcement of virtuous ends.

John F. Kennedy

There are two educations. One should teach us how to make a living and the other how to live.

John Truslow Adams

CASE STUDY

Is There a Duty to Lie?

Barbara Gonzales is a special procedures nurse at a medium-sized community hospital. She enjoys her position as it allows her to spend additional time with the patients who have come in for cardiac stress tests. In fact, she enjoys almost all aspects of her job with the exception of dealing with Dr. Jones, who is invariably late for procedure appointments. Barbara understands that physicians have full schedules and often must take additional time with some patients, which makes them late for all other appointments that day. However, in this case, it is not a professional problem that is delaying the physician but rather a personal one. It is widely known among the hospital staff that he is having an affair with a nurse from the critical care unit. Barbara does not care who Dr. Jones is having an affair with and feels that it is not her business to judge. However, she resents being brought into the matter, as the doctor has directed her to tell his waiting patients that he is being held up in an emergency.

1. Is nurse Gonzales making a big deal over a small matter?

2. Does she have a duty to protect her colleague?

3. How would you address this issue?

4. What best serves the patients?

PROFESSIONAL CODES OF ETHICS

Historically, the essential characteristics of the learned professions (education, clergy, law, health care) are self-regulation, a specialized body of knowledge, standards of education and practice, a fiduciary relationship with those served, and the provision of a particular service to society. Most often the professional groups operate under a legal practice act and develop a code of ethics to assist in self-regulation.

Codes of ethics are common within the many specialties of the health professions. The language within these codes is usually vague as to levels of expected performance, and therefore the fair enforcement of the rules is difficult. In addition to set statements listing minimum criteria for ethical performance, codes usually include a section outlining the profession's mission and objectives. It is toward these ideals that the profession moves. Common problems associated with professional codes are:

- Vagueness as to duties and prohibitions
- Incompleteness as to duties
- Excessive concern with promotion and prestige of profession
- Vagueness in regard to self-regulation and peer enforcement
- Excessive concern with financial and business interests

Although most health education curricula have course work that examines ethical issues, the stress placed on this area is generally less than the technical aspects of the field. Yet it is often the human elements contained within ethical practice that are the most difficult to master. When we review the profession's code, we often fail to find a solution to the problem among the listed rules and must turn to ethical theory and reason for answers. Professional codes are often as much concerned with professional etiquette as with matters of important ethical concern. This is not to say that the codes of our professions do not have a legitimate place. They have as a purpose the binding of a group of practitioners and the expressing of the aims and aspirations of that group. They speak to our better selves in the area of personal integrity, dedication, and principled behavior.

As a member of a health profession, you take upon yourself the obligation to be a peer to others on the health care team. Part of these obligations can be considered gatekeeping functions whereby you look out for the interests of the profession and of others in a similar practice. These obligations flow naturally as a result of our professional obligations and education, which lead to a strong sense of collegiality with others in our practice.

This sense of collegiality and mutual support is found in the earliest of codes when new practitioners undertook obligations to their teachers and the professional guild. The following statement is found in the standard English translation of the Hippocratic Oath.

I swear by Apollo Physician and Asclepius and Hygieia and Panaceia and all the gods and goddesses, making them my witnesses, that I will fulfill according to my ability and judgment this oath and covenant:

To hold him who has taught me this art as equal to my parents and to live my life in partnership with him, and if he is in need of money to give him a share of mine, and to regard his offspring as equal to my brothers in male lineage and to teach them this art if they desire to learn it without fee and covenant; to give a share of precepts and oral instruction to all the other learning to my sons and to the sons of him who has instructed me and to pupils who have signed the covenant and have taken an oath according to the medical law, but to no one else.

The new practitioner, in taking the oath, bound himself to share knowledge only with those within the guild and to treat other practitioners equal to members of one's own family. From these early practices have come a series of traditions within the professions: to avoid the disparagement of other practitioners, share new therapies and technologies, offer professional courtesy for services, avoid sexual and other conflicts of interest, and look after the general welfare of the profession and those in practice.

DISPARAGEMENT OF PROFESSIONAL COLLEAGUES

In practice, allied health and nursing personnel have long known that our physician colleagues were very loathe to criticize other physicians and practiced **gatekeeping** as part of their professional duties. This gatekeeping function, whereby one looks out for the interests of the profession or of others in a similar practice, comes as a result of our professional obligations and training, which lead to a strong sense of collegiality with others in our practice.

Yet as health care providers, we are often faced with the question raised by Cain: "Am I my brother's keeper?" As a member of a health profession the answer is often yes! Not only are we responsible for our actions in regard to the patient but we are also charged with the duty to ensure that the rest of the health team is practicing appropriate care. The patients who are served have a certain vulnerability and dependence that is not usually found in other professional occupations. It is the essence of the therapeutic relationship and the trust that it inspires that makes individuals feel so betrayed and outraged when abuses occur.

Although some health care practitioners are independent entrepreneurs, the principle of caveat emptor (buyer beware) cannot be allowed to govern the interactions between clients and health care providers. To protect vulnerable patients from exploitation, regulatory licensing mechanisms, legal remedies, and peer review systems have come into being. The code of ethics that is part of each of our professions does more than set forth a series of ethical rules for the membership. It symbolizes that this group of professionals is differentiating itself from the broader group of occupations and technical careers. One of the essential characteristics of a profession is that the members generate a code of ethics and are willing to become self-regulating. It is true that sometimes codes of ethics serve rather crude ends, such as limiting competition, restricting advertising, and promoting a particular image, especially during the initial stages of professional development. The first American physician code, written in 1847, was directed as much toward separating orthodox practitioners from homeopaths, empirics, Thomsonians, and neuropaths, as it was toward regulating ethical conduct. Even in the modern codes of ethics, there is often a vagueness in both what one should do and what is to be avoided. Internally, there are often conflicts between the various prescriptive rules, and unresolved questions in regard to peer review and enforcement in which conduct is found to be inappropriate. Still, the main importance of a code of ethics is to affirm that the professional is an autonomous, responsible decision maker, not someone who just follows orders. There is an implied promise that the practitioner will not pursue his own interests at the expense of the client or patient. This implied promise then obligates the practitioner to the maintenance of professional gatekeeping in a great number of areas.

In the early 1980s, an allied health educator became disturbed by the number of ill-advised resuscitation efforts being called for in the local hospitals. In order to bring attention to the practice and to bring about needed reforms, the therapist wrote the following article for his local society newsletter:[1]

> A month or so ago, a young lady who had had two heart surgeries and a couple of (cardiac) arrests during the past two years, which resulted in hypoxic brain damage that had left her feeble minded and with a convulsive disorder, arrested again at home one evening because of a failed pacemaker. She was resuscitated and brought into the hospital, with no oxygen in the ambulance. There in the medical intensive care unit where everyone knew her from prior admissions, she arrested AGAIN about an hour later. Since she was not red-tagged, we were obliged to resuscitate her AGAIN, and put her on a ventilator. There she literally rotted away for three or four weeks (they had promptly fixed her pacemaker so that her heart wouldn't be able to stop again), until in spite of hell (which included dialysis for renal failure for over a week) she finally managed to "die."
>
> Now, if one of the male staff had jumped into her bed and raped her, this would have been regarded as a criminal assault, and everyone would have been outraged, right? But what we did was far more damaging physically, far more protracted, and not one whit less immoral. Just the same, in the eyes of our curious social system, it was OK. Some system!
>
> Another time recently I was privileged to attend a code blue on a patient who had arrested during cobalt therapy! That was only one of a whole series of resuscitations done routinely on terminal cancer patients at that hospital.
>
> Why, when such patients have literally nothing going for them, must we be so hell-bent on interfering with this perfectly natural process which would relieve them of their hopeless suffering? Have our physicians taken complete leave of their senses? These are outrageous prostitutions of the art and science of resuscitations.

Resuscitation is the most literally lifesaving act the therapist performs. It is the noblest, loftiest, most heroic, and should be the most God-like thing one mortal can do for another. But everytime I am called to one of these grossly inappropriate codes, I am sick in my soul at this UN-godly, beastly business. The dictum that we are required to resuscitate ANYbody who arrests if he is untagged, no matter what's wrong with him or how long before he has been found the arrest may have occurred, really sticks in my craw. It is just reckless irresponsibility of the most irrational and immoral sort.

What's behind this tragedy? NEGLECT! Nobody talked with the patient or his family about whether he (they) wanted him resuscitated if he should arrest. Doubtless the rule always to do so in the absence of a no code order was put there because of the policy that nobody but a physician should make this decision. This can, of course, be construed as protecting nonphysicians from being accused of not resuscitating a patient who was in their judgment nonsalvageable.

But we all know of all too many instances where the doctor has specified NOTHING either way, and where the wishes of the patient or his family have NOT been explored. This situation is, of course, inescapable when there is no time; but usually the subject was just plain avoided because it was too unpleasant.

I think we should complain about this to our medical directors, and try to get them to use their influence on medical staffs to face this responsibility squarely, and then definitely to red tag or no code all patients who are either (a) not regarded as salvageable, or (b) who have expressed their desire to be allowed to die in peace. Actually, hospitals could relieve doctors of some of this unpleasantry by making this question a part of the admissions interview with either the patient or the next of kin.

The etiquette of not **disparaging** (talking ill of) fellow practitioners becomes the issue here. The therapist, while perhaps in the right, was guilty of professional disparagement of his colleagues. The end result of the therapist's article as applied to inappropriate resuscitation was not a great change in clinical practice but rather harm to his own distinguished career. The point of the matter was not whether his account was untrue, or even whether he had an absolute right and perhaps a duty to bring it to the attention of the professional community. The problem lay in the manner of his presentation. Often, in questions of morals, we feel so intensely about what we consider to be right that we consider those who are in opposition to our point of view not merely wrong but evil. In the article, the therapist goes well beyond presenting a legitimate problem and likens the physicians' practice to criminal assault and rape. In assigning reasons for why the practice continued, his only rationales were that perhaps the physicians had taken leave of their senses, or were neglectful or recklessly irresponsible. It is not likely that such a manner of presentation would have gained him willing listeners among those he accused.

There are many problems in modern health care practice that need to be addressed, and the allied health practitioner and nurse have an important part to play in these discussions. The effectiveness of our input—that is, the willingness of others to listen and to cause positive change—will have a great deal to do with the collegiality of our presentation and the positive nature of our proposals.

GAMING THE SYSTEM

Gaming the system is a term that has been widely used since the advent of prospective payment systems and managed care. The term as it is commonly used means that the diagnosis or clinical condition is described in such a manner that the process stretches the truth or is fraudulent in order to get the plan to pay for a test that is not strictly covered or to pay at a higher rate. In the early days of prospective payment, some companies created software to assist in the process of gaming the system. Today, in the managed care arena, gaming is most often done to get around the time-consuming process of challenging the rules and applying for an exception to the rules for a particular patient.[3]

For our purposes however, we will use *gaming* in a more general sense in which the practitioner is attempting to get around the system and is willing to lie in the process. Often the gaming is not even done for the practitioner's benefit but is being done in behalf of a patient or at a patient's request. The therapist who creates a paper trail that provides the basis for a longer period of rehabilitation therapy than would be allowed given the actual situation of the patient, or the physician assistant who certifies that an elderly patient with bunions needs a handicapped parking sticker, when in fact the severity of the problem does not meet the standard for authorizing the sticker, are both gaming the system.

It would seem that it would surely be more acceptable to game the system on behalf of the patient rather than for one's own benefit. Given the world in which we practice, where institutional rules and health care policy plans are not always fair, where our duties to third-party obligations are surely less binding than our obligation to the patients we serve, perhaps some think that we may have a duty to game. Does the health care provider's obligations to the patient's health or to the patient-provider relationship outweigh our duty to the principle of veracity?

As tempting as the thought is, health care practitioners have a fundamental responsibility to be truthful, to keep promises, and to be fair. Giving that gaming (on behalf of patients) seems in most cases to be a rather innocuous practice and given the myriad incentives to game, it is easy to have deception become the standard way of doing business. In her article "Gaming the Rules, Dodging the System," Morreim outlines several basic harms based on utilitarianism that come about as a result of these deceptive practices.[4]

- Lying inevitably undermines a person's credibility. Even when you are doing gaming at the request of the patient, as in the example of the handicapped parking sticker, you may in fact erode the trust between you and the patient. A patient who observes you lying *for* him cannot help but wonder whether you would be willing to lie *to* him.

- If an individual clinician is found to be lying, this can have a harmful effect on the entire health care profession. Much of the good we do is based on the trust we receive from the public and patients. If the public were to perceive us as unworthy of the trust, our ability to serve them would be lessened.

- Gaming can harm other patients. In a world of finite resources, if you somehow manage to get more resources for your patient, you may in fact be taking needed resources away from an equally or more needy patient. In the example of the parking sticker, when the handicapped slots are filled, someone has to walk farther. This may seem trivial but would not seem so for a patient needing an intensive care bed, only to find all beds full because another physician gained the bed for her patient by describing a stable angina as an unstable one. This practice would surely seem to offend distributive justice.

The principle of veracity has a long tradition in health care ethics that goes beyond the utilitarian seeking of a balance between good and harm. Philosophers such as Immanuel Kant held that truth is a fundamental duty for all individuals at all times and that those who lie offend human dignity. Whether you are comfortable with an absolutist view such as that of Kant or with assessing and weighing outcomes, the end result is the same. Within health care, there is a general assumption that deception is problematic even if it is motivated by good intentions.

CONFLICTS OF INTEREST

Under no circumstances may physicians place their own financial interests above the welfare of their patients. The primary objective of the medical professions is to render service to humanity; reward or financial gain is a subordinate consideration. For a physician to unnecessarily hospitalize a patient, prescribe a drug, or conduct diagnostic tests for the physician's financial benefit would be unethical. If a conflict develops between the physician's financial interest and the physician's responsibility to the patient, the conflict must be resolved to the patient's benefit.

Council on Ethical and Judicial Affairs 1996[2]

Recently, in the literature, health care provider **joint-venturing** and **self-referral** practices have been questioned. Most of these criticisms have been directed toward physicians who have joint-ventured into health care services such as physical therapy, diagnostic imaging centers, ambulatory surgical centers, and durable medical equipment companies. Simultaneously with these joint business interests has come an increase in outpatient costs, which appears to be linked to the practice of self-referral. Surveys in regard to this practice show that there is an apparent link between self-referral and increased costs, increased utilization, and reduced quality of care.[5] As a matter of fiduciary good faith and pragmatic practice, any commercial relationship between a practitioner and a company, in which the practitioner has a material interest that could form the basis for a conflict of interest, this relationship should be spelled out in a disclosure statement. Examine the case study of the hard-working therapist in the light of conflicts of interest.

CASE STUDY

The Hard-Working Therapist

Sheryl is a respiratory therapy technician in a small town in Michigan. The town has a small hospital and a small durable medical supply company. Sheryl is known locally as an entrepreneur ball of fire and has managed to become both the head of the hospital respiratory care department and the owner of the small durable medical supply company.

1. In that most of the referrals from Sheryl's department for home care equipment are to Sheryl's home care business, does this represent a conflict of interest?

2. What should Sheryl do?

Obviously, in some or even a majority of these instances, the patients are well served. In some cases, these joint ventures create a competitive atmosphere and may even provide services to a community that might otherwise be unavailable. In these instances, the joint ventures serve a patient-centered health care ethic, and perhaps **safe harbor rules** need to be put into place to allow these clinics to continue to function.[6]

However, whether it serves a patient-centered ethic or no, self-referral is suspect and causes a credibility gap that is hard to overcome. From the outside, joint venturing appears to be a practice "where one comes to do good and winds up doing well." In response to these criticisms, the American Medical Association recently adopted a new policy against physician self-referral. The policy holds that, in general, physicians should not refer patients to health care facilities in which they have an investment interest but do not themselves provide direct medical service.[7]

It seems clear that to self-refer to an establishment in which you do not provide service but have an economic interest is at least suspect and perhaps unethical. Yet there are other equally serious situations of conflict of interest that are more subtle. What of the pens, writing pads, free texts, medical equipment, and drug samples that at times seem a normal part of the delivery of health care? Does the fact that the gift is small make it more ethical to receive? Millions of dollars are spent each year by drug companies to influence physicians in regard to their purchases. Where does this process of receiving goods from drug firms or equipment companies cease to be good advertisement and begin to be unethical? If you were invited to a free seminar held on a cruise ship—where your travel, housing, food, and entertainment were picked up by a company—would this be unethical or continuing education? In one case, physicians were asked to participate in a drug study. The drug that was being studied offered no substantive therapeutic advantage over other drugs of its class and was somewhat more expensive. The doctors were reimbursed $125 for each patient they enrolled in the study, to cover their time and expenses.[8] Did that represent a bribe or gratuity, or was it a legitimate reimbursement to otherwise busy professionals who had done the company a service and participated in important research? Do these practices affect patient care in regard to what companies the patients were referred to or what pharmaceuticals were used? If the practices did change the behavior on the part of the health care practitioner, was the change brought about on the basis of new information gained or favors granted? The very fact that such questions can be asked should cause professional concern.

Although much has been written in regard to the joint venturing practices of physicians and their relationships with drug companies, it is very difficult to determine exactly where the line should be drawn. Reflections on these same practices can be found in the dealings of nursing and allied health professionals. How many of the national, state, and local meetings that these practitioners attend are underwritten by commercial companies? To stem the practice of therapists' referring their recently hospitalized patients to local durable medical equipment companies and receiving a finder's fee, the respiratory care national association (AARC) has been vigorous in its condemnation of referrals whereby the practitioner had monetary gain. Figure 6-1 outlines the AARC statement.[9] Conflict of interest is not limited to the practice of physicians and is equally suspect as a practice whoever the health care provider is. A practitioner who changes his way of practice through any motive other than patient benefit has embarked on a slippery slope of compromised ethics. As a patient care provider, each professional needs to evaluate and prioritize to determine the point at which a service or provided gift ceases to be merely good advertisement or continuing education, and begins to be a favor offered to compromise the client-centered nature of our health care practice.

The Code of Ethics of the AARC applies to all respiratory care practices regardless of the environment in which care may be delivered. In general, the following definition of conflict of interest is provided:

Under no circumstances should any respiratory care practitioner engage in any activity which compromises the motive for the provision of any therapy procedures, the advice or counsel given patients and/or families, or in any manner profit from referral arrangements with home care providers.

FIGURE 6-1 AARC Statement Regarding Ethical Performance of Respiratory Home Care

SEXUAL MISCONDUCT IN HEALTH CARE PRACTICE

Whatever houses I may visit, I will come for the benefit of the sick, remaining free of all intentional injustice, of all mischief and in particular of sexual relations with both female and male persons, be they free or slave.

Hippocratic Oath

It is generally held among all health care providers that sexual relations between practitioners and patients are unethical. This is true because the relationship between practitioner and patient is always unequal. The nature of the practitioner-patient relationship places the practitioner in a position of advantage in the critical areas of knowledge, power, status, and personal vulnerability. Often, very intimate relationships are formed on the basis of our roles, and these can be powerful and intense for both patient and practitioner alike. Moreover, these normal, caring relationships developed between provider and patient frequently evoke strong and complicated feelings. These emotions of admiration, caring, and trust can be misunderstood, and patients are especially vulnerable when they are experiencing intense pressures or major traumatic life events.

Because of these inequalities of position, sexual relations under these situations cannot be considered, nor can they be understood as representing the true consent on the part of the patient. Inasmuch as practitioners have an obligation to treat the needs of the patient first, their own personal gratification cannot become a consideration. The therapeutic relationship rests on the patient's belief that the health care provider is dedicated to her welfare and that there are no other motives or considerations. Sexual relations, by their very nature, create emotional factors that interfere with the therapeutic relationship and the needed objective judgment. Whether due to a temporary failure to manage the therapeutic relationship or to crass exploitation of a professional situation, these relationships are neither ethically excusable nor condonable. Examine the case study on the next page in regard to romantic attachments to patients.

When the practitioner feels that a potential for misunderstanding is possible or that there is the potential for mutual feelings of romantic interest, it is time to end the professional relationship. In that the patient's feelings formed during a time of illness often extend beyond the health care situation, the termination of care does not in itself provide an ethical basis for such a relationship to blossom into sexual contact. If the practitioner is exploiting the feelings of regard, respect, trust, and vulnerability gained as a result of the patient-provider relationship, the ethical propriety of such action is still suspect. In regard to the obvious question of how long is an acceptable period of interruption of the association, the answer is whatever time it takes until the emotions derived from the relationship cannot be misused or manipulated.

CASE STUDY

An Old Friend, a New Relationship

Jason is a twenty-four-year-old respiratory care practitioner who works the evening shift. One of his patients is a woman near his age named Gabriela who is in the hospital for acute asthma. Jason knows her age because he and Gabriela went to the same high school together although she was in the class below his. He had not seen her since high school.

During the week that she is hospitalized, he and Gabriela talked about the old high school days and he feels they have a lot in common. Jason feels that Gabriela is feeling some affection toward him. but he keeps their relationship friendly but professional. On her last night in the hospital prior to her checking out, he hugs her and kisses her on the cheek, and she asks him to give her a call.

1. Now that Gabriela has gone home is it okay for Jason to take her out?

2. Does the fact that they were acquaintances prior to the hospitalization make any difference?

3. Assuming that he wants to call her, how long should he wait?

Scope of Practice

All allied health and nursing personnel work within a **scope of practice**. This scope of recognized duties for our professions is usually set by the traditions of our specialty and by state legislation that enables our practice. Figure 6-2 lists the elements usually found in a scope of practice act. Practitioners who stray outside the scope of legitimate duties not only call upon themselves censorship from their peers and colleagues but also may face loss of legal credentials or litigation. The principle of **role fidelity** requires that we remain within our scope of legitimate practice. In most cases, the scope of practice is clear, and one does not cross the line without willful intention. For example, the nursing or allied health practitioner who is performing physicals and pretending to be a physician has not made an honest error. However, traditions and practices change, and sometimes the line is not as clear as one might suppose.[10] The following case outlines the problems that can occur as a result of being unclear as to specific duties, especially during a period in which there is a shift of traditional roles.

Practice acts will vary in emphasis but the majority will address the following elements:

    a. Scope of professional practice

    b. Requirements and qualifications for licensure

    c. Exemptions

    d. Grounds for administrative action

    e. Creation of an examination board and processes

    f. Penalties and sanctions for unauthorized practice

FIGURE 6-2   Basic Elements of a Practice Act

In the mid-1970s, a nursing educator in Idaho had contact, through a student, with a female client who had chronic myelogenous leukemia. This form of leukemia can often be managed for years with little or no chemotherapy. The woman had done well for twelve years and had ascribed her good health to health foods and a strict nutritional regime. However, her condition had turned for the worse several weeks before, and her physician had advised her that she needed chemotherapy if she was to have any chance of survival. The physician had also advised her of the potential side effects associated with the therapy, including the loss of hair, nausea, fever, and immune system suppression with the increased potential for infection.

The woman had consented to the therapy and signed the appropriate forms, but later had begun to have second thoughts. The nursing educator and student had given the patient one dose of therapy when she began to cry and to express her reservations in regard to the treatments. She questioned the nurse about alternative treatments to the use of chemotherapy. The patient related that she had agreed to the therapy because her son believed that this was the best treatment, but she also related that she had not questioned the physician about alternatives, as he had already told her that chemotherapy was the only treatment indicated. The nurse did not discuss the patient's concerns with the physician, and later that evening returned to the hospital to talk to the patient about alternative therapies. In the discussion, rather non-traditional and controversial therapies were covered, including reflexology and the use of laetrile. The woman's son and daughter-in-law were present at the time of these discussions. During the talk, the nurse made it very clear that the treatments under discussion were not sanctioned by the medical community.

The patient's feelings toward alternative therapies were strengthened by the evening's conversation, but she nevertheless decided to go ahead with the chemotherapy. The treatments, however, did not bring remission to her crisis, and she died two weeks later. The son who had been present during the discussion regarding alternative therapies related the conversation between his mother and the nurse to the doctor.

The physician brought charges against the educator for unprofessional conduct and interfering with the patient-physician relationship. The Board of Nurse Examiners for the state of Idaho charged her with unethical conduct and removed her license to practice. An appeals court later overturned the decision on the basis that the nursing standards used by the board to judge her conduct were too vague, and therefore it was an injustice to remove her license. Although she was somewhat vindicated by the court of appeals decision, the three years of struggle had cost the nurse her teaching position and harmed her career.[11]

Who was right in this case: the nurse, who acted upon the changing role of nursing to function as a patient advocate, or the physician, who, following his professional code, could not truly advocate uproven alternative therapy? Had the physician done so, he would be violating the rule that physicians only practice medicine having a scientific basis.

What is meant by the term **patient advocate** in a situation such as this? Does it extend to excluding the physician from conversations that potentially affect the patient's medical decisions? The role of the nurse is changing, but even as late as 1985 two other nurse-patient relationship models beyond patient advocate were still being discussed. Under both of these, the bureaucratic model (in which the emphasis is on the maintenance of social order at the expense of the individual patient's welfare) and the physician advocate model (in which the goal is to enhance the authority of the physician), the nurse's actions could have been considered contrary to good order.[12]

But what if the appropriate model were that of patient advocate, and the nurse knew that the physician would not have been willing to talk to the patient about her concerns even if she had asked him? Would that have made the situation different? Would the nurse then have had a legitimate right to provide the information under the requirements of informed consent? Does informed consent require that you discuss treatments without scientific basis?

The fact that the nurse did not discuss the situation with the physician and came back during off-duty hours to discuss the matter with the patient indicates that perhaps she knew that the scope of practice line was being breached. Whether her patient advocate role was such that the decision was necessary is a matter that individual practitioners must answer for themselves. There is a truism that runs, "You must not die for principle every day," but every once in a while, an issue arises that is of such importance that the professional must not back away even at the cost of her practice. The question for all of us is, When is this?

Impaired Colleagues

The practice of health care is often very stressful, and it is not surprising that certain providers have found themselves susceptible to alcohol and drugs. It is estimated that 6–8 percent of the nurses in the United States today are addicted to alcohol or other drugs, and in one state study more than 90 percent of the disciplinary hearings for nurses within the state were related to substance abuse.[13] These are often very bright, hard-working practitioners who are ambitious and hold responsible positions. What is to be done when you find that a colleague is impaired? Impaired colleagues place clients at risk. The nature of substance abuse is such that even fine practitioners begin to experience behavioral difficulties such as absenteeism, illogical decision making, and excessive errors. Guided by the principle of nonmaleficence, the question that must be faced is not whether the practitioner has a duty to intervene, but rather the manner of the intervention.

The normal questions that one asks oneself are:

- Do I have all the facts?
- Am I sure?
- Is this my problem?
- Who am I to judge?
- Should I ignore the situation?
- What might it cost me if I confront the situation?
- Is it worth the trouble?

The problem with these rather legitimate and normal questions is that they often do not lead to the correct answer. It is too easy to say "How terrible! I'm sorry about _____, but it's not my job to tell anyone." The problem with this approach is that it is very enabling and does not assist the impaired provider. Equally problematic is the muttering to friends about "poor old Joe," as that is not effective in stopping the behavior and is destructive to the individual's reputation and to the reputation of all health care specialists.

Suppose you saw a colleague administer only one-half of a dose of narcotic, place the syringe in his pocket, and leave for the restroom. To make the case clearer, suppose you later found a bloody, empty syringe in the restroom wastebasket. What should you do? What if you confronted the individual and he denied the whole thing? Addicted individuals often seem to have an infinite supply of rationalizations, prevarications, and subterfuges to convince others that the truth is untrue. It is hard to imagine a more unpleasant task than confronting a colleague about substance abuse, but—pleasant or no—the health care provider must be confronted and be made to seek effective assistance. Where possible, it is best that the individual be encouraged to seek the help independently; where not possible, help must still be obtained in order to protect the patients and salvage the practitioner. Regardless of how the process goes, the basic elements are that the practitioner receives effective help and that those with knowledge of the situation treat the impaired colleague humanely, as we would any patient who needed our assistance.

WHISTLE-BLOWING

Whistle-blowing in cases where we find colleague or institutional misconduct that must be addressed is often very painful and not always appreciated by the institution one serves. In her book *Secrets,* Sissela Bok states that the elements of dissent, accusation, and breach of loyalty, common to the nature of whistle-blowing, combine to create an almost natural negative reaction toward the whistle-blower.[14] Hospitals are usually hierarchical and bureaucratic institutions that often do not respond well to whistle-blowing, especially if the complaint is lodged against someone in a high professional position. Correction of the problem may often cost money, embarrass individuals or the institution, and change the status quo. In that no one likes problems, the messenger is often given as much grief as the person who was the actual problem. Harassment, avoidance, demotion, or termination have sometimes been the fate of those who have reported unpleasant but true instances of misconduct.[15] Because of these potential ramifications, the professional must be very sure of her ground, gather all the facts, and be able to describe the situation in very concrete terms before taking the problem through appropriate internal channels. Figure 6-3 offers guidance on when whistle-blowing is justified.[16]

Regardless of risk, the professional must also recognize that not to report serious misconduct is to become an accessory to the conduct. Whistle-blowing is a process of gatekeeping, a function of role duty and professionalism that cannot be ignored. Peter Raven-Hansen, an attorney, has outlined a series of defensive strategies for those who have decided that an exercise in whistle-blowing is necessary.[17]

- Write a clear, short summary of the situation, describe what it means and why action is necessary. Once the process is started, meticulous documentation of who said what, to whom and when, is necessary.
- Avoid personalization; focus on the nature of the incident.
- Where possible, have your statements verified by other health care providers. Sticking to the incident will assist you in avoiding libel and slander charges.
- Make every effort to settle the matter internally. In most cases the media are the last, rather than the first, channel to use.
- Do not believe that you can remain anonymous. The nature of the incident and the details of the disclosure will more than likely reveal who blew the whistle.
- Expect a slow process. The nature of bureaucratic institutions creates an inertial barrier to change.
- Expect retaliation. Disclosures of this nature often are embarrassing and costly to those involved. The whistle-blower must expect to face characterizations of being a snitch and a disloyal problem causer. The whistle-blower must be prepared to live with these attitudes or move on to another position.

- The wrongdoing in question is grave and has created, or is likely to create, serious harm.
- The professional who is contemplating blowing the whistle has appropriate information and is competent to make a judgment about the wrongdoing.
- The professional has consulted others to confirm his information and judgment.
- All other internal resources to resolve the problem have been exhausted.
- There is a good likelihood that the whistle-blowing will serve a useful purpose.
- The harm created by the whistle-blowing is less than the harm done by a continuation of the wrongdoing.

FIGURE 6-3   Justification of Whistle-Blowing

Whistle-blowing is not a task that should be entered into casually. Even under the best of circumstances, the individual must understand that, though necessary, the position of whistle-blower is high risk, often lonely, and rarely appreciated. A quotation from attorney Joseph Rose, whose career was initially placed on hold as a result of whistle-blowing, provides some understanding of the nature of the process.

> Gandhi said that noncooperation with evil is as much a duty as cooperation with good; Edmund Burke said that the only thing necessary for the triumph of evil is for good men to do nothing. Both concepts are still viable . . . although expensive.[18]

Often practitioners are faced with moral distress in that they know what is right but seem unable to follow the correct path. This distress is common among allied health practitioners and nurses, as these health care providers are responsible to many masters. The most commonly perceived constraints are physicians, fear of lawsuits, hospital policies, habits of professional socialization that require the following of orders, and fear of loss of security.

There is a natural ambiguity to the practice of health care that seems to create a certain amount of moral distress. Providers, however, can reduce this by asserting more control over their situation. The first and perhaps most essential form of this self-assertion is to interview potential employers as to their attitudes toward important issues prior to signing on as an employee. Quite often we look only to the pay, fringe benefits, or distance from home in making employment decisions. Equally important would be the institution's policies in the areas of abortion, euthanasia, incompetent patients, religious matters, living wills, organ procurement, codes, and team medicine.

INSTITUTIONAL ETHICS COMMITTEE

One of the important issues of role duty is the obligation that each practitioner has in maintaining not only a high level of technical practice but also maintaining the common field in which all health specialists practice. There is a great and deep well of respect that is afforded each practitioner, which has been filled by those who have practiced before us. Our conduct in representing our specialties, the humanity of our service to the patients, the respect we afford other practitioners, and the service we provide to the community are important aspects of a professional career, and it is these activities that maintain the area of common practice that surrounds us.

One growing area of potential service is the opportunity to serve as a member of an institutional ethics committee. An institutional ethics committee (IEC) can be defined as an interdisciplinary body of health care providers, community representatives, and nonmedical professionals who address ethical questions within the health care institution, especially on the care of patients. The impetus for such a committee came from the high-profile cases involving Karen Ann Quinlan and Baby Doe.[19] The President's Commission for the Study of Ethical Problems in Medicine and Biomedical and Behavioral Research advocated research into ethics committees.[20]

Often ethics committees are seen as alternatives to court litigation. Health care providers were struggling with new issues that came as the result of previously unimagined life-saving medical technology and team medicine in which literally hundreds of practitioners were responsible for some aspect of the care. The committees were seen as a way to safeguard the patient's interests by serving on a consultative basis to analyze ethical dilemmas; educate health care providers, patients, and families; and guide hospital policy. Figure 6-4 lists the most common functions associated with ethics committees. Note that decision making is not one of the functions listed. These committees play an advisory role.

In 1992, the Joint Commission on Accreditation of Healthcare Organizations (JCAHO), the accrediting agency for hospitals and other health care organizations, required the establishment of organizational mechanisms for addressing conflicts within the health care setting. In most organizations covered by JCAHO, this has meant the development of ethics committees.[21] The modern committee is often a multidisciplinary group that includes physicians, nurses, social workers, philosophers, laypersons, lawyers, administrators, and religious leaders. In recent years, health care providers have become increasingly sophisticated regarding ethical issues and processes through readings, conferences, seminars, and so forth. In that ethical training is increasing in all health care programs, in the future more allied health and nursing professionals will be prepared to participate in IECs.

Often the philosophy of the committee reflects the nature of the institution. For example, a Catholic hospital will generally reflect the tenets of that faith. The refinements in policies con-

- Policy and procedure development
- Educational role
- Case consultant
- Retrospective case review

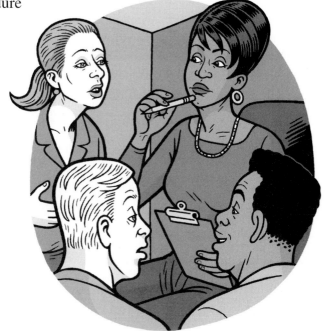

FIGURE 6-4   Common Functions of Ethics Committees

cerning brain death determinations, do not resuscitate (DNR) orders, and patient rights have been a great strength of the ethics committees. Given our movement toward health care reform and the use of market forces to assist in cost containment, it is likely that new areas of policy will include issues involving care of the uninsured, care for the medically indigent, organ procurement, rights of the incompetent elderly patient, and problems of premature discharge.

CONCLUSION

Regardless of the level of practice, the ability and opportunity to participate in the provision of health care is an awesome and wonderfully engaging enterprise. The health professions are meaningful professional careers. To enter the practice of health care is to enter into a social contract with other practitioners, patients, and the community in general. This social contract calls not only for a particular set of clinical skills but also appropriate ethical, legal, and social behaviors.

Like any other professional endeavor, the common area of practice belongs to each of us. It is unthinkable and unwise to believe that some other group of specialists such as physicians will maintain the health care arena. The obligations of ethical conduct, community service, and the refinement of knowledge are not the obligations of the few but the many. Health care is a team effort, and the team is responsible for the outcomes. It is a common field where we labor, and like any other field, it requires that all those involved in the harvest maintain the space so that we can come again, and when we have finally finished, leave it to others who will replace us in the labor.

We are in a time of great change for American health care. Rapid technological and social change has pushed the frontiers of health into uncharted territory. Many of the legal and ethical issues faced by health care providers are new. To make matters more complicated, this is also a time of legislative reform to the health care system where at times it seems the only thing that is truly stable is change.

This is a litigious age. Out patient populations have come to expect miracles that cannot always be delivered. Practitioners at times find themselves seemingly between two forces: unhappy patients, aggrieved relatives, and their lawyers versus the risk management departments, other health care providers, clinical institutions, and insurance companies. Practitioners are expected to conduct themselves in a manner that protects the patients and the institutions they serve.

This chapter has dealt with several functions that can be listed under the headings of "small ethics." While they do not deal with the great life-and-death issues such as euthanasia, justice, or withholding or withdrawing life support, they are the daily stuff of modern practice. They come to us as a function of our role duty and are the price we pay for being professionals. As practitioners of health professions we have an obligation to our patients, our colleagues, and our professions to perform these necessary, albeit unpleasant, gatekeeping tasks.

KEY CONCEPTS

- Self-regulation is one of the key elements of profession. Professional codes of ethics are important documents in the process of self-regulation.
- Disparagement and improper bad-mouthing of other health care providers serves neither our profession nor our patients.
- Care must be taken to manage the therapeutic relationship so that patient exploitation is avoided.
- Under no circumstances may the practitioner place his financial interests above the welfare of his patients. The primary objective of the health professions is to render service to humanity. Reward or financial gain is a subordinate consideration.

- Gaming the system even for the benefit of the patient is a suspect practice that harms the health professions.

- All clinicians must understand and remain within the constraints of their professional practice act.

- Gatekeeping within role duty and fidelity requires that individual practitioners be responsible not only for their standard of practice but work to protect the community, patients, and our specialties from abuses of other practitioners.

REVIEW EXERCISES

A. On an ethical basis, going beyond your scope of practice, having sexual relations with patients, and self-referrals are problems. Write a short paragraph for each of these practices using a legitimate moral rationale (excepting "that's how I feel") indicating why these practices do harm to the professions, the practitioners, and the patients we serve.

1. Going beyond scope of practice

2. Sexual relations with patients

3. Self-referral

B. In the article (found in the chapter) regarding inappropriate resuscitation, the therapist was attempting to bring about legitimate change in practice. What he wanted was the establishment of guidelines such as:[22]

1. DNR orders should be documented in the written medical record.

2. DNR orders should specify the exact nature of the treatment to be withheld.

3. Patients, when they are able, should participate in DNR decisions. Their involvement and wishes should be documented in the medical record.

4. Decisions to withhold CPR should be discussed with the health care team.

5. DNR status should be reviewed on a regular basis.

6. DNR is not equivalent to medical or psychological abandonment.

   With the above guidelines in mind, first underline the sections within the article that appear inflammatory and devoid of collegiality. Second, rewrite the article so that it is less inflammatory and more persuasive. Third, decide upon a plan (Who, What, Where, Why, When) on how you are going to go about bringing your ideas in regard to changing the resuscitation policy so that it comes into line with the above guidelines.

C. The story in regard to the nursing educator from Idaho was essentially true. Indicate whether you think the nurse or the Board of Nursing was correct. In deciding, use the decision-making model proposed by M. C. Silva:[23]

1. Gather the facts.

2. Identify the dilemma in concrete terms.

3. Explore all options and rules or principles governing each option.

4. Make a decision, and be prepared to reflect on the decision.

D. Use the following decision-making format for the following case involving an impaired coworker. (Take each step as a separate exercise and work through the problem)

Steps to Problem Solving

1. Problem sensing—gather information, review facts.

2. Formulate and state the problem.

3. List all solutions of initial credibility.

4. Evaluate each solution in terms of its consequences for the individuals involved.

5. Evaluate solutions in terms of upholding or sacrificing the basic principles of health care.

6. Select the solution with the best consequences and least sacrifice of basic ethical principles.

7. Prepare a defense for your choice.

You and Ben have been friends since you met in physical therapy school. Following graduation you both took positions within a local clinic. Lately Ben has been going through a difficult and emotional divorce. At work he has begun to act erratic, often talking a mile a minute and at other times appearing withdrawn and quiet. You wonder if he has begun to abuse drugs.

One day Ben confirms your fears when he tells you that he is needing to take pills to go to sleep and that he takes others in the day to stay awake. He feels that he is not abusing the drugs in that he has prescriptions for all of them provided by a variety of physician friends. He asks you as his friend not to tell anyone, and tells you that he will be able to get a handle on his problems once the divorce is settled.

The next morning during report, Ben appears to fall asleep. After report, your supervisor, who knows that you and Ben are friends, comes to you and asks, "What is the matter with Ben?" How do you respond?

NOTES

1. James Whitacre, "Ole Nincompoop Says: Help Stamp Out Inappropriate Resuscitation," *Newsletter of the Missouri Society for Respiratory Therapy* (1980): pp. 11–12.

2. Council on Ethical and Judicial Affairs, *Code of Medical Ethics: Current Opinions and Annotations.* (Chicago: American Medical Association, 1996).

3. Jeremy Sugarman, *Ethics in Primary Care* (New York: McGraw-Hill, 2000).

4. E. H. Morreim, "Gaming the System, Dodging the Rules," *Archives of Internal Medicine* 151 (1991): pp. 443–447.

5. Elton Scott and Mark Ahern, "Effects of Joint Ventures on Health Care Costs, Access and Quality," *Nursing Economics* 10, no. 2 (March–April 1992): pp. 101–109.

6. Jean Mitchell and Elton Scott, "New Evidence of the Prevalence and Scope of Physician Joint Ventures," *Journal of the American Medical Association* 268, no. 1 (July 1992): pp. 80–84.

7. Mitchell and Scott, "New Evidence of the Prevalence and Scope of Physician Joint Ventures."

8. Jerome Freeman and Brian Kaatz, "The Physician and the Pharmaceutical Detail Man: An Ethical Analysis," *Journal of Medical Humanities and Bioethics* 8, no. 1 (Spring–Summer 1987).

9. American Association for Respiratory Care, "AARC Statement in Regard to Ethical Performance of Respiratory Home Care," Judicial Committee, AARC.

10. Gerald Winslow, from "Loyalty to Advocacy: A New Metaphor for Nursing," *Hastings Center Report* (June 1984), pp. 32–39.

11. *In re Tuma,* Supreme Court, State of Idaho case 12587, 1977.

12. W. J. Pinch, "Ethical Dilemmas in Nursing: The Role of the Nurse and Perceptions of Autonomy," *Journal of Nursing Education,* 24, no. 9 (1985): pp. 372–376.

13. Sharon Ross, "Chemically Impaired Nurses," American Association of Critical Cases Convention, Orlando, FL, 2004.

14. Sissela Bok, *Secrets* (New York: Vintage Books, 1983).

15. Morton Glazer, "Ten Whistle-Blowers and How They Fared," *Hastings Center Report* 13, no. 6 (October 1983): p. 33.

16. Amy Haddad and Charles Dougherty, "Whistle-Blowing in the OR: The Ethical Implications," *Today's O. R. Nurse* (March 1991): pp. 30–33.

17. Peter Raven-Hansen, "Do's and Don't's for Whistle-Blowers: Planning for Trouble," *Technology Review* (1980): pp. 34–44.

18. Joseph Rose, as quoted in Glazer, "Ten Whistle-Blowers and How They Fared."

19. Valerie Glesnes-Anderson and Gary R. Anderson, *Health Care Ethics* (Rockville, MD: Aspen Publication, 1987).

20. President's Commission for the Study of Ethical Problems in Medicine and Biomedical and Behavioral Research (Washington, D.C.: U.S. Govt. Printing Office, 1982).

21. Brandon Minogue, *Bioethics: A Committee Approach* (Boston: Jones & Bartlet Publishers, 1996).

22. Stuart Younger, "Do Not Resuscitate Orders: No Longer a Secret But Still a Problem," *Hastings Center Report* 17 (February 1987): pp. 24–35.

23. Mary C. Silva, *Ethical Decision Making in Nursing Administration* (Norwalk, CT: Appleton and Lange, 1990).

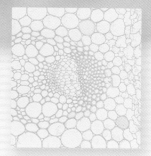

CHAPTER 7

Autonomy vs. Paternalism: A Contest Between Virtues

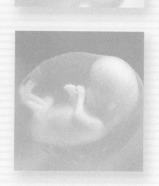

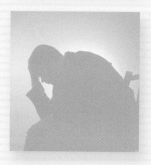

GOAL

To outline the nature of the conflict between autonomy and paternalism, and to discuss the requirements and elements of informed consent. A secondary goal is to investigate the nature of competency determination.

OBJECTIVES

Upon completion of this chapter, the reader should be able to:

1. Define paternalism.

2. Describe how paternalism is, in its best sense, a result of physician beneficence.

3. List and describe the four models of physician-patient interaction as outlined by Robert Veatch. Explain why the contractual model seems best suited for today's practice.

4. Define and list the elements of informed consent.

5. Differentiate between the professional community standard and the reasonable patient standard, and explain how the latter better serves the needs of the autonomous patient.

6. Explain why a more subjective standard than the professional community standard or the reasonable patient standard may be needed to protect patient autonomy.

7. Define *therapeutic privilege*, list the situations in which it is used, and explain the problems of benevolent deception.

8. List several groups in our society that would have limited autonomy.

9. Outline the major elements of competency determination.

10. Explain how the First Amendment to the U.S. Constitution protects the autonomy of religious individuals who have beliefs that conflict with current medical practice.

11. Outline the requirements of EMTALA.

12. Provide definitions for *qualitative* and *quantitative futility*.

KEY TERMS

Ad litem	**EMTALA**	**Professional autonomy**
Authentic decision	**Futile care**	**Professional community**
Brain dead	**Material risk**	**standard**
Competency	**Patient-centered standard**	**Reasonable patient standard**
Do not resuscitate order	**Persistent vegetative state**	

VALUE PREFERENCE AS THE BASIS OF HEALTH CARE DECISIONS

The objection of some of the laymen concerned about the problem has been to what they call the "Father Knows Best," authoritative, paternalistic attitude of physicians. In fact, if "Father" didn't know best, he ought to retire from the case.

Noted Surgeon

CASE STUDY

Who Is the Patient?

In a recent pediatric case presentation, a physician described a situation in which a fourteen-year-old boy is brought to the clinic. The teenager is described by the physician as having one of the most severe cases of attention deficit disorder (ADD) that he

(*continues*)

Who Is the Patient? (cont.)

had seen in practice. During the session, the boy fidgeted, did nonstop hand gestures, and did leg swinging and tapping. According to the mother, the boy would not pay attention to any adult attempting to engage him and was in jeopardy of flunking ninth grade. The mother wants the physician to write a prescription for Ritalin. Given the boy's condition, the request seems reasonable although not without some potential side effects, such as tics and sleep disturbances.

The boy, however, does not want the medication, stating that when "I take that stuff, I zone out. I'm like a log. Ritalin ruins my life!" He describes life without the medication as being in a room in which all the newest videos are playing and trying to watch them all. When he is not on medication, he feels that he is more alive, that he can crack great jokes, and fellow students like him. Given that adolescence is the time when we want young people to find out who they are, is it right to medicate him and not allow him to express what he sees as being his true self? It is clearly the mother, not the boy, who wants the prescription.

1. Should the physician write the prescription?
2. Explain how you reached the decision (duty, consequence, virtue, or divine command reasoning).
3. What basic principles did you consider in your decision process?

If the health care practitioner is the expert and if health is a universal good, it would seem that the patient, who is a stranger to this specialized world of medicine, would just lie there and allow the medical team to work on his behalf. The problem with this reasoning lies in the fact that although health is a universal good, it is not the only one. The good life, however we define it, contains many goals beyond health—which at times have a higher personal value. A hypothetical case that looks at how a variety of factors interplay to shape decisions is that of an author who contracts a terminal disease. His physician knows of a drug that, if taken, will extend the author's life by ten years. Without the medicine, the prognosis is two to three years. Following the physician's recommendation, the author takes the medication and starts what he anticipates will be his greatest work. Unfortunately, the medication leaves his mind clouded, and he loses his creative ability to write. He is faced with the problem of taking the medication and extending his life to ten rather cloudy, noncreative years or not taking the drug and shortening his life by seven or eight years. Without the drug, however, during his remaining two to three years he would be clear minded, which would potentially allow him to finish his greatest work.

In this hypothetical case, the author discontinues the treatment against his doctor's recommendations. The desire to complete what he considered to be his greatest literary accomplishment had a higher personal value than did an extended nonproductive life. The example shows that health care decisions are matters not only of medical expertise, but also of individual value preferences. When the client's personal value preferences, uncoerced by pain, depression, lack of maturity, or other factors that limit **competency**, lead her to an **authentic decision** regarding a personal health care choice, it is an important part of patient autonomy and the health care provider's duty to patient advocacy to support the decision when possible.

From Paternalism to Patient Autonomy

An irony of health care is that in an earlier age, when practitioners had less to offer by way of scientific evidence for their cures and nostrums, society allowed them a greater role in medical decision making. Now, when every treatment is subjected to scientific method and scrutiny, the patient is demanding and receiving a greater role in the decision-making process. The scope of the distance we have come in this process from physician paternalism to patient autonomy can be seen from two excerpts—one from the *Code of Ethics of the American Medical Association* (1848) and the other from the American Hospital Association's *A Patient's Bill of Rights.*

1848 Code, Section 6

The obedience of a patient to the prescriptions of his physician should be prompt and implicit. He should never permit his own crude opinions.[1]

Patient's Bill of Rights.

4. The patient has the right to refuse treatment to the extent permitted by law and to be informed of the medical consequences of his action.[2]

Health care practitioners down through the ages have prescribed faith and obedience as essential aspects of the cure. Roughly speaking, *paternalism* consists of acting in a way that is believed to protect and advance the interests of another even though the actions may be against the desires, or may in fact limit the freedom of action, of the individual. At its best, paternalism comes into being when the desire to honor the principle of beneficence comes into conflict with the patient's autonomy.

Autonomy vs. Beneficence

The most eloquent statement and defense for personal autonomy is found in the essay *On Liberty* by John Stuart Mill. In this work, Mill holds that the only purpose for which power can be rightfully exercised over any other member of a civilized community against his will is to prevent harm to others.

His own good, either physical or moral, is not a sufficient warrant. He cannot be compelled to do or forebear because it will be better for him to do so, because it will make him happier, because, in the opinion, to do so would be wise or even right. These are good reasons for remonstrating with him, but not for compelling him or visiting him with any evil in case he does otherwise.[3]

The issue is more complex than who is in charge or even who knows best. The real issue is which of the basic ethical principles holds supremacy in a given situation. Should it be the personal liberty of self-determination under the principle of autonomy even at the expense of forcing the health care provider to do less than could be done, or should it be under the principle of practitioner beneficence, in which care is provided even in cases in which the patient wishes to be left alone?

Should alert, rational patients be allowed to refuse reasonable care if that decision sacrifices their lives or health? A secondary question is, "What duty do health care providers have in this choice?" Can the practitioner assist after the patient has made a decision that is medically incorrect and, if followed, would lead to personal harm?

What of the practitioner's professional autonomy? Can a patient's desire to be treated in a particular way overcome the autonomy of the health care provider? For instance, if a patient demands an abortion from a physician with a pro-life view, whose autonomy should prevail? In general, the practitioner is not required to act contrary to basic personal values and beliefs. However, if a patient-provider relationship has been established and the practitioner feels that he must withdraw services, care must be taken to ensure that the patient is not abandoned and is referred appropriately.

The attitudes of some practitioners toward patient autonomy can be brought into focus by considering what is meant when we say, "Mr. Jones is a good patient," or "Physicians and nurses do not make good patients." Often what is meant is that Mr. Jones follows orders but that physicians and nurses are assertive and noncompliant. In this light, "good" indicates an individual who allows the medical staff to make all the decisions.

The arguments for and against paternalism have led to disagreements in regard to when practitioner beneficence can validly overcome a patient's autonomous action. Can the health care provider, under the guise of doing good, force a patient to receive lifesaving care, even against his will? Children and the elderly often find their autonomy limited in that they are held to be incompetent and incapable of assessing risk to themselves.

PROVIDER-PATIENT RELATIONSHIP

Robert Veatch, former director of the Kennedy Institute of Ethics, proposed a series of hypothetical models used for the examination of the physician-patient relationship. In these models the relationships take four basic forms:[4]

Engineering Model

In this pattern, the physician acts as a scientist who deals only with facts. The physician gathers the information, explains the material to the patient, and then divorces himself from the decision. The physician allows the patient to make the decision and follows the dictates of this choice. Although this model allows for a high level of patient autonomy, it permits no professional determinism. The practitioner would not be allowed to exercise personal values, and if called upon would perform duties that might possibly be personally abhorrent.

Priest Model

This is a highly paternalistic model, where the physician operates from the moral position of knowing what is best for the patient. It often takes the form of, "As your physician I recommend. . . ." The patient is led to believe that her opinion is not of the same value as that of the learned physician. This form of paternalism goes well beyond paternalism based on the concept of beneficence, and is more a matter of personal control.

Collegial Model

This model suggests that the physician and patient should see themselves as colleagues solving the common problem of eliminating illness. Mutual trust and confidence drive the model as the two work toward the shared and common goal in a collegial, harmonious atmosphere of equality. While this model may have some element of reality in the radical health movement or in free clinics, it has limited usage in other medical arenas.

Unfortunately, due to ethnic, class, social, or value differences between patients and their physicians, a collegial atmosphere of equality is more a pipe dream than a reality. The physician as our pal is not a picture that most of us hold for any period of time.

Contractual Model

This is a shared decision-making model in which the patient is accorded the right to make decisions and to have control over his own life whenever significant decisions are to be made. Once the highly value-laden decisions are made, the patient relies on the technical experience and skills of the medical team for most of the decisions in regard to care. Both the physician and patient have the option to reopen the contract and to leave the relationship if the decisions of one run contrary to the value systems or are abhorrent to the other. The contractual model allows both individuals to interact in an atmosphere of both obligations and expected benefits.

INFORMED CONSENT

It is from the struggle between paternalism and autonomy that the basis for the doctrine of informed consent has been derived. This moral and legal doctrine is a product of the last half of the twentieth century as judges have sought to protect the patient's right to greater freedom of choice. Informed consent binds the physician to an adequate disclosure and explanation of the treatment and the various options and consequences. Simply stated, informed consent requires that before any risky or invasive procedures can be performed, the health care practitioner must inform the patient of pertinent details about the nature of the procedure, its purpose, potential risks, and any reasonable alternatives that might be chosen. The elements of informed consent found in most definitions include:

1. Disclosure: The nature of the condition, the various options, potential risks, the professional's recommendation, and the nature of consent as an act of authorization.

2. Understanding: In the United States, most states require that the physician provide information at a level that a hypothetical reasonable patient would understand.

3. Voluntariness: No efforts toward coercion, manipulation, or constraint are allowed. The patient must be in a position to practice self-determination.

4. Competence: Decisions in regard to competence usually take into account experience, maturity, responsibility, and independence of judgment.

5. Consent: An autonomous authorization of the medical intervention.

Examine the following case study in relation to the need to gain informed consent and how it might be provided.

CASE STUDY

Locked-In Syndrome and Informed Consent

Some patients following a massive cerebrovascular accident (stroke) survive the loss of function within their brain stem and suffer a condition known as locked-in syndrome. Paralyzed from head to toe, they are locked in their body and unable to move, but their mind remains intact. In this particular case the only means the patient had to communicate was by blinking the left eye.

(continues)

Locked-In Syndrome and Informed Consent (cont.)

Unable to effectively clear secretions, these patients often are subject to life-threatening aspiration pneumonia. In order to gain informed consent for a do not resuscitate order should the aspiration pneumonia become severe, the physician and patient decided on the mechanism of one blink for yes and two for no.

1. Do you need to have an informed consent when the patient has this level of limitation?
2. Can this patient be considered competent to make the decision?
3. Can informed consent be given with a blink of an eye?

It is important to understand that informed consent does not require full understanding or full voluntariness to be in place. If these criteria were truly to be required, autonomous action would be a rare event. The courts have held that a patient suing under the principle of informed consent must prove the physician failed to inform him of a material risk. Unfortunately, there is no bright line that separates material from immaterial risk. In general, a risk is material if it would be likely to affect a patient's decision.

Consent may take many forms, including oral, implied, written, general, and special consent. Oral consent is as binding as written consent as there is no general legal rule that consent must be provided in written form. However, oral consent requires collaboration and therefore is difficult to prove when there is disagreement.

Implied consent is often used in cases in which immediate action is required to save a patient from death or permanent impairment of health. In the case of an unconscious patient in the emergency room, consent is presumed when inaction may cause greater injury or would be contrary to good medical practice. It should be noted, however, that if a patient were to refuse a particular treatment and then become unconscious, her prior autonomous decision must be respected. Similarly, autonomous alert patients in emergency room situations may refuse lifesaving treatments.

Another form of implied consent that occurs outside the emergency situation is when the patient voluntarily submits to a treatment and implies consent. As an example, an individual noticed a line of passengers on a ship receiving injections. The person entered the line and submitted to the injection without giving prior authorization. His autonomous act of entering the line and remaining there to receive the injection constituted implied consent.

Written consent is the preferred form of consent. The consent form provides legal, visible proof of the patient's intentions in the matter. Physicians have a legal obligation to inform their patients regarding any procedures they are ordering and to gain consent. This obligation to gain consent from patients should not be delegated to others on the health care team.

Often when a patient is admitted to the unit, a general consent form is signed. These general statements are worded in such a way as to permit the health care providers to perform almost any medical or surgical procedure that is deemed medically necessary in the patient's best interest. These forms, however, do not provide a unit with carte blanche authority but are used to provide consent to routine services and routine touching by the health care staff. They are not designed and do not provide authorization for specific high-risk procedures or treatments.

Specific high-risk procedures or treatments that expose the patient to an unusual risk require the completion of a special consent form. Often a listing of procedures and treatments that require special consent is maintained by the unit along with the forms. The special consent form is usually signed, dated, and witnessed at the time the physician explains the procedure or treatment. In order for these forms to be truly effective, they should be signed within a reasonable time prior to the procedure or treatment.

STANDARDS OF DISCLOSURE

It is informed consent that allows autonomous self-determination. The main struggle in the courts has been to determine what standards should govern the level of disclosure. Two standards have been proposed, the professional community standard and the reasonable patient standard.[5]

Professional Community Standard

The health care provider is bound to provide the amount of information that would be expected from other reasonable practitioners within the community in similar situations. This formed the basis of the decision in the 1906 *Natanson* v. *Kline* case,[6] which set forth what a physician must disclose in regard to the side effects of cobalt therapy. This standard was based on the concept that the practitioner and patient were bound in a special fiduciary relationship in which the difference in levels of information and patient trust binds the professional to act in the patient's behalf without allowing any conflict of interest. The amount of information provided and the nature of the information would be determined by the traditions of the practice and the professional community. The application of this standard seems to generate a great number of problems, since the focus is not on patient understanding but rather on the physician's standard of practice. Since there is often a wide gap between the social, economic, and educational level of the physicians and their patients, even given the best of intentions this standard does not necessarily lead to a level of communication that allows for true patient autonomy.

Reasonable Patient Standard

This holds that the amount and kind of information needed is that which a hypothetical reasonable person would need in order to understand the nature of the condition and the various options. This standard was articulated in the 1972 *Canterbury* v. *Spence* case, in which the court ruled that "true consent to what happens to one's self is the informed exercise of a choice, and that entails an opportunity to evaluate knowledgeably the options available and the risks attendant upon each."[7] The rationale for this standard is that the type and amount of information needed must be at the patient's level if he is truly to be autonomous as a decision maker. This idealized person should not be equated to the ordinary person or average person. The reasonable person is one who is never subject to irrational fears or personal idiosyncrasies. One legal text described the reasonable person:

> He is not to be identified with an ordinary person, who might occasionally do irrational things; he is a prudent careful person, who is always up to standard.

One criticism of the reasonable patient standard is the nature of the hypothetical person. Who is to say that this person is anything like the patient in regard to beliefs, cognitive abilities, and social background?

Patient-Centered Standard

What perhaps is needed is a patient-centered standard that relies on the unique nature and abilities of the individual patient to determine the amount of disclosure needed to satisfy the requirements of informed consent. This more subjective standard would allow a greater differentiation based on patient reference. A patient who values a pain-free life is very different from one who values an extended life regardless of pain or, as in the case of the would-be great author, a person who values a life with full faculties above all other considerations is possibly quite different from some hypothetical reasonable patient.

In practice, the courts have not provided clear direction, inasmuch as they can be seen at various times to be forceful proponents for both autonomy and paternalism. In several landmark cases, an absolute need for individual self-determination, with the requirements of informed consent, has been outlined; in others, the doors have been opened for therapeutic privilege and professional determination. *Therapeutic privilege* is the legal exception to the rule of informed consent, which allows the caregiver to proceed with care without consent in cases of emergency, incompetence, and in which, due to depression or instability, the patient could be harmed by the information. The latter case is a rather controversial form of therapeutic privilege, as the decision to withhold information based on "sound medical judgment" opens the door for professional determinism at the expense of patient autonomy.

This shifting in position can be highlighted in the difference between the early cases of *Pratt* v. *Davis* (1905)[8] and *Schloendorff* v. *The Society of New York Hospital* (1914),[9] as well as later cases such as *Canterbury* v. *Spence* (1972). In the two early cases, the courts outlined a rigid respect for personal autonomy: "Under a free government at least, the free citizen's first and greatest right which underlies all the others—the right to the inviolability of his person, in other words, his right to himself."[10] This right to self was supreme even if the physician was attempting to do good. Doing good was not enough if the good was performed without the consent of the patient. In the *Schloendorff* case, a woman had refused surgery but had allowed the physician to examine her under ether. During the examination, the surgeon had found fibroid tumors that needed to be removed, and proceeded to remove them, feeling that the care was medically expedient. In his review, Justice Cardozo wrote:

> Every human being of adult years and sound mind has a right to determine what shall be done with his own body; and a surgeon who performs an operation without his patient's consent, commits an assault for which he is liable in damages.[11]

In later cases, the courts moved away from a rigid defense of autonomy and allowed for a level of benevolent deception. *Canterbury* v. *Spence* case involved a nineteen-year-old male who underwent a laminectomy for severe back pain. After the surgery, he attempted, without assistance, to get up to urinate. In his attempt, he fell and suffered a setback that led to paralysis from the waist down. Although he had been warned about moving without assistance, he sued on the basis of negligent failure to warn him of the risk of paralysis.

Although the court was deeply sympathetic to the young man, it held that the physician had not been negligent in failing to explain the risk of paralysis, and that if, in his medical judgment, the patient was better served by the deception, under the empowerment of therapeutic privilege the physician could limit the amount of disclosure.

> It is recognized that patients occasionally become so ill or distraught on disclosure as to foreclose a rational decision, or complicate or hinder the treatment, or perhaps even pose psychological damage to the patient. . . . The critical inquiry is whether the physician responded to a sound medical judgment that communication of the risk information would present a threat to the patient's well being.[12]

The courts have not provided a consistent presentation of what is required in regard to informed consent, at times seeming to shift from full disclosure to the allowance of paternalism. Critics such as Jay Katz have likened informed consent to a fairy tale.[13] He argues that, although the doctrine is enchantingly appealing in its simplicity, it does not live up to its promise of delivering decisional authority to the patients. The reality of current medical practice does not fulfill the promise, and is often perfunctorily performed, not so much to convey information and open dialogue between physicians and patients as to comply with the legal letter of the law. Katz argues that "once kissed by the doctrine, frog-patients" do not become "autonomous princes."

COMPETENCY DETERMINATION

What, then, is the basis of the medical judgment that overcomes and limits patient autonomy? As a general rule, the practitioner must respect and abide by the decisions of an autonomous patient. This general rule, however, cannot apply when the patient's decision is based on incomplete information, lack of understanding, or external controlling influences that preclude independent judgment.

In general, a competent adult has the absolute right to refuse medical treatment even if the refusal is life threatening. At question is patient autonomy, which is positively confirmed by being able to answer yes to two questions: (1) Does the patient understand the nature of the illness and the consequences of the various options that may be chosen? and (2) Is the decision based on rational reasoning? The decision itself need not be rational, but the reasoning process should be. Given First Amendment protections for religious belief, the second question in regard to the need for rational processes needs to be modified to include the protection of decisions based on faith, that is, "a belief held to be true, in regard to things unseen." A corollary question needs to be added in these cases: (3) Is this seemingly irrational thinking based on a religious belief acceptable and entitled to First Amendment protections? In order to be protected, a belief must be held by a sufficient number of people, for an extended time period, or be sufficiently like other beliefs that are held by other groups that are considered orthodox.

In regard to the Jehovah's Witness faith, the courts have provided a rather inconsistent picture as to honoring the decision not to accept transfusions. Orthodox Jehovah's Witnesses believe that in the Old and New Testament Scriptures, the Lord declares that His followers should not partake of blood:

> For it is the life of all flesh: the blood of it is for the life thereof; therefore I said unto the children of Israel, Ye may not eat of the blood of no manner of flesh; for the life of all flesh is the blood thereof; whosoever eateth it shall be cut off. (Leviticus 17:14)

> But that we write unto them, that they abstain from pollution of idols, and from fornication, and from things strangled, and from blood. (Acts 12:50)

To Witnesses, the acceptance of a transfusion places them in a situation in which they may indeed prolong their life here on earth, but places them in jeopardy of being eternally cut off from their God.

The decision to honor decisions of this nature is not based on whether an individual's faith is rational to the health care provider, but rather on whether the decision is being made by an autonomous adult. In a 1965 Chicago case in which a woman repeatedly told her physician that she understood the consequences of her actions, but as an act of faith could not take a transfusion, the courts held:

> Even though we may consider the appellant's beliefs unwise, foolish or ridiculous, in the absence of an overriding danger to society we may not permit interference . . . in the waning hours of her life for the sole purpose of compelling her to accept medical treatment forbidden by her religious principles and previously refused by her with full knowledge of the probable consequence.[14]

The decision by an autonomous Jehovah's Witness patient not to accept a lifesaving blood transfusion could be honored. We would do so on the basis that she understands the nature of the condition and the consequences of her options, thereby satisfying question 1. She would need to rely on First Amendment protection of her rights, as the decision is not a matter of reason but faith, using the corollary to question 2. It is interesting that if the patient appealed not to a protected orthodoxy but rather to someone like the "First Poo Baa of Mu," who dwells under Mt. Shasta, we would consider the decision delusionary and would limit the autonomy in order to protect the patient.

Even in protected beliefs, however, patients must satisfy the requirements of question 1, in that they must understand the nature of their condition and the consequences of the options. An individual who states that by failing to be treated, he knows that he will be healed and not face death, has not met the requirements of knowing and accepting the potential consequences of his actions. This is a much different case from that of another person who tells you that she understands that she may die as a result of her decision to refuse treatment, but feels that the need to follow the dictates of her particular faith is such that she will place her fate in the hands of God.

The autonomy of members of the Jehovah's Witness faith or other orthodox religion that restricts medical care does not extend to the refusing of medical care for their children. The courts have held that parents no longer exercise the power of life and death over a child.

> Parents may be free to become martyrs themselves. But it does not follow that they are free . . . to make martyrs of their children before the children reach the age of full and legal discretion when they can make that choice for themselves.[15]

In these cases the courts will usually appoint a guardian **ad litem** for the specific and limited purpose of making treatment decisions on behalf of the child. The child is usually not removed from the home or control of the parents except for the limited area of medical decision making.

In nursing homes across the United States, there are estimated to be 100,000 patients with some level of dementia. Most of them, following our guidelines, would be determined incompetent to make decisions about their medical care. In the acute hospital setting, about 50 percent of the decisions not to resuscitate if the patient begins to fail involve incompetent patients. The question of competency determination and who makes the decisions when incompetence is determined is a problem that will continue to bedevil modern medical care until systems are developed to handle these cases. The outlines of such a system will be explored in later chapters.

> ## CASE STUDY
>
> ### Refusal of Lifesaving Therapy
>
> A thirty-five-year-old pregnant woman was taken to the hospital following an accident in the home. At the hospital, it was determined that the near-term fetus was not getting sufficient oxygenation. According to medical opinion, both mother and child needed a blood transfusion. The woman, a member of the Jehovah's Witness faith, refused the blood on the basis of her religion.
>
> It is clear that the woman had the right to refuse the blood for herself, but the situation is complicated by the fact that her choice adversely affected the child, who was delivered by cesarean section. After the birth, the father refused a blood transfusion for the child, indicating that he did not want to go against his wife's wishes in the matter.
>
> The baby nevertheless was given a transfusion over the decision of the father, but by the time he received it, he was already too compromised and died shortly after.
>
> 1. Should the clinical staff have accepted the father's wishes? Provide the rationale for your decision.

INFORMED DEMAND FOR FUTILE TREATMENT

In recent years, the frustrating problem of patient demand for futile care has become an ethical dilemma for health care providers. What is to be done when the health care providers make the decision that all further efforts with regard to treatment are futile and yet there is a demand for a continuation of therapy? In 1991, the American Thoracic Society provided the following statement in regard to the obligation of health care providers in cases when all continuance of life-sustaining therapy appears futile.

> A physician has no ethical obligation to provide life sustaining intervention that is judged futile . . . even if the intervention is requested by the patient or surrogate decision maker. To force physicians to provide medical interventions that are clearly futile would undermine the ethical integrity of the medical profession.[16]

Although it may not be an ethical obligation to provide life-sustaining care that is determined to be futile, the courts have not always been willing to allow for the discontinuance of the therapy. In January 1990, an eighty-five-year-old woman was taken from a nursing home to a medical center for emergency care. Helga Wangele required emergency intubation and was placed on a ventilator. During a weaning attempt, the patient suffered a cardiac arrest and had to be resuscitated. Following the arrest and resuscitation event, the patient was in a persistent vegetative state. The attending physicians concluded that nothing further could be done and that the continuation of life support was futile in that no treatment could reverse the underlying disease processes or restore the woman to a state of acceptable function. Although continued treatment was considered futile, the patient was not brain dead.

The physicians approached her husband in regard to removing the ventilator from his wife. During the conversation, he informed them that although his wife had not given her opinion regarding the matter, he wanted everything done and that the physicians could not play God. It was the husband's opinion that his wife was not better off dead and that removing the ventilator was just another sign of the decay within the culture.

It seemed to the health care staff that the request was entirely consistent with rational health care and the need for cost containment. Although the costs for the continued care of Mrs. Wangele were being borne by Medicare, the physicians felt that the case had already consumed a fair share of the resources that had been pooled for the benefit of the community. An editorial in the *Minneapolis Star Tribune* summed up the matter:

> The Hospital's plea is born in realism, not hubris. They (the physicians) should be free to deliver and act on, an honest time-honored message: "Sorry, there is nothing more we can do."[17]

Given the impasse between what appeared to be medically rational to the health care providers and the husband's clear authentic choice, the matter was decided in the courts. On July 1, 1991, the court agreed with the husband and appointed him to represent his wife's interests. Three days later the patient died of multisystem organ failure.

Futility and Baby K

In October 1992, Baby K was born. The diagnosis of anencephaly was made prenatally. Anencephaly is usually associated with a failure of the neural tube to fuse; it results in minimal development of brain tissue and absence of skull bone. It is a tragic and untreatable condition, and infants typically survive only a few weeks, with palliative care. Despite the physician's prognosis, the mother made the decision to carry the baby to term. Upon birth, the infant was intubated and placed on ventilatory support. The case was brought to the institution's ethics committee, which agreed with the physician recommendation for a do not resuscitate order. The mother rejected the recommendation, and the infant eventually was weaned from the ventilator.

Individuals make decisions in cases of apparent futility for a host of reasons:

- Denial
- Unrealistic expectations based on the hope that medicine can provide miracles
- Feelings of helplessness, guilt, and a desire not to abandon the patient
- Belief and or hope that the prognosis is incorrect
- Placing trust in God and a higher power
- Faulty reasoning
- Belief in entitlement

Due to the continuing disagreements regarding the care for Baby K, it was decided that the infant would be transferred to another hospital. All hospitals in the area were contacted; none with pediatric intensive care units was willing to accept the infant. Finally, the mother agreed to have the baby transferred to a nursing home under the condition that the hospital would readmit her should necessity require. Over the next several months, the hospital readmitted Baby K on several occasions for respiratory distress and apnea.

At six months of age, Baby K was again readmitted to the hospital, and a tracheotomy was performed. The hospital filed a motion in federal court for appointment of a guardian and a declaratory action that would allow them to provide only palliative care. The appointed guardian agreed that aggressive treatment should be stopped.

The district court disagreed with the hospital's decision and ruled that the institution was legally obligated to provide ventilator management to Baby K under the requirements of the Emergency Medical Treatment and Labor Act (EMTALA), the Rehabilitation Act of 1973, and the Americans with Disabilities Act. Figure 7-1 provides an overview of EMTALA.

The hospital appealed the ruling based on its view that it was the anencephaly, not respiratory distress, that was the foundational problem. Ventilator support was essentially futile in these cases, and only palliative care should be provided. It was the hospital's view that any care beyond palliative care was both quantitatively and qualitatively futile, and therefore it should not be required to provide life-sustaining support. (Figure 7-2 provides a description of quantitative and qualitative futility.) The appeals court ruled against the hospital, stating that the EMTALA did not make exceptions for other terminally ill patients when they presented to the hospital in respiratory distress even when their underlying condition was foundational to the symptoms and that it was not the job of the courts to ignore established law.

Baby K spent many months in the hospital's pediatric intensive care unit at a minimum cost of $1,140 per day. Nursing home costs were estimated at approximately $100 per day. All treatment was covered by private insurance and Medicaid. The child died in April of 1995 of cardiac arrest at two and a half years of age. The mother, who visited her child daily, said that "God, and not other humans, should decide the moment of her daughter's death." She felt that she had "the right to decide what is in her child's best interests."

Hospitals must

1. Provide a medical screening examination to all patients who seek emergency care

2. Stabilize the patient's condition if necessary

3. Maintain an accurate on-call directory for physicians

4. Provide medically appropriate transfers, which include:

   • Completing a transfer form certifying that the medical benefits of the transfer outweigh the transfer difficulties

   • Obtaining written consent from the patient or a person acting in the patient's behalf for the transfer

   • Obtaining agreement of the receiving unit to accept the transfer

   • Transfering in an appropriate vehicle, staffed by qualified transport personnel to meet the level of needed care

   • Sending copies of medical records and radiographs with the patient

FIGURE 7-1 Emergency Medical Treatment and Labor Act Requirements

Qualitative futility—When it is decided that a treatment is futile based on consideration of reported empirical data (such as the treatment has been found to be useless in the last 100 cases), or similar personal experience, or experiences shared with colleagues.

Qualitative futility—A futility decision based on an assessment that the treatment will merely preserve biological life such as permanent unconsciousness or a treatment that cannot end dependence on intensive medical care.

FIGURE 7-2 Qualitative and Quantitative Futility

The concept of futility is often linked to the use of massive resources at the end of life. Anyone who has worked in acute care provision knows that often these last-stand situations involve an avalanche of ever more expensive interventions. Some feel that futile situations are perhaps the place to start rationing health care, and at some level, this has a certain appeal. However, rationing is a matter for societal discussion and consensus. The bedside of a tragically ill infant does not seem to be an ethically appropriate venue to begin this discussion.

Futility choices are at best difficult, and the courts have for the most part demonstrated a reluctance to compromise patient autonomy. The passage of the federal Patient Self-Determination Act in 1990 further increases the rights of patients and their families to determine the course of their medical treatment. Medical futility would seem to be an issue clearly that falls under the umbrellas of the federal Patient Self-Determination Act. As a result, most of the court rulings have supported the idea that medical futility questions involve judgment about the quality of life and that this judgment does not belong solely to health professionals. In cases in which there has been disagreement between the practitioners and the families, the courts have most often supported the idea that end-of-life decisions are better made by loving families.

Communicating Futility

Concepts of great importance such as futility care are often bedeviled by definitions. There are so many stages between health and death that it would seem necessary for those seeking solutions, such as families making desperate choices, clinicians making judgments in practice, and those looking at cases from the vantage of law, to have a common set of definitions from which to begin. As an example, the physician who tells a patient that cardiopulmonary resuscitation (CPR) would be futile probably means that the procedure would have a low chance for success, while the patient hearing these words might interpret the meaning as the CPR having no chance of success. The very fact that we use the term *medical futility* in different ways without clarification can lead to miscommunication and mask value judgments, which may become a subtle form of paternalism. In its broadest form, medical futility refers to medical care that prolongs suffering, does not improve the quality of life, or fails to achieve a good outcome for the patient. However, if we are to make rational judgments regarding futility in a particular case, it would seem that we need to narrow the definitions.

It is clear that these are difficult decisions that attempt to balance the moral integrity of the health care providers against our obligations to enable and allow the autonomous and authentic choices of patients and their families. On the surface we are again arguing autonomy versus beneficence.

How much do we limit autonomy if we begin by limiting the patient's right to demand futile treatment? Upon examination, a right to demand futile treatment in and of itself does not fit the health care environment. In health care, while we have obligations to help rather than hurt and to work unceasingly on behalf of the patient, this is not an equivalent to "the customer is always right." A patient with chest pain does not have the right to demand an unnecessary cardiac bypass.

Yet futility questions go beyond the correct decisions of technical medicine. These are value-laden decisions, and in value-laden cases, generally the values of the patient rather than the practitioner should prevail. In one case, a physician was counseling a patient in regard to a do

not resuscitate order and indicated that CPR would only give the patient a one in one thousand chance of survival. The patient replied by asking what her chances would be if CPR was not provided. Who determines what chance of life is too remote to consider?

It is clear that we have not come to a resolution regarding futility. Professional integrity would seem to require that futile treatment be suspended with or without agreement of the patient or the surrogate or, if this is not possible, that at least the professional be allowed to withdraw from the case.

AUTONOMY RECONSIDERED

It is clear that in modern health care practice, the principle of autonomy has been considered more important than paternalism, even when the paternalism is based on the principle of beneficence. Some voices in the society at large suggest that we have moved too far in the protection of individual autonomy and that there is a proper use of coercion and constraint in a liberal society.[18] According to this view, the emphasis on autonomy has become perverted, and we have developed a misguided reverence for individual freedom and have denied the community the right to demand a certain level of conduct from its citizens. Cited in the assertion that we have moved too far in the direction of individual freedom are the following examples.

- The right of the mentally incompetent homeless to refuse shelter, which essentially allows them the right to live, freeze, and die on the streets of our cities.
- The expanded right of privacy that allows a pregnant woman the right to refuse testing for AIDS, thereby needlessly denying the newborn available protection against this disease.
- The suppression of a successful program that provided teenage girls a dollar a day to avoid pregnancy. The program was considered coercive and abandoned on the basis of autonomy.
- The demand for health care providers to provide futile care.

The writings that call for an examination of our movement toward individual freedoms, with the intent to find a new balance, are persuasive given that individuals are the building blocks of the community, and the community must function. It may be that in the future, we will see individual autonomy become less dominant in the discussion and placed in a more rational balance with other principles.

CONCLUSION

The provision of health care is a shared practice in which the expert and the patient both work to be sure that what is delivered is satisfactory to each. As the expert, the practitioner knows what is needed in a pure medical sense, but does not know how the value preferences of the patient will affect what part of the care will be accepted.

Since there is general agreement that, through the exercise of personal autonomy, the patient has the right to decide the nature of care, it is vital that the practitioner make sure that the decision is based on appropriate information. Informed consent is required for all invasive or risky procedures that have potential for harm. The physician must disclose pertinent details about the nature and purpose of the procedure, its risks and benefits, and any reasonable alternatives to the recommended treatment.

There have been several standards for this disclosure of information, but today most practitioners recognize the reasonable patient standard, which requires that the information be explained in such a manner that a hypothetical reasonable person could understand and make decisions. Because all of us are unique in what we value, it may be time to develop a more subjective standard than that of a "reasonable person."

While there is general agreement that the autonomous adult has the right to decide these issues, there are times when the autonomy of the patient is limited by pain, trauma, age, or mental competency. Competency is usually established in the ability to answer two questions in the affirmative. First, does the patient understand the nature of the condition and the various options available; and, second, is the decision-making process rational? The second question is somewhat modified when the decision is based on a protected religious faith, rather than reason.

Paternalism in its best sense is based on the principle of beneficence and a desire to do well for the patient. In modern health care, this desire to do good is not a justification for overcoming a competent patient's personal autonomy.

KEY CONCEPTS

- Over the historical period of American health care practice, we have moved away from the principle of paternalism to the acceptance of patient autonomy.
- The patient-provider model of interaction that seems to fit modern health care practice best is one where competent adult patients are accorded the right to make the significant decisions regarding their personal health care.
- Informed consent includes information regarding the pertinent details of the proposed procedure, its purpose, potential risks, and any reasonable alternatives that might be chosen.

- Competent adults have an absolute right to refuse medical treatment even if the refusal is life threatening.

- Competency is generally granted following the positive affirmation to two basic questions. (1) Does the patient understand the nature of the illness and the consequences of the various options chosen? (2) Is the decision based on rational reasoning? In cases where the decision is faith based, a corollary question needs to be added. (3) Is the decision based on a religious belief acceptable and entitled to First Amendment protection under the U.S. Constitution?

- In modern health care practice, the desire to do good (beneficence) should not be used as a justification for overcoming a competent patient's personal autonomy.

- Informed demand for futile care is an increasing problem in health care. Further discussion and debate are required for the development of societal consensus in this area. The courts have in general found for the patient and family in cases where the disagreement seems to be a matter of value differences in goal outcomes between the health care provider and the patient.

REVIEW EXERCISES

A. Often decisions in regard to accepting or rejecting health care are dependent not on medical expertise but rather on the value preferences of the patient. The following list of values in regard to health might cause very different decisions in regard to care. Rank-order the list in terms of importance to you personally.

1. "I want to live as long as possible." _____

2. "I wouldn't want to live if I were on a ventilator." _____

3. "If I can't live an active life, I don't want to live at all." _____

4. "I don't care what you do, or what condition I'm in, as long as I don't suffer from any pain." _____

5. "I would rather die than live a life that doesn't allow me to be me." _____

In regard to the case of the author with a terminal disease, which of the above values best express his decision? _____

B. The following cases are examples of the struggle between patient autonomy and the directive to do good and avoid harm. State what you think should be done in each case.

1. A young woman in the early stages of pregnancy has a mild but not disfiguring case of acne. She has recently read that a new medication will cure the condition and requests a

prescription. By consulting the Physicians' Desk Reference outlining the effects of the medication, the physician finds that the drug has the potential for teratogenic effect and might harm the fetus. He informs the patient of the problem; however, the woman wants to take the chance and demands a prescription for the new medication.

2. Mr. Liu, a middle-aged man with a family history of heart disease, including the untimely death of his father and uncles, begins to become short winded upon moderate exercise. He is very frightened and has a morbid fear that perhaps he is beginning to have the same problems as his relatives.

   After Mr. Liu has been examined by his physician, he tells her that he does not want to know the truth if the results are bad. The examination results show that, indeed, he has serious problems and will likely suffer a major heart attack unless he agrees to immediate surgery and a change in lifestyle.

3. Mrs. Smith, a young woman thirty-two years of age with two children, is a member of the Jehovah's Witness faith. After a serious automobile accident, she has internal bleeding that appears to be life threatening. The physician wishes to transfuse the patient in order to stabilize her so that exploratory surgery can be done and the bleeding halted. The patient refuses the treatment, based on her belief that it would be against the will of God.

   Following are two ways in which the patient's decision might be framed. One would be acceptable in regard to competency determination and the other would not. Decide which could be honored as an authentic autonomous decision, and which could not. Defend your decision.

   (a) "I refuse this blood, as it is against my religion. I feel that the taking of blood is against the will of God. I understand the consequences of this decision and am willing to place my fate in the hands of my God, who will bless me and be merciful."

   (b) "I refuse this blood, as it is against my religion. I feel that the taking of blood is against the will of God. I know that if I am faithful to His will, He will bless me with a long life and the opportunity to raise my children."

   We can see similar reasoning in the decision in the *Department of Human Services* v. *Northern* case (563 S.W.2d 197, 1978), where a lucid, intelligent, seventy-two-year-old female patient expressed the desire to both live and keep her gangrenous foot. In that keeping the gangrenous foot was not compatible with living, the court held that she was delusional and ordered protective services on her behalf.

4. Mr. Jones is an active, elderly man (eighty years of age) in a nursing home who has no close relatives except a young nephew. During a walk one day, he receives a puncture wound to the leg that becomes infected and gangrenous. As a result of his illness, Mr. Jones has a high fever and becomes unresponsive to questions. The physician decides that the only way to save his life is to remove his leg. The nephew tells the physician that

he does not think his uncle would want to live if his leg were amputated. The patient has left no advanced directives in regard to what he would wish in such a case.

- Before you come to a conclusion in this case you will need to investigate all the facts— usually of the who, what, why, when, and how variety. In making your decision in regard to Mr. Jones, list the questions you would like answered and the individuals you would like to discuss the case with (for example, the head nurse of the unit).

- When you question Mr. Jones's lawyer, you are told that the nephew is his only heir and that he is very wealthy. Does this change your decision?

- Once all the facts of the case have been examined and the motivations of the individuals explored, the next phase of decision making is to generate all the solutions of initial credibility. In regard to Mr. Jones, list these. Now estimate how each of your solutions would affect each of the following individuals: Mr. Jones, the nephew, the physician.

- State your decision and evaluate it in regard to the basic principles involved. Does it promote them or sacrifice them?

C. You are a radiographer doing an ultrasound examination on a pregnant patient, and the woman wants the test to determine the week of gestation so that she can determine whether she can legally request an abortion. If your personal view is that of "pro-life," would you need to perform the test? What place does your professional autonomy play?

D. What information needed to be explained to the nineteen-year-old in the *Canterbury* v. *Spence* case to ensure that the requirements of informed consent had been complied with?

E. In the legal case *Stepp* v. *Review Board of the Indiana Employment Security Division* (521 N.E.2d 350, (Ind. Ct. App. 1988), a laboratory technician was found to have been properly dismissed from her job for refusing to perform chemical examinations on vials with AIDS warnings attached. If professionals have the right to professional autonomy, shouldn't the technician have been allowed to refuse to provide the service? Whatever your opinion, defend your position.

F. In recent years, progressive scoring systems (including the Acute Physiology and Chronic Health Evaluation, known as APACHE) have been developed to help health care providers determine which of their patients are most likely to benefit from life-sustaining treatment. These scoring systems use databases to predict the hospital mortality of patients who receive critical care. The values have been shown to correlate well with clinical judgments and outcomes in most cases (positive predictive value of 80 percent, negative predictive value of 90 percent). Given that much of the controversy over futility decisions is based on the perceived subjective decisions making of health care providers, would you feel comfortable in creating a system in which the computer would make these decisions?

NOTES

1. American Medical Association, *Code of Ethics* (1848).

2. *A Patient's Bill of Rights,* statement issued by the American Hospital Association and affirmed by the AHA House of Delegates on February 6, 1973.

3. John Stuart Mill, *On Liberty,* ed. Gertrude Himmelfarb (New York: Penguin Books, 1974), pp. 68–69.

4. Robert Veatch, *A Theory of Medical Ethics* (New York: Masik Books, 1986).

5. Gary Anderson and Valerie Anderson, *Health Care Ethics* (Rockville, MD: Aspen Publications, 1987), pp. 199–200.

6. *Natanson* v. *Kline,* 186 Kansas 393 P.2d 1093 (1960).

7. *Canterbury* v. *Spence,* 464 F.2d 772, at 785–787 (D.C. Cir 1972).

8. *Pratt* v. *Davis,* 118 Illinois App. 161 (1905).

9. *Schloendorff* v. *New York Hospital,* 211 New York 125, 105 N.E., 92, 93 (1914).

10. *Schloendorff*

11. *Schloendorff*

12. *Canterbury*

13. Jay Katz, "Informed Consent—A Fairy Tale?" in T. Beauchamp and L. Walters, *Contemporary Issues in Bioethics* (Belmont, CA: Wadsworth Press, 1982), pp. 191–197.

14. *In re Estate of Brooks,* 32 Illinois 2d 361, 205 N.E. (1965).

15. *Prince* v. *Mass.* 321 U.S. 158, 166 (1944).

16. American Thoracic Society, "Withholding and Withdrawing Life Sustaining Therapy," *North American Review of Respiratory Disease,* 144 (1991): p. 728.

17. *Minneapolis Star Tribune,* May 26, 1991, p. 18A.

18. Willard Gaylin and Bruce Jennings, *The Perversion of Autonomy* (New York: Free Press, 1996).

CHAPTER 8

Justice and the Allocation of Scarce Resources

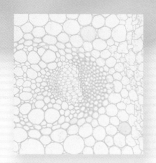

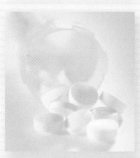

GOAL

To gain an understanding of our current national health care crisis and to examine potential solutions under the principle of justice.

OBJECTIVES

Upon completion of this chapter, the reader should be able to:

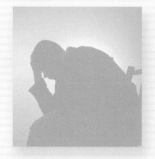

1. Differentiate between Medicare and Medicaid as national programs.

2. Discuss how the prospective payment and diagnostic related groups were an attempt to contain health care costs in the United States.

3. Identify three forces in our society that have tended to cause the dramatic inflation of health care costs in the United States.

4. Define and differentiate between micro allocation and macro allocation as they relate to health care.

5. Define and differentiate between formal and material justice.

6. State how the fair opportunity rule relates to material justice.

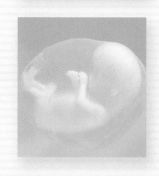

7. Define and differentiate between the theoretical positions of utilitarianism, egalitarianism, and libertarianism as they relate to distributive justice.

8. Define and give examples of how medical and social utility are used in the micro allocation of scarce resources.

9. Discuss the process of "lifeboat ethics" and relate it to our dealings with Third World nations.

10. Discuss the process of triage, and relate it to the micro allocation of beds in intensive care units.

11. List the mechanisms used by managed care to contain costs.

12. List the mechanisms used by managed care to contain costs that appear to interfere in the patient-provider relationship and cause ethical concern.

KEY TERMS

Distributive justice	**Managed care**	**Social utility**
Egalitarianism	**Material justice**	**Triage**
Formal justice	**Medical utility**	**Utilitarianism**
Libertarianism		

HEALTH CARE IN THE UNITED STATES

A strong America cannot neglect the aspirations of its citizens—the welfare of the needy, the health care of the elderly, the education of the young. For we are not developing the nation's wealth for its own sake. Wealth is the means, and the people are the ends. All our material riches will avail us little if we do not use them to expand the opportunities of our people.

John F. Kennedy

We have come to ever more desire what we cannot any longer have in unlimited measure—a healthier, extended life—and cannot even afford to pursue much longer without harm to our personal lives and other social institutions.

Daniel Callahan, cofounder of the Hastings Center

Perhaps the most common characteristic of the "good life" as it is defined by any of the world's people is good health. Health is valued above almost all other factors, such as wealth, education, or social status. Perhaps the most common characteristic of the "good life" as it is defined by any of the world's peoples is good health. In the recent World Health Organization Quality of Life Survey, people across the world listed the top four elements of a good life as:

1. being able to go about one's life independently and free of physical burden

2. being able to see and hear well

3. having energy

4. having mobility

These basic indicators of good health were more highly prized than body image and appearance or even satisfaction with one's sex life. Even in the most materialistic of the societies surveyed, most of us seem grateful for the basic physical functions that allow us to live and breathe day by day.[1]

Advances in health technologies and therapeutics during the second half of the twentieth century brought the practice of health care from nostrums to magic bullets. One after another of the dreaded plagues were brought under control and, in the case of entities such as smallpox, eradicated. It was an age of doing things better: better nutrition, better sanitation, and better vaccines. All of these rather inexpensive health initiatives combined to create better health conditions for all Americans. Following the advent of antibiotics, for a period of time society gained control over bacterial infections, and pneumonia ceased to be feared as a killer of children and the aged.

In many areas of the economy, American industry and applied science have been eclipsed by our competitors, but medical science and technology is nowhere better developed than in our superb urban tertiary centers. Our National Institutes of Health is one of the world's premier biomedical research organizations. We have more physicians per capita than most other industrialized nations, and health issues such as weight, smoking, exercise, drinking, and personal hygiene, are daily fare for our print and electronic news media. Although this generation of Americans is the healthiest ever, the actual improvement in health has not been matched by a subjective sense of better health. We live longer and better, yet as a nation we report more frequent and longer episodes of serious acute illness than citizens in the past. It appears that we have lowered the threshold for mild disorders and now are quicker to see in minor discomforts the signs of serious disease. We have become, in some sense, a nation of the worried well.

HEALTH CARE CRISIS

The cost of American health care is staggering by any measure. Currently, society spends 15.3 percent of the gross domestic product on health care. This amounts to more than $1.7 trillion each year. Over the last half of the twentieth century, per capita medical costs increased by over 1,000 percent. The demographics of the future include an aging population who will place an even greater burden on an already stressed system. While the use of high technology in medicine has been and continues to be dazzling, these miracles come with a heavy economic price.

In health care, unlike most other industries, technology has not brought about a decrease in personnel needs. In fact, the opposite has occurred. Often when a new technology such as sonography is developed, this has initiated the need for a whole new group of technical specialists to provide the services. Unless major cost reduction systems are put into place, by about the year 2030, when the baby boomers reach their seventies and eighties, the estimated costs for health care are expected to grow to $16 trillion dollars and account for over 30 percent of the gross domestic product.

It is difficult to imagine spending over 30 percent of the gross domestic product on health care. While health is a priority, it is not the only priority. Even in the face of clear evidence as to the negative effects on personal health, there are competent adults who drink too much, eat too much, smoke too much, and exercise too little. If, in fact, health was viewed as the primary value, this would not be the case. Good health, while a universal positive value, is just one of the competing values to which society must attend. To allow health care costs to spiral out of control is to allow it to consume money needed for education, rapid transit, roads, bridges, new investments, social welfare, and military defense. Society is reaching a funding crisis in regard to health care that must be faced.

Among the modern industrial nations, the United States is unique in that it alone treats health care as a commodity to be distributed according to an ability to pay rather than as a social service to be distributed according to medical need. A job change, a downsizing, an insurance exclusion for a particular medical condition, or the seemingly ever-present rise in premiums can all lead to a loss of insurance. It is estimated that on any given day, over 45 million individuals have neither public nor private health care insurance coverage. Even those Americans who are covered today cannot be sure that a change in fortunes will not place them in the ranks of the uninsured tomorrow. Over half of all Americans say they worry that they will lose coverage sometime within the next five years. In general, the health care insurance crisis is largely a middle-class problem, as the poor are covered by Medicaid. Working adults and their dependents constitute the vast majority—84 percent—of the uninsured.[2]

Being uninsured causes a fiscal problem and also affects health care outcomes. Children in families without health insurance often do not receive the preventive care, hearing, vision, and developmental screening needed for early intervention. Even for children without chronic health problems, there is a tendency to miss or delay recommended immunizations that places them at greater risk of acute and chronic illness.[3] Adults unable to afford coverage will often ignore ailments and forgo routine care that might detect and cure a problem in an early stage. As a result, uninsured adults often access the health care system late in the process when their conditions have reached an advanced state and the remaining solutions are expensive. As a group, they are twice as likely as insured patients to be at risk of dying prior to reaching the hospital.

Another negative characteristic of the American health care system is a maldistribution of access. For the urban poor, the problem is that of poverty, and they face the same problems in gaining access to health care as they do to other goods and services. For rural populations, the problems go beyond just poverty and are complicated by the low physician-to-population ratio, which is much lower than that found in urban areas. In regard to critical incidents, such as heart attacks and cerebral vascular accidents, in which early treatment is often vital, a patient in a major urban area can expect to receive emergency care within the first few minutes. In contrast, a patient in some rural sites may wait hours prior to receiving vital emergency assistance.

An important aspect of the maldistribution problem has been the historical shift of physicians from general to specialty practice. Prior to World War II, the typical physician was in a general fee-for-service practice working alone and delivering a variety of services, from pediatrics to geriatrics. Now there is a shortage of general practitioners, and most physicians are specialists, confining their attention to a particular branch of medicine or a particular age group. The earlier individual practices are now outnumbered by physicians who practice in groups, are salaried employees of hospitals, or have joined some other nontraditional delivery mode.

As Americans, we are uneasy about our health care system. Although the media are replete with stories such as the discovery of new drugs and therapies, which brilliant researchers and clever physicians use to reduce brain damage following stroke, facilitate conception of infertile couples, and provide prenatal diagnosis for the high-risk fetus, there is still a general feeling of crisis. Too many dollars are being consumed by a health care system that is spiraling out of control, yet for all our spending, too many citizens lack basic health care coverage and must depend on emergency rooms as their primary health care access point. Somehow, two seemingly contradictory things must be accomplished: cut back on health care costs while widening health care access.

Middle-class citizens find themselves in a situation in which personal income is dropping in a relative sense for most families, and both husband and wife must now work outside the home to maintain a stable quality of life. These citizens live in fear of catastrophic illness or a change in work status that would reduce their insurance and place them outside the health care lifeboat. It is in this atmosphere of uncertainty that questions regarding health care distribution are being debated. There is a general feeling that we are entering a watershed period of change, but no consensus has yet been achieved.

GOVERNMENT INVOLVEMENT

Throughout most of the nineteenth century, the government took a laissez-faire position toward private enterprise, including the practice of health care. This hands-off policy was superimposed on a religious and philosophical foundation that idealized hard work, thrift, and personal responsibility. The effects of this pro-growth policy was a remarkable increase in material goods and services. However, the invisible hand, as described by Adam Smith, did not distribute these goods and services equally and the system produced a form of social Darwinism that promoted the strong, and perhaps predatory, at the expense of the weak and disorganized.

As the nation entered the twentieth century, public sentiment decried the harshness of laissez-faire principles. Government was called on to curb rampant individualism and adopt a positive role in providing services to the population. If in the nineteenth century there was a general view that the government had no responsibility for the individual, some intellectuals of the twentieth century proclaimed that the individual had no responsibility for resolving his own difficulties and that collective action was required to solve most problems. Many voices called for a right to health care, but few voices called for individuals to live their lives in such a way as to make the provision of health care less necessary.[4]

A right to health is an interesting concept, as it supposes that somewhere in society there is a supply of health that can be distributed, and that if the society could organize itself appropriately, it could deliver this service to its citizens. This becomes even more difficult to imagine when we realize that there is no unified definition of exactly what constitutes health. Certain groups such as the World Health Organization (WHO) define it in the broadest terms: "a state of complete physical, mental, and social well being, and not merely the absence of infirmity."[5] Whereas it is difficult to imagine a right to health or the distribution system that could deliver it, it is less difficult to image a right to health care. Within this area of thinking, there are several questions that should be considered. If health care is a right, does it create an obligation for citizens to use it? If health care is a right, who has the duty to pay for its use?

Society is bedeviled by the fact that even in instances where access to preventive care measures such as early childhood vaccinations is available and free, many children remain unprotected. Can a society require changes in personal behavior to use it? Should parents be punished if they fail to take a child to a free clinic to receive standard vaccinations? Can a liver transplant be denied to someone who has destroyed his or her original organ through alcohol abuse? Before signing on too quickly to a system that punishes those who actively participate in their own ill health, consider the great number of individuals who eat too much, drink too much, smoke too much, and drive too fast. What is to be done with them? Even if society decided that it would be correct to somehow deny benefits to smokers, drinkers, or overeaters, what about those who eat too much red meat, mountain climb, hunt mushrooms in the wild, or do all sorts of interesting things that may have an unfavorable impact on health?

During the twentieth century, the government assumed an increasing role in the provision of health care for the society. Figure 8-1 provides a review of governmental programs designed to increase the access to health care.

Although there is a general feeling that the health care system in the United States is in crisis, there currently appears to be no national will to create change. Most congressional initiatives regarding health care are being taken at the margins of the problem, such as providing portability of insurance for citizens between jobs and minimal prescription benefits.

1935	Social Security Act included funding for maternal and child health grants and support for the disabled. This was the first federal acknowledgment of a positive role in the provision of health care to the public.
1959	The Federal Employees Health Benefits Program was established to provide basic hospital and major medical health insurance to active federal employees and their families.
1965	Medicare and Medicaid authorization. Medicare provides assistance to pay for health services for people sixty-five and older and for persons receiving Social Security disability benefits after two years. Medicaid (Title XIX of the Social Security Act) authorizes federal matching funds to assist the states in providing health care for certain low-income groups at or near the federal poverty line. Both Medicare and Medicaid are entitlement programs and provide benefits automatically to all individuals who qualify.
1983	The Medicare prospective payment system was initiated under which program rates were set in advance for each medical diagnosis. Because payments for a given illness were predetermined and fixed, health care facilities had a powerful incentive to contain costs.
1993	President Bill Clinton appointed the Task Force on National Health Care Reform, headed by First Lady Hillary Rodham Clinton, to devise a plan for overhauling the health care system. The efforts of the task force appeared overreaching to most Americans and were defeated in Congress.
2003	Medicare Prescription Drug Improvement and Modernization Act: The act added new prescription benefits for the elderly, people with disabilities, and those with end-stage renal disease.

FIGURE 8-1   U.S. Government Health Care Programming

The crisis in health care is not a problem that will go away. The costs of American health care are at present too high and rising. Ways must be found to maintain quality, increase access, and control costs. Whether these changes occur as a result of government intervention or by market forces is a real issue that must be addressed.

MICRO AND MACRO ALLOCATION OF HEALTH CARE

The United States faces questions involving health care distribution at both the macro and micro allocation level. Macro allocation is usually the province of Congress, state legislatures, insurance companies, private foundations, and health organizations as society attempts to determine how much should be expended and what kinds of goods and services will be made available. Macro allocation problems are demonstrated in such questions as: What kinds of health care will be available? Who will get it, and on what basis? How will the costs be distributed? Who will deliver the services? Who controls these issues? Micro allocation is the more personal determination of who will receive scarce resources, such as intensive-care beds, advanced technology, or organ transplants.

FORMAL AND MATERIAL JUSTICE

The fair and equitable division of scarce goods and services is usually considered an issue of **distributive justice**. The requirements of **formal justice**, as attributed to Aristotle, are that in distribution, "equals must be treated equally, and unequals must be treated unequally." Formal justice does not attempt to provide any criteria for the determination of equality and does not state in what respect equals are to be treated, except that they must be treated equally. Under formal justice, any criteria could be used; age, sex, marital status, land ownership, provided the criteria was applied equally in all similar cases. Principles that specify relevant characteristics or determine morally relevant criteria in regard to treatment are said to be material principles and form the basis of **material justice**.

Society has used a wide variety of criteria for the distribution of resources. Figure 8-2 lists the common methods, but certainly does not exhaust the list of possible criteria.[6]

- To each person an equal share

- To each person according to need

- To each person according to merit

- To each person according to contribution

- To each person according to effort

- To each person according to social worth

TABLE 8-2   Common Methods for Distribution of Goods and Resources

The ethically least acceptable rationing schemes would be those that placed individuals or groups disadvantaged by poverty or incapacitated by illness in the lowest priority. "Discrimination between classes of people is morally justified only if properties of the groups are the moral responsibility of the group members or if they are the sort of properties that can be overcome."[7] The attempt to treat all equally is formulated in the fair opportunity rule, which holds that no persons should be granted social benefits on the basis of undeserved advantage and no persons should be denied social benefits on the basis of undeserved disadvantages. Under the fair opportunity rule, sex, race, IQ, national origin, sexual preference, and social status would be ruled out as relevant criteria for material justice in the moral distribution of health care.

CASE STUDY

"You Play, We Pay?" A Matter of Personal Choice

Utah and Nevada, which lie side by side in the West, are similar in climate, levels of income, level of health care delivery, and many other aspects. Yet Utah residents are reported to be among the healthiest in the United States and Nevada residents among the least healthy. At least on the surface, this difference appears to result as a function of lifestyle choice. Utah is inhabited primarily by Mormons, who by religious doctrine avoid alcohol, cigarettes, and illicit drug use and often live in large, stable families. Alcohol and cigarette consumption is higher in Nevada, and family structure there appears less stable.

1. In regard to health care benefits, should individuals be made responsible for lifestyle choices? For example, would you favor a risk analysis component for health insurance deductibles? A person who is a heavy smoker or drinker or a divorced adult would pay higher premiums or deductibles, in the same way that those with poor driving records pay higher auto insurance rates.

2. What prohibitions would you consider putting in place to curb alcohol, cigarette, and drug use?

3. What incentives might be considered to promote stable families, as this seems to have a positive impact on health care costs?

THEORIES OF JUSTICE

In the debate over the allocation of health care resources, several theoretical positions have been advanced. Some have called for a total abandonment of governmental intervention, with goods and services being distributed by the invisible hands of a free market. They argue that the increases in health care costs, even in the face of massive governmental efforts to contain expenditures, threaten to break the back of the U.S. economy. These free-market disciples feel that the interventions themselves are the root of the problem and that if the government ceased all efforts to manipulate the market, the price of health care would find its natural level. They point to research done by groups such as the Rand Corporation that seems to indicate that persons who have access to free health care use significantly more care than those who paid at least 25 percent of the costs.[8]

On the other extreme are those who argue that an affluent society such as ours must find a way to pay health care costs. This group holds that members of the society are bound in a social contract and that the presence of human need in the form of illness creates a moral obligation on the whole of the society. The society then has a collective obligation to provide these goods and services to the extent of its available resources.

Both of these positions—whether to place distribution in the hands of the free market, or to collectively provide services on the basis of social responsibility—borrow aspects from one or more of three theoretical positions: egalitarianism, utilitarianism, or libertarianism.

Egalitarian Theories

Egalitarian theories emphasize equal access to goods and services. Egalitarian thinkers believe that an affluent society such as ours must find a way to provide universal health care to all its citizens. It is within the egalitarian end of the spectrum that the advocates of a right to health care are most comfortable. Egalitarian proponents often point to socialistic universal access health care systems, such as those found in Canada and the United Kingdom, as models worth emulation. In its most extreme form, these thinkers hold that any deviation from absolute equality in distribution is unjust. Some take a romantic view to the health care problem and fail to take into account the scarcity of resources relative to human wants. They see the barrier to free and available health care to all in unlimited quantities as being caused by human error and organization rather than to basic human choices that must be made between health care and other needed goods and services. When confronted with the inevitable gap of tragedy between available resources and human desires, the romantics often point to human error such as waste, fraud, or a stingy political system, claiming that these are the real barriers, thus protecting their illusion that no scarcity exists.

A useful formulation of egalitarianism can be found in the contract theory of John Rawls, who holds that a social arrangement is an agreed-on contract to advance the good of all who are in the society.[9] In this communal effort, all would work toward the equal distribution of goods and services, unless an unequal distribution would work to everyone's advantage. Beauchamp and Childress have argued that this collective social protection and the fair opportunity rule form the basis of a right to health care.[10]

Utilitarian Theories

These theories emphasize a mixture of criteria so that public utility is maximized. Public utility is defined in the phrase "the greatest good for the greatest number." Utilitarians generally accept political planning and intervention as methods of redistributing goods and wealth to bring about public utility. The public health policies of many Western nations have been formulated according to utilitarian theory. If our resources are limited and choices need to be made, does it make sense that in many of our cities, the most technologically advanced area is the hospital and the least advanced our public schools?

Authorities such as Daniel Callahan, cofounder of the Hastings Center, feel that even in times of moderate shortages of goods and services among societies, health care must be rationed and provided only to those who will benefit most and denied to those who will benefit less, such as the elderly. An example of this approach can be seen in Great Britain, where there exists a social, political, and medical consensus that allows practitioners to deny frail or severely demented elderly patients hospitalization or intensive care, even for such treatable conditions as pneumonia. It is considered reasonable, however, in Great Britain to provide extensive home care and geriatric day care. Not all theorists agree that health can be considered as other goods, and many agree with Paul Ramsey that in a pluralistic society such as ours, placing health in conflict with better roads, schools, and bridges would be "almost, if not altogether, incorrigible to moral reasoning."[11]

One example of how a utilitarian rationing system might work has been proposed by Daniel Callahan and is known as the *natural life span argument*.[12] He feels that such a rationing scheme is necessary to stave off the ever-widening gap between resources and our expanding health needs caused by the flaws in our current system, as well as the increased needs generated by an aging population. Callahan argues that a natural life span is one that ends with a natural death and that this occurs at the end of the life cycle. Figure 8-3 lists the criteria used to establish the end of a natural life cycle. Using this theory, one can imagine allocating resources for oneself over the whole of one's life. One could devote, say, 10 percent to one's prenatal care, 10 percent to birth and early childhood, 10 percent to adolescence, 10 percent to years twenty through forty, and so on. We can see that such an allocation could be argued as rational and moral. Possibly it can be determined, for example, that money spent on the early years of one's life can make one's medical costs much less in later life. But one might also wish to concentrate one's expenditures in the twilight years to better "rage against the dying of the light," in the words of Dylan Thomas. If one could imagine allocating health care funds in this way for

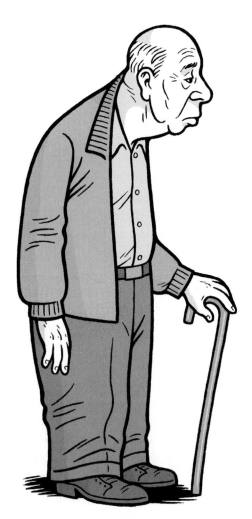

- One's life work is completed.
- One's moral obligations to people one is responsible to have been discharged.
- One's death does not seem to others an offense to sense or sensibility or tempt others to despair and rage at human existence.
- The process of dying is not marked by unbearable and degrading pain.

FIGURE 8-3   The End of a Natural Life Cycle

oneself, then it is not a large step to say that government would be justified in allocating health funds in a similar fashion. Indeed, it is quite likely that government could do a good job of allocating these funds, given all the statistical analysis that is available for health care expenditures over time.

We concentrate the largest portion of our health care dollar in the last years of people's lives. According to national health statistics for 2003, 1.7 trillion dollars, 15.3 percent of the GDP was spent on health care, which outpaced growth in the overall economy by 3 percentage points.[13]

It is estimated that within the population served by Medicare, over 30 percent of the dollars spent were consumed by enrollees who died in that year.[14] We might decide that this is the best policy for humane reasons, but we might also decide that this is an inefficient use of limited health care funds.

Natural life, then, would culminate in natural death (most often between seventy-eight and eighty-two years), natural death should be accepted, and no life-extending technologies should be instituted. Callahan offers the following principles for practice: (1) After a person has lived out a normal life span, medical care should no longer be oriented to resisting death. (2) Medical care following a natural life span would be limited to relief of suffering. (3) The existence of technologies capable of extending life beyond a normal life span creates no technological imperative for its use.

Those who have argued against the natural life span argument have done so using several lines of reasoning. First, there are questions in regard to the artificiality of setting a certain age range as constituting the natural life span, and, second, Callahan has been somewhat vague in regard to what constitutes life-extending technologies. Under the model, a patient who was receiving a life-extending drug such as insulin prior to entry into the selected age group could continue until death. However, someone who began to need the drug in order to extend life— after completion of a natural life span—would have it denied.

For all its faults, the life span model may be ethically persuasive if it operates as a closed system, in which all savings gained from the limitation of technology at the end of life would be used to enhance health during the other phases of natural life. The closed-system approach would assist in diminishing our current problems of intergenerational inequity, in which one age group seems to benefit at the expense of others. As an example, our current federal expenditure for children is only one-fifth the outlay for the elderly, even though a greater number of children live in poverty.

With a closed system, money saved from not providing life-extending technologies could be used to invest in childhood health and provide better maintenance for the elderly.

Libertarian Theories

Libertarians emphasize personal rights to social and economic liberty. They are not as concerned with, nor do they outline the requirements of, how the material goods and services are to be distributed, only that the choice of allocation system be freely chosen. In the United States outside of our charity, social welfare, and military medical services, we have chosen for the most part to allocate goods and services using the free-market approach. Figure 8-4 provides one humorous vision of a libertarian future under "managed competition." The free-market approach has recently been criticized, as it has created not a unified system of health care delivery within our nation but a whole series of micro systems, some of which work well and others that appear broken.

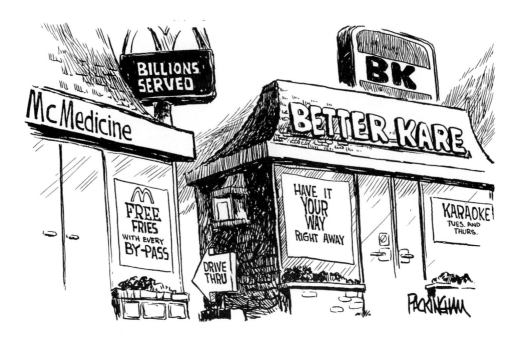

FIGURE 8-4   Managed Competition?

Our free-market system that operates on the material principle of ability to pay usually invokes some form of libertarianism as its justification. Given our national penchant for personal liberty and individuality, it is quite likely that some aspects of the free market will coexist within any national health care plan we evolve.

MANAGED CARE

Most recent health care reform efforts have been in the area of **managed care** systems, which attempt to bring free-market restraint to spiraling health care costs. Essentially, *managed care* is an umbrella term for plans that coordinate health care through primary care generalists. In that this is a very dynamic period of health care in which change is occurring at a dizzying rate, it is difficult to say exactly what managed care is. Because of the diversity of systems, one author has described managed care as a modern Jekyll and Hyde, saying the term *managed care* does not necessarily tell you what you are getting.[15] As Victor Cohn, of the Washington Post remarked, "If you've seen one managed care system, you've seen one managed care system."[16] Table 8-1 lists the major types of managed care plans.

TABLE 8-1
Major Types of Managed Care Plans[17]

Preferred provider organizations (PPO)	Usually fee-for-service organizations with incentives for the beneficiary to stay within a defined pool of providers. Providers discount their rates in exchange for a guaranteed steady stream of clients.
Exclusive provider organizations (EPO)	Similar to a PPO but with tougher restrictions on out-of-network services. There may be stricter utilization review mechanisms and no coverage at all for out-of-network services.
Health maintenance organizations (HMO)	These organizations receive a set monthly premium for each patient enrolled. Enrollees designate a primary care physician and subsequently pay a small fixed fee for each office visit. Some HMOs provide some benefits for use of out-of-network providers. Network physicians are compensated on a claims-submitted basis (usually at a previously contracted discounted rate).
Individual physician association model (IPA)	The HMO contracts with a network of physicians to provide services on a discounted fee-for-service basis. There may be incentives such as year-end bonuses or penalties such as reduced-fee schedules depending on whether the aggregate cost-control goals are being met.
Staff model HMO	Hospital- or clinic-based HMOs whose health care providers are salaried employees working almost exclusively with HMO enrollees.

Figure 8-5 provides an interesting attempt in applying managed care cost containment techniques to an orchestra concert. From the cost containment processes described, it is easy to see why many health care providers, at all levels of practice, find the trends unsettling. Because physician activities account for 60 to 80 percent of the expenditures within the hospital, the following discussion will focus primarily on managed care as it affects physician practice. Managed care systems use a variety of approaches to alter the practice behaviors of physicians and other health care providers. The use of case managers to coordinate care, financial incentives to conserve resources, and health care protocols to guide the delivery of care all seek to bring about changes in health provider behavior with a lower expenditure of funds. Case managers may review health care records and deny physicians payment for unnecessary health care services and seemingly ration certain services provided within the plan. The results of managed care activities have been to lower the rising costs of health care. During the early phase of managed care, HMOs enjoyed high capitation rates based on historical costs under fee-for-service structures. They also had the benefit of being able to enroll younger, healthier patients. As managed care market penetration increases, these two forces, which provided a cushion for profitability and cost containment, will decrease. Managed care services will be forced to enroll a broader mix of people, including costlier, sicker patient populations, and their capitation rates will more accurately reflect the cost of providing reasonable services. There are those who argue that previous profits and cost containment benefits were gained from the cushion of enrollee selection and inflated historical costs. Once these are gone, it is feared that dollars allocated for business profits will compete directly with patient care.

The media also carry disquieting stories of conflicting interests between managed care participants. The American Medical Association expressed its concern regarding the potential deleterious effects of managed care on the physician-patient relationship and have offered the following four guidelines regarding physician practice within the system.[18]

1. The duty of patient advocacy is a fundamental element of the patient-physician relationship that should not be altered by the system of health care delivery. Physicians must continue to place the interests of their patients first.

2. When health care plans place restrictions on the care that physicians in the plan may provide to their patients, physicians should insist that the following principles be followed.

   a. Any broad allocation guidelines that restrict care and choices—which go beyond the cost/benefit judgments made by physicians as part of their normal professional responsibilities—should be established at a policy-making level so that individual physicians are not asked to engage in bedside rationing.

   b. Regardless of any allocation guidelines or gatekeeping directives, physicians must advocate for care they believe will materially benefit their patients.

The president of a large California health insurance company was also the chairman of the board of his community's symphony orchestra. He could not attend one of the concerts and gave his tickets to the company's director of health care cost containment. The next morning he asked the director how he enjoyed the performance. Instead of the usual polite remarks, the director handed him a memorandum that went like this. "The undersigned submits the following comments and recommendations relative to the performance of Schubert's Unfinished Symphony by the Civic Orchestra as observed under actual working conditions:

- The attendance of the orchestra conductor is unnecessary for public performances. The orchestra has obviously practiced and had the prior authorization from the conductor to play the symphony at a predetermined level of quality. Considerable money could be saved by merely having the conductor critique the orchestra's performance during a retrospective peer review meeting.

- For considerable periods, the four oboe players had nothing to do. Their numbers should be reduced and their work spread over the whole orchestra, thus eliminating peaks and valleys of activity.

- All twelve violins were playing identical notes with identical motions. This is unnecessary duplication; the staff of this section should be drastically cut with consequent savings. If a larger volume of sound is required, this could be obtained through electronic amplifications, which has reached very high levels of reproductive quality.

- Much effort was expended playing 16th notes. This seems like an excessive refinement as most of the listeners are unable to distinguish such rapid playing. It is recommended that all notes be rounded up to the nearest 8th. If this were done, it would be possible to use trainees and lower-grade operators with no loss of quality.

- No useful purpose would appear to be served by repeating with horns the same passage that has already been handled by the strings. If all such redundant passages were eliminated, as determined by a utilization review committee the concert could have been reduced from two hours to twenty minutes, with still greater savings in salaries and overhead. In fact, if Schubert had attended to these matters on a cost containment basis, he probably would have been able to finish his symphony."

Source: Anonymous.

FIGURE 8-5 Musings on Managed Care

c. Physicians should be given an active role in contributing their expertise to any allocation process and should advocate for guidelines that are sensitive to differences
among patients. Health care plans should create structures similar to hospital medical
staffs that allow physicians to have meaningful input into the plan's development of
allocation guidelines. Guidelines for allocating health care should be reviewed on a
regular basis and updated to reflect advances in medical knowledge and changes in
relative costs.

d. Adequate appellate mechanisms for both patients and physicians should be in place
to address disputes regarding medically necessary care. In some circumstances,
physicians have an obligation to initiate appeals on behalf of their patients. Cases
may arise in which a health plan has an allocation guideline that is generally unfair in
its operations. In such cases, the physician's duty as patient advocate requires not
only a challenge to any denials of treatment from the guidelines but also advocate at
the health plan's policy-making level to seek an elimination or modification of the
guideline outside the plan when the physician believes the care is in the patient's best
interests.

e. Health care plans must adhere to the requirement of informed consent that patients
be given full disclosure of material information. Full disclosure requires that health
care plans inform potential subscribers of limitations or restrictions on the benefits
package when they are considering entering the plan.

f. Physicians also should continue to promote full disclosure to patients enrolled in
health care plans. The physician's obligation to disclose treatment alternatives to patients is not altered by any limitation in the coverage provided by the patient's health
care plan. Full disclosure includes informing patients of all of their treatment options,
even those that may not be covered under the terms of the health care plan. Patients
may then determine whether an appeal is appropriate, or whether they wish to seek
care outside the plan for treatment alternatives that are not covered.

g. Physicians should not participate in any plan that encourages or requires care below
minimum professional standards.

3. When physicians are employed or reimbursed by health care plans that offer financial incentives to limit care, serious potential conflicts are created between the physicians' personal financial interests and the needs of their patients. Efforts to contain health care
costs should not place patient welfare at risk. Thus, physicians should accept only those
financial incentives that promote the cost-effective delivery of health care and not
the withholding of medically necessary care.

4. Physicians should encourage both that patients be aware of the benefits and limitations
of their health care coverage and that they exercise their autonomy by public participa-

tion in the formulation of benefits packages and by prudent selection of health care coverage that best suits their needs.

There is frustration among health care providers that managed care has placed others between them and their patients—others who make decisions as to what type of care can be provided. Health care providers must assume greater responsibility in determining the nature of managed care systems. As a result of the fiduciary relationship between the patient and provider, the patient has a right to expect that his interests will be protected. These expectations contain the important elements of professional competence, professional autonomy, respect for persons, continuity of care, beneficence and nonmaleficence, patient advocacy, confidentiality, and, perhaps most important, no conflicts of interest.

TWO-TIER SYSTEM AND THE DECENT MINIMUM

One interesting position in regard to the macro allocation of health care goods and services is that of the two-tier system. Under this approach, everyone would be guaranteed coverage for basic care and catastrophic health needs. This coverage of a decent minimum of care would be distributed on the basis of need, with everyone being ensured equal access to basic and catastrophic services. The second tier, based on the ability to pay, would provide expanded and perhaps better care at private expense. This blending of utilitarian and libertarian values may have real appeal in the United States as we attempt to increase the services for those citizens who do not compete well in the marketplace.

One plan that is approaching the concept of a two-tier system is the Oregon rationing system, which was put into place to extend the benefits of health care to a wider population. In 1983, in response to a desire to expand the number of Oregonians who received an acceptable level of medical care, the state began to hold public meetings in regard to health policy. These meetings culminated in the formation of a group known as the Citizens Health Care Parliament, which produced two reports: "Society Must Decide," and "Quality of Life in Allocating Health Care Resources." The Oregon Health Services Commission, using complicated cost-benefit analysis, set out to assess the relative value attached to each medical service by the citizens of the state. Each service was ranked on three factors: the public's perception of value, the effectiveness or outcome, and cost. The prioritization was to have the effect of denying some medically important treatments to Medicaid recipients. By decreasing the expenditures, the cost savings could be used to increase the number of people who could be served. The services considered most valuable on the basis of public perception, effectiveness, and cost were prenatal care, and those least valued were those involving infertility and cosmetic surgery. The goal was to expand the number of citizens eligible for care by not providing every conceivable service of modern medicine. The 1988 legislature acted on these initiatives, making Oregon the first jurisdiction to explicitly decide on a rationing system for health care in the United States.[19]

In truth if we were to allow our desire to have everything for everyone, we could pour our complete gross domestic product into health care in pursuit of the perfect outcome. In time, we would no longer be troubled by the common cold, low back pain would vanish, and our lives might even be extended to equal those of Methuselah and the early patriarchs of the Bible. This might not be worth the effort and resources expended, given what we would have lost in the process. Health is but one of the goals of a good life, not the only one. The question of rationing is not really whether we will ration our health care resources but whether we will do so ethically and rationally. The Oregon plan is at least a rational attempt to achieve this aim. We currently ration health care in many different ways that seem to be neither rational nor ethical. Figure 8-6 provides a listing of a few of the less explicit methods by which we currently ration health care in the United States.

Perhaps the most disturbing of our rationing methods has to do with the fact that cultural and social barriers still bar the way for many of our citizens to receive health care. Studies show that even in programs such as Medicare, where one would suppose equality of access, significantly fewer procedures, diagnostic tests, and therapies are performed on black than white beneficiaries, even under the same presenting circumstances. Black Americans receive fewer services than whites whether they live in Maine, Mississippi, or Montana. One could imagine several acceptable methods by which to ration health care, but to ration by prejudice is not among them.[20]

- Controls placed on access by pricing

- Differing and arbitrary payment methods

- Variations in practice patterns

- Insufficient emphasis on practice patterns

- Language and cultural barriers

- Insufficient numbers of minority health professionals

- Lack of information about available health services

- Social class membership as a deterrent

- Limited organ supply for transplantation

FIGURE 8-6   Nonexplicit Rationing Methods

LIFEBOAT ETHICS

In 1842, the American ship the *William Brown* struck an iceberg near Newfoundland and began to sink. The crew and half the passengers managed to leave the vessel in two overcrowded lifeboats. After twenty-four hours, one of these vessels began to founder in the high seas. The crew became concerned that all the lives would be lost unless they decreased the numbers in the boat. The decision was to give priority to married men and all women. Under this system, fourteen single men were thrown overboard, and two young women, sisters of men in the water, chose to join them. Several hours later, the survivors in the lifeboat were rescued by passing vessels.

Upon their return to Philadelphia, all of the crew—with the exception of Seaman Holmes—disappeared. Holmes was brought before the court to face trial for murder of the individuals thrown overboard. The defense argued that the actions were needed to save lives and that there were no volunteers to enter the water. The defense justified the decisions using the utilitarian value of keeping families intact and the duty-oriented value of protecting helpless females. The court, using a different duty-oriented approach based on the sacred nature of each life, stated that a lottery would have been the only ethical method, and Seaman Holmes was convicted.[21] This view that a random selection among equals is the best approach has been forcefully restated in the works of the ethicist Paul Ramsey:

> The equal right of every human being to live, and not relative personal or social worth, should be the ruling principle. When not all can be saved and all need not die, this ruling principle can be applied best by random choice among equals.[22]

Lifeboat ethics, which take their title from this episode, have often been used to describe the situation of the industrialized Western nations and their relationship to much of the Third World. With seemingly more and more of the world's population living in conditions of famine and pestilence, we can see an analogy to a lifeboat afloat on a human sea of tragedy. Who shall be saved from drowning, and what will be the criteria for our selection?

Similar in some aspects to lifeboat ethics is the process of **triage**. This process of allocating scarce resources has been commonly practiced and justified in the crises of war or disaster. When used in time of war, the practice is usually to divide the wounded into three groups. The first group is the walking wounded, who have received superficial wounds that require minimal care. These soldiers are often ignored during the first few minutes or patched up immediately if they can be sent back to the battlefield. The second group are the fatally wounded, who are given available narcotics to ease their pain but are not treated for their injuries. The third group are the seriously wounded. These are treated immediately, as their care will bring about the highest percentage of survivors. Examine the following case in the light of allocation of intensive care unit (ICU) beds.

> ### CASE STUDY
>
> ## A Problem of Space
>
> It is a busy night at the emergency room and the ICU is down to two open beds. At two in the morning, the ambulance pulls up to the emergency room door with three patients who had been involved in a shoot-out.
>
> Apparently, a sting operation had gone bad during a drug deal, and an undercover policeman and two drug dealers had been wounded. All three men appear to be in critical condition and need the services of the ICU.
>
> 1. Consider how you would decide which of the three men receive the ICU beds.
>
> 2. Given that the policeman was hurt in the line of duty, is this a time when social utility is an appropriate method for micro allocation of scarce resources?

Similar principles to triage are used in the allocation of ICU beds when there is overcrowding. One criterion often used and very similar to those employed on the battlefield is that of best prognosis or **medical utility**. Which patient is most likely to survive? It is from this criterion that questions emerge as to whether patients with a DNR order truly belong in intensive care, if in fact we do not intend to treat them intensively.[23] A second common principle is **social utility**—which patient has the greatest social worth. When the president of the United States is in any major U.S. city, critical trauma specialty areas are held in reserve in case of an emergency. His value to us as a society gives him a first call on these resources, based on the principle of social worth. However, both social utility and medical utility have inherent problems. Medical utility, or best prognosis, is often difficult to assess; and social utility, or social value decisions, seems to invite problems of racism, ageism, sexism, and bias against the retarded and mentally ill. Perhaps the most neutral system is that of "first come, first served," or random selection that treats all patients as essentially equal.

One interesting (although disturbing) experience with micro allocation through the criterion of social worth was the use of anonymous committees to determine who could be placed on kidney dialysis in the early 1960s, when the need for the therapy far outstripped the number of units available. In Seattle, these committees used factors such as age, sex, marital status, number of dependents, net worth, income, educational background, future potential, and emotional stability to make their decisions. It was interesting to note that if the individuals were later divorced, became alcoholics, or had financial downturns, they were not taken off the therapy, although they then did not match the criteria. Due to the lack of neutrality of the criteria, the committees' choices favored males, caucasians, and the middle class or above. One critique quoted by Ramsey called the selection "a disturbing picture of the bourgeoisie sparing the bourgeoisie," and held that the "Pacific Northwest is no place for a Henry David Thoreau with bad kidneys."[24]

Although not as blatant as the Seattle experience, the difference between the moneys available for cardiac and pulmonary rehabilitation seems to be the result of social-worth criteria. The patient who suffers a cardiac arrest is usually younger than the pulmonary patient. Once cardiac patients have completed rehabilitation, they often return to their positions and again produce work and pay taxes. Pulmonary patients, however, are usually beyond their working years, and once rehabilitation is complete, patients may lead a better quality of life, but usually not one productive in work output or active in the payment of taxes. Both forms of rehabilitation seem needful and beneficial to the patients; however, cardiac rehabilitation is more available, better funded, and more likely to receive third-party-payer support.

CONCLUSION

In the United States, although we have a very high standard of health care, inflationary rises in costs due to increased demands for services and the use of expensive life-extending technology threaten to overwhelm the system. In 2003, we were spending about 15.3 cents out of every dollar of the gross national product on health care, and the trend indicates increases in the foreseeable future. These costs have escalated, even in the face of massive governmental intervention. The end result of our seeming inability to contain costs has been to place an ever-increasing number of our citizens outside our health care system, without money to purchase care, insurance, or health benefits to cover costs. A feeling of crisis permeates the nation in regard to health care issues as we struggle to decide who is entitled to what and who is to pay.

National discussions in regard to the micro and macro allocation of health care resources have centered around the principle of justice. Proponents of egalitarian, libertarian, and utilitarian theories of justice have put forward a variety of rationing schemes. The options range over the full spectrum of political philosophy. There are those who argue for a capitalist approach, whereby costs are contained by the invisible hands of a free market. Others see the need for a utilitarian system, with government distributing care so as to provide the best for the most by restricting access of certain therapies to selected patient groups. Still others admire egalitarian proposals, by which everyone has equal access to all the care available consistent with resources.

Several mixed models for the macro allocation of health care resources have been put forward. They call for a two-tiered system that provides a decent minimum level of basic and catastrophic care available to all citizens, using the criterion of need, and a second tier of more complete care available to those who can afford to purchase it. The concept of a two-tiered system, providing a decent minimum of care, forms the basis of the Oregon plan.

On the micro allocation level, groups have struggled with the allocation of such diverse resources as mechanical hearts, fresh organs, and intensive care beds. Several systems have been put forward, looking at a variety of triage schemes, with criteria based on such concepts as social and medical utility, ability to pay, first come first served, and the lottery. Whatever system is finally selected, to be ethically sound it must not fall more heavily on the socially disadvantaged or those incapacitated by illness. The weighing of one class of treatments or technologies against another must take place in a closed system. When beneficial care is denied to one group, it must be because there is a better use of those resources elsewhere in the system. The criteria for making decisions of what constitutes "better use" should be in accordance with the principle of material justice and the fair opportunity rule. These are difficult decisions and unfortunately Figure 8-7 accurately reflects our current state as we prepare to enter the next century.

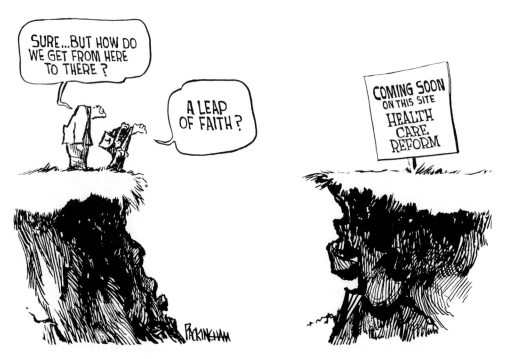

FIGURE 8-7

KEY CONCEPTS

- Medicare and Medicaid are national health care programs. Medicare primarily serves the elderly, and Medicaid serves indigent populations.

- Increased technological advancements, increased health care utilization, and a system with unclear priorities that promotes waste and competition between classes of citizens for available dollars have created a $1.2 trillion health care system that still leaves over 45 million citizens uninsured.

- Micro allocation of health care deals with the personal determination of who will receive scarce resources such as an intensive care bed. Triage systems that evaluate medical utility issues (such as best prognosis) seem more acceptable than systems such as social utility, in which there is a subjective determination of an individual's worth in making these decisions. Macro allocation deals with the larger societal issues of what kinds of health care will be provided to the citizens as a whole. Macro determinations are generally the province of the U.S. Congress or state legislatures.

- Material justice requires that the criteria used to distribute a scarce resource be morally relevant. In this sense, it is more useful than formal justice, which requires only that the criteria be applied equally. A useful formulation to satisfy the requirements of material justice is the fair opportunity rule.

- It is clear that some form of rationing system will need to be considered if we are to provide health care services to all citizens. Efforts such as the Oregon plan offer some direction as we attempt to create a rational and ethical system.

- *Managed care* is an umbrella term for plans that coordinate health care through primary care generalists in an effort to restrain soaring health care costs. Care is needed to ensure that the patient remains the important consideration as we move to constrain costs.

- Epidemics in some nations of the Third World threaten to overwhelm their resources and bring to mind the issue of lifeboat ethics.

REVIEW EXERCISES

A. Our society has chosen several methods of resource allocation, such as need, ability to pay, merit, potential worth, past contribution, and equal share. All of these could form the basis of distribution according to formal justice (as long as equals are treated equally, and unequals unequally). Which do you think is best suited for the requirements of material justice? Defend your answer.

If you chose "need" as the basis for resource allocation, consider the following rejection of need as a criterion for just distribution drawn from the works of Ayn Rand.[25] "A morality that holds need as a claim, holds emptiness—nonexistence—as its standard of value; it rewards an absence, a defect: weakness, inability, incompetence, suffering, disease, disaster, the lack, the fault, the flaw, the zero. Who provides the account to pay these claims? Those who are cursed for being nonzero, each to the extent of his distance from that ideal. Since all values are the product of virtues, the degree of your virtue is used as the measure of your penalty; the degree of your fault is used as the measure of your gain."

The emphasis of Ayn Rand's statement is similar to the reasoning used against providing welfare payments for able-bodied persons, as they seem to be getting "something for nothing," while those who work are penalized for their efforts. What gives anyone the right to the services of health care providers, given that we do not claim any rights to the services of the butcher, banker, or baker?

Some 40 to 50 percent of Americans—the aged, children in poverty, the dependent poor, and those with chronic disabilities—require larger amounts of health care than they have the financial resources to purchase. Does their need provide a reasonable justification for their demand for service? Defend your answer.

B. With managed care, the charges that can be made for a particular condition are often predetermined and fixed; hospitals make or lose money depending on whether they are able to treat the patient within the confines of the predetermined payment. This has resulted in pressure on health care providers to reduce staff, reduce length of hospital stay, and reduce services provided. Can a health care provider serve both the society's need for cost containment and yet be the advocate for the patient as required by the basic principles of role duty and beneficence?

C. On September 21, 1971, an infant was born with severe combined immunodeficiency disease (SCID). The family and physicians involved, knowing that the baby had an even chance of having the fatal illness, had the child delivered by cesarean section and then sealed in a plastic chamber. Frequent newspaper reports on "David the bubble boy" continued through the years, as he was moved to larger and larger chambers. The absolute devotion of his family, coupled with approximately $200,000 per year in research grants from the National Institutes of Health, and extraordinary and imaginative technology, allowed David to remain free from contact with organisms and to celebrate his twelfth birthday. After attempted treatment of bone marrow previously treated using monoclonal antibodies, David died on February 22, 1984.[26]

If David were born next week instead of in 1971, do you think that we should begin the ever-more-demanding bubble process? Whatever your answer, defend it using some rational ethical criteria.

D. The National Commission to Prevent Infant Mortality points out that for every $1 invested in prenatal care, $3 to $10 is saved on postnatal care. The nation spends over $2 billion a year on hospital care to keep low-birth-weight babies alive, and many of those who survive are left with a lifetime of medical disability. For a quarter of the cost spent on low-birth-weight babies, prenatal care could be provided to all pregnant women who now go without care.

Assuming that you could use the money saved by not providing for low-birth-weight babies on prenatal care for all women, as well as better "well baby" care for all infants, would you make the choice? Whatever your answer, defend it based on some criteria of justice.

E. In the Oregon rationing system, the commission attempted to rank-order over 700 differing health care services on the basis of perception of value, effectiveness, and cost. Rank-order the following 20 services using these criteria. First, rank-order the list individually; then rank-order them as a group. In that some of the services may be of equal value to you, give them the same ranking (e.g., it will be possible to have more than one service in first or second place).

Once we have rank-ordered the list, we can often get a better discrimination between items by giving our choices a weight factor. This is done by first adding all of the individual rankings and then dividing this number by the total number of items, which in this case is 20. Each individual ranking is then divided by the factor to discriminate between items.

	Rank Order	Weight Value
1. Prenatal care	_____	_____
2. Neonatal intensive care	_____	_____
3. Mammography	_____	_____
4. Cardiac rehabilitation	_____	_____
5. Nursing home maintenance	_____	_____
6. Genetic screening	_____	_____
7. Pulmonary rehabilitation	_____	_____
8. Well baby care	_____	_____
9. Drug rehabilitation	_____	_____
10. Liposuction	_____	_____
11. Cosmetic surgery	_____	_____

(continues)

	Rank Order	Weight Value
12. Organ transplants	_____	_____
13. Burn centers	_____	_____
14. Fertility clinics	_____	_____
15. Primary care services	_____	_____
16. Dietetics	_____	_____
17. Sports medicine	_____	_____
18. AIDS treatment centers	_____	_____
19. Chemotherapy	_____	_____
20. Dental and orthodontics	_____	_____

Look at your top five weighted items and your bottom five weighted items. What, if anything, does it say about your perception of value? Would you say you were more favorable to any age group? Would you say that you had a bias toward social utility? How did drug rehabilitation and AIDS patients fare?

F. You have a four-bed intensive care unit and seven patients who need a bed. The following is a short description of the seven patients. You cannot select on the basis of first come, first served, as they showed up at your door at exactly the same time.

1. Mr. Jones, a seventy-five-year-old pulmonary patient with chronic emphysema. He is retired and has a DNR order.

2. Ms. Cho, a twenty-seven-year-old hemophiliac patient with AIDS contracted from a transfusion of contaminated blood.

3. Mr. Rogers, a sixty-five-year-old retired general with congestive heart failure.

4. Mrs. Rankin, a fifty-two-year-old housewife, an alcoholic with acute liver disease.

5. Ms. Reubin, a twenty-three-year-old college student in a persistent coma following an alcohol/drug overdose at a party.

6. Carlton Child, a twelve year old with head trauma and in a persistent vegetative state, following a beating by his stepfather.

7. Joey Scoy, a severely retarded Down syndrome teenager with a mental age of five years. He is suffering from aspiration pneumonia.

Select your four patients, and state what criteria you used to exclude the other three.

G. Do patients with DNR orders belong in intensive care if there is a bed shortage? How would you make the decision as to who stays and who goes? Would you use medical utility, social utility, or an egalitarian first come, first served?

H. Singapore has adopted a system that seems to have the benefit of increasing the individual's responsibility for personal health and utilization, increasing physician attentiveness to patients, retarding utilization of resources, and yet providing health care services for all at about 3 to 4 percent of the GDP.

In this system, the government provides health insurance that covers preventive services and serious hospital (catastrophic) care. All preventive care must have a scientific basis of benefit to be covered. All citizens have a primary care physician who works in an outpatient setting and is mostly paid for his services by the patient. In that patients are paying for this service out of pocket, they will shop around for the most attentive physicians and not go unless they truly feel unwell. A patient who wishes to see a specialist must cover that cost also, although there are some supplemental insurance policies that can be bought.

1. Do you think that such a system would work in the United States? If not, why not?

I. Some authorities, such as Daniel Callahan, argue that as long as we continue to focus on the individual's needs and desires for health care resources, we are doomed to failure as there is seemingly no end to what we individuals may require in postponing the inevitability of our mortality. If we as a society provided health care on the basis of what was needed for a healthy society, we might gain control over the expenditures for health.

Outline what you think might be a requirement for a healthy society—for example, "A healthy society needs enough workers to work well and hard to take care of their own needs and the needs of our society." In your answer, be sure that you provide for the national defense, democratic institutions, and an educated citizenry.

Given your descriptions of society's needs, would we need to provide heart transplants to those over fifty-five or neonatal care for infants under 500 grams? Would the society benefit in any real sense by medical technology extending our life expectancy from the current seventy-seven years to ninety-five? Do you feel that moving from an individual needs–based system to a societal needs–based system makes sense? Write what you feel about such a proposal. Defend your ideas.

J. In this exercise, you will find three value statements in regard to health care delivery. Write three more statements that you can agree with.

1. The principle of justice should prevail in the distribution of health care.

2. Society has a moral obligation to care for the suffering.

3. Any system of health care delivery selected must not fall more heavily upon those least able to afford care.

K. The "Musings on Managed Care" (Figure 8-6) is an anonymous evaluation of managed care. Is the criticism fair? List the problems associated with managed care experienced by allied health and nursing personnel. Defend or criticize the "Musings on Managed Care."

NOTES

1. Camille Chatterjee, "It's Small World After All." *Psychology Today* (May/June 2000).

2. Carmen DeNaves-Walt, Bernadette Proctor, and Robert Mills, *Income, Poverty, and Health Insurance Coverage in the United States: Current Population Reports*, Publication 60-226 (U.S. Census Bureau, 2003).

3. James Reschovsky and Peter Cunningham, *Chipping Away at the Problem of Uninsured Children*, Issue Brief 14 (Washington Center for Studying Health System Change, August 1998).

4. *Congressional Digest* (October 1994): pp. 226–232.

5. Preamble to the Constitution of the World Health Organization (1946).

6. Gene Outka, "Social Justice and Equal Access to Health Care," in *Ethics and Health Policy* (New York: Ballinger, 1976), pp. 79–91.

7. Tom Beauchamp and James Childress, *Principles of Biomedical Ethics* (New York: Oxford University Press, 2001).

8. Newhouse, Corris, et al., "Some Interim Results from a Controlled Trial of Cost-Sharing in Health Insurance," *New England Journal of Medicine,* 305 (1981): pp. 1501–1507.

9. John Rawls, *A Theory of Justice* (Cambridge: Harvard University Press, 1971).

10. Beauchamp and Childress, *Principles of Biomedical Ethics.*

11. Paul Ramsey, *The Patient as a Person: Exploration in Medical Ethics* (New Haven: Yale University Press, 1970), p. 240.

12. Daniel Callahan, *Setting Limits: Medical Goals in an Aging Society* (New York: Simon and Schuster, 1987).

13. Center for Medicare and Medicaid Services, National Health Statistics, 2003.

14. N. Levinsky et al., "Influence of Age on Medicare Expenditures and Medical Care in the Last Year of Life," *Journal of the American Medical Association,* 286, no. 11 (2001): pp. 1349–1355.

15. C. M. Clancy and H. Brooks, "Managed Care—Jekyll or Hyde?" *Journal of the American Medical Association* 274, no. 4 (1995).

16. Victor Cohn, "A Map of the Health Care Maze," *Washington Post,* May 30, 1995.

17. Malcolm Sparrow, *License to Steal* (Boulder, CO: Westview Press, 2000).

18. "Ethical Issues in Managed Care," *Journal of the American Medical Association,* 273, no. 4 (1995): pp. 330–335. Updated June 2002.

19. Barbara Combs, "Two Ethics Compete in Debate on Health Care Rationing," *Critical Care Nursing* (1990).

20. George Lundberg, *Severed Trust* (New York: Basic Books, 2000).

21. *United States* v. *Holmes.* 26 Fed. Case 360 (C.C.E.D. Pa. 1842).

22. Ramsey, *The Patient as a Person,* p. 256.

23. Barbara Edwards, "Does the DNR Patient Belong in the ICU?" *Critical Care Nursing Clinics of North America* 2, no. 3 (September 1990): pp. 473–479.

24. Ramsey, *The Patient as a Person,* p. 256.

25. Ayn Rand, *Atlas Shrugged* (New York: Signet Books, 1975), p. 958.

26. "Bubble Boy," *Journal of the American Medical Association,* 253, no. 1 (January 4, 1985).

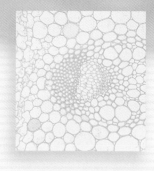

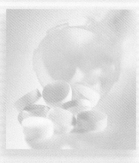

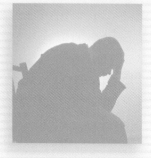

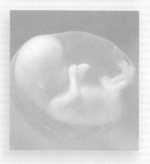

Withholding and Withdrawing Life Support

GOAL

To understand the various arguments used and the types of patients involved in the issues of withdrawing and withholding life support.

OBJECTIVES

Upon completion of this chapter, the reader should be able to:

1. Differentiate between "life" as defined in either a biological or biographical sense.

2. State the necessity for redefining death beyond that of a loss of cardiac and pulmonary function, which in many circumstances can be sustained by modern technology.

3. Define the concept and criteria of brain death.

4. Outline the rationale for the proposal to redefine death with a neocortical definition.

5. Define PVS and state the characteristics of the syndrome.

6. Differentiate between the "best interest" and "substituted judgment" standards as they relate to proxy decisions.

7. Define the difference between "ordinary" and "extraordinary" care.

8. Outline the problems associated with the standard differentiations given for ordinary and extraordinary care.

9. Differentiate the various lines of reasoning and arguments needed to decide the following types of cases in regard to withdrawing or withholding care:

   a. Persistent vegetative state cases

   b. Profoundly retarded patient cases

   c. Baby Doe cases

   d. Informed nonconsent cases

10. Outline the arguments for personhood criteria and state how they could be used in withdrawing care determinations.

11. Define what is meant by the "clear and convincing evidence" standard.

12. Explain the difference between the two major types of advanced directives: living wills and durable power of attorney.

13. Differentiate between active and passive euthanasia.

14. State how a communitarian approach might hold a solution to a scarcity of organs for donation.

KEY TERMS

Advanced directives

Best-interest standard

Biographical life

Biological life

Born Alive Infant
   Protection Act

Clear and convincing
   evidence standard

Cognitive sapient state

DNR (do not resuscitate) orders

Euthanasia

Ordinary and extraordinary care

Parens patriae

Patient Self-Determination)
   Act of 1990 (PSDA)

Personhood

Substituted-judgment
   standard

Xenografting

BIOLOGICAL AND BIOGRAPHICAL LIFE

I cannot but have reverence for all that is called life. I cannot but have compassion for all that is called life. This is the beginning and foundation of morality. . . . It is good to maintain and cherish life; it is evil to destroy and check life.

Albert Schweitzer

Possibly . . . no contemporary superstition is so stupid and pernicious as the indiscriminate adoration of the word life, used without any definite meaning but effectively hiding the fact that life includes the most loathsome forms of disease and degradation. Sanity and wisdom consist not in the pursuit of life but in the pursuit of the good life.

Morris Cohen

Of all the problems that can be considered life and death ethics,[1] none has caused the same level of moral anguish as that of withholding and withdrawing life-support systems. The attitudes and values expressed in the quote by Dr. Schweitzer are a positive affirmation of life, and it is often sentiments such as these that bring individuals to the practice of health care. Today, however, the practitioner is faced with the frustrating problem of available technology that allows for life extension but cannot restore the patient to a life free of pain and misery—or even, in some cases, to an awareness of the environment. This frustration often leads to a new attitude toward life, one that finds expression in statements like the one above by Morris Cohen. The practitioner's duty to respect life and preserve it where possible may at times come into direct conflict with the duty to alleviate pain and suffering. The Hippocratic Oath binds physicians to take upon themselves the duty to adopt practices that shall benefit the patients and protect them from hurt or wrong. What is to be done when the care we offer appears to have no value to the patient? What is to be done when the quality of life restored has a negative value, when life itself appears to be an added injury?

REDEFINING THE CONCEPT OF LIFE

It has been suggested that what is needed is a restatement of what is meant by the word *life*. In the common use of the term, we often mean two very different things. In one sense we use the word living to differentiate the things of our world into two basic categories: one of bugs, bushes, deer, and humans, which are considered living things, and the other of air, water, and minerals, which are nonliving things. With the question, "Is there life on other planets?" we are

Brain death cases are often very problematic to families, as the patient appears to have natural warmth and color, the EKG may be in sinus rhythm, and the chest rises and falls with each cycle of the ventilator. Families view these as signs of life and need time to be brought to an understanding of the true condition. During this period of counseling, the practitioners will often broach the question of consent in order to arrange for the harvest of valuable organs for transplantation.

At these times, a natural shift occurs; nothing more can be done for the brain-dead patient, who is deceased. The support of the family in this time of personal loss becomes the major concern of the health care practitioner. In a real sense the family become the patients with whom the health care practitioners are involved. Great care and sensitivity must be taken as equipment is removed. Often the devices are turned down slowly so that cardiac failure takes place to simulate death. The removal of the equipment, however, is not an act of "allowing to die," as, in fact, a corpse (as defined by brain death) cannot be thought to die. Out of respect to the families or out of fear of legal issues, practitioners may delay the removal of life-sustaining equipment, but no consent is required for unhooking a ventilator from a dead body.

One interesting formulation of what constitutes death is an attempt by Thomas Furlow to look at death not as an event but rather as a process of withdrawal (Figure 9-3).[4] According to this model, the process of dying can be likened to three concentric circles. The outermost ring is made up of one's interpersonal relationships and is called the *social life*. Being outermost, this is the most vulnerable of the aspects of our being and usually is the first to die. The individual then withdraws to the middle circle, which represents human *intellectual life*, that part of ourselves that separates us from the rest of the biological world. Consciousness and interaction, deriving from the highest level of the brain or the cerebrum, characterize this level. Once dying has claimed this region, biographical death has occurred and only the innermost ring is left—*biological life*, controlled largely by the brain stem. As we have said, this form of life is not uniquely human because it shares common features with nonhuman life forms. Loss of function in this region constitutes biological death. Some authorities have argued that the time is near when medicine will need to revise the definition of death beyond the brain-dead criterion to include neocortical death.[5] A person would be considered dead by this criterion if only the higher brain centers, and not the entire brain, had lost function irreversibly. Under this criterion many patients in a PVS who have the potential for years of vegetative life would be judged dead. However, some real problems are involved as patients have come back from a PVS. In brain death, the body ceases to function once ventilatory support is discontinued. With PVS, the patient would continue to breathe once devices now considered ordinary care were removed. The adoption of this standard necessitates additional movement toward active euthanasia, for which, at present, we have no consensus.

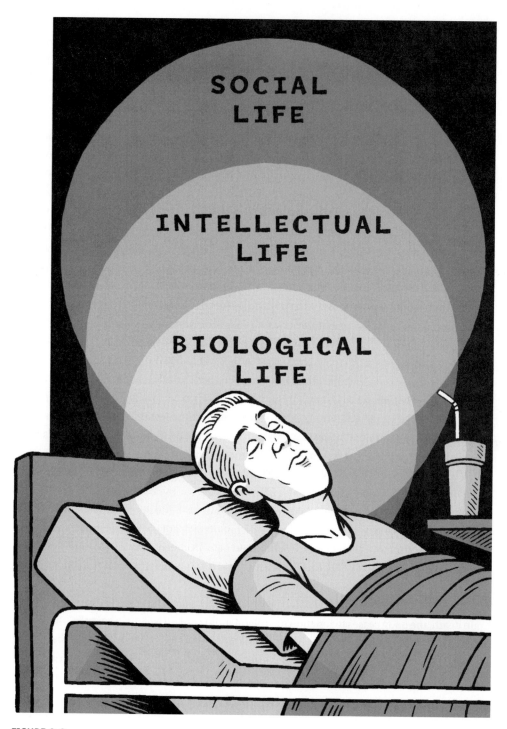

FIGURE 9-3

PERSISTENT VEGETATIVE STATES

In April 1975, a twenty-one-year-old female, while with friends, ingested an undetermined amount of alcohol and tranquilizers. She was brought to the hospital in a coma, having suffered two periods of apnea (not breathing) lasting for at least fifteen minutes. This resulted in brain damage with the diagnosis of PVS, in which she had no recognizable cognitive function. PVS is characterized by a permanent eyes-open state of unconsciousness. The patient is not co-matose; she is awake but unaware. The eyes are often vacant, and often the patient assumes a severely contracted body position. Clinically, PVS suggests the irreversible loss of all neocorti-cal function. Generally, brain stem functions remain, and patients can breathe on their own. They do not, however, match the criteria of brain death, inasmuch as they have elicitable re-flexes, spontaneous respirations, and reactions to external stimuli. Recovery from PVS is rather remote. Using the guidelines of waiting three months in cases of PVS following cardiac arrest, six months for patients under forty with head injuries, and twelve months for patients under twenty-five with head injuries, the chance of any sort of recovery is less than one in a thousand.

The twenty-one-year-old patient remained in this state for a period of seven months, being sustained by a ventilator and feeding tubes. At this time, the physicians in the case indicated to the family that it was their opinion that there was no hope she would ever regain consciousness and that she would die if ventilatory support was removed. After hearing this grim prognosis, the family requested the ventilator be removed. It was their religious conviction that this was in keeping with God's will, and they felt that their daughter would not have wanted to live this way. However, in that the patient did not match the criteria for brain death, the physicians refused to remove the ventilator and the family took the matter to court.

The press exposure from this early case made Karen Ann Quinlan a name recognized by everyone and brought increased awareness of the need for a procedure whereby extraordinary care could be withdrawn from patients.[6] In the lower court decision, the family was refused per-mission to have the ventilator removed. However, on appeal, the New Jersey Supreme Court overturned the lower court decision and appointed Karen's father as her guardian for purposes of discontinuing the ventilator. The court ruled that when an individual has no chance of re-covering a cognitive sapient state, the argument for the protection of life weakens and the in-dividual's right to privacy may call for discontinuance of burdensome life support, as determined by a guardian. Karen's nurses, understanding that the court might grant the family permission to remove the ventilator, began to wean the patient from the device, so that when it was finally removed, she continued to breathe. Karen remained in a persistent vegetative state for an additional ten years. In June 1985, she contracted acute pneumonia and died. Antibiotics that might have been used to continue her existence were not used.

During the additional decade of her life following her removal from the ventilator, Karen was sustained by feeding tubes and IV fluids. Had these been removed along with her ventilator, she would have died ten years earlier. The case of Karen Ann brings up many ethical problems in regard not only to removal of ventilators from patients with no chance of recovering but also what constitutes **ordinary and extraordinary care**.

ORDINARY AND EXTRAORDINARY CARE

It is generally held that one can ethically forgo extraordinary means of continuing life but is obliged to continue ordinary means of care. In the 1957 encyclical, "Prolongation of Life," by Pope Pius XII, this view was reaffirmed that in the prolongation of life, "one was held to use only ordinary means—according to circumstances of persons, places, times, and culture—that is to say, means that do not involve any grave burden to oneself or another."[7] Although not binding as a statement of practice, the encyclical was important given that the source could be expected to be on the conservative side of the sanctity of life issue.

Questions regarding what constitutes ordinary and extraordinary care have generally resulted in classification of items such as oxygen, antibiotics, and IV fluids listed as "ordinary," while ventilators, extracorporeal oxygenators, and dialysis devices are "extraordinary." This analysis has two basic problems: it does not take into consideration technological advancement or patient reference. For example, in the United States, we had a critical shortage of dialysis devices in the 1960s, and therefore the treatments were considered extraordinary. Today, through technological advancement and resource allocation, we have an adequate supply of equipment, and kidney dialysis has become ordinary care. The second problem is the lack of patient reference. What might be extraordinary care for a ninety-two year old with terminal cancer, might be considered ordinary for a thirty-year-old postappendectomy patient. A good example of lack of patient reference was the nasogastric feeding and IV fluids given to Karen Ann Quinlan. Under normal conditions, these are considered ordinary; however, their continuance forced Quinlan to continue a life without personal value for another decade following the removal of the ventilator. In that the procedures offered no reasonable hope of benefit, perhaps they also were extraordinary care.

Figure 9-4 gives a formulation provided by Father Gerald Kelly, S. J., for ordinary and extraordinary care that allows for consideration of costs, pain, inconvenience, and potential benefit. Under this definition, the problems of technological change and patient reference are satisfied. Any form of care can be extraordinary if it offers no hope of benefit. Under this definition, IV fluids and nasogastric feedings would qualify as extraordinary care in patients with PVS as they offer no potential benefit.[8] With this line of reasoning, the focus is placed on the usefulness and burdensomeness of care rather than on any characteristic of the treatment itself. There are other scholars, however, who would argue that food and water are not in a real sense medical care at all but rather "the sort of care that all human beings owe each other" as a function of our

> **Ordinary means** are all medicines, treatments, and operations that offer a reasonable hope of benefit and that can be obtained without excessive expense, pain, or other inconvenience.
>
> **Extraordinary means** are all medicines, treatments, and operations that cannot be obtained or used without excessive expense, pain, or other inconvenience or that, if used, would not offer a reasonable hope of benefit.

FIGURE 9-4   Ordinary vs. Extraordinary Means

common humanity.[9] The removal of food and water seems more causally related to the death of the patient than just standing aside and allowing her to die.

PERSONHOOD

One rather controversial line of reasoning that seems appropriate for cases involving patients in a PVS with no hope for recovery is the examination of the requirements of personhood. While we generally agree that human beings have certain rights and privileges, and that these rights are not extended to rocks, trees, or animals, what is the essential difference? What types of beings can be thought of as bearers of rights? What types of beings can be thought of as persons?

Philosophers such as Joseph Fletcher[10] and Joel Feinberg[11] have attempted to define characteristics that a being must possess in order to be considered a bearer of rights. Among the suggested criteria are:

1. One who could be said to have interests; a person for whom something can be said to be good for his or her own sake.
2. One who has cognitive awareness; a being of memories, expectations, and beliefs.
3. One who is capable of relationships. Interpersonal relationships seem to be at the very essence of what we idealize in truly being a person.
4. One who has a sense of futurity. How truly human is someone who cannot realize there is a time yet to come as well as a present? The words, "What do you want to become," make sense only in relation to a person.

If these criteria were accepted as being necessary for one to be considered a bearer of rights (a person), then patients in PVS do not meet the criteria. Whereas Karen Ann Quinlan, prior to her accident, may have had the right to vote, right to freedom of speech, and many other rights, it becomes incomprehensible to consider her as a possessor of these rights once she irreversibly lost neocortical function. These patients cannot be thought of as beings for whom rights make sense—either the right to life or the right to die. Since patients who have become irreversibly co-matose cannot be thought of as having interests, nothing we do to them can run counter to their interests. In this sense, what we do or don't do is rather dependent on the interests of others—society, family, health care practitioners—who can be considered bearers of rights. The pa-tients themselves can be left out of the equation. Some have suggested that personhood should replace brain death as the legitimate criterion for death. For others, the personhood argument is a rather slippery slope that could allow some monstrous wrong to be perpetrated against a helpless minority in the future. The historical precedence of one group denying others the clas-sification of personhood and then using this argument to justify slavery or sterilization rings frighteningly true and appalling. What can militate against such a philosophy is that the crite-rion being used for personhood is currently very basic. As long as the definitions remain at the level of self-awareness, no potential group of targeted and persecuted minorities could be ex-cluded. Denying personhood to those with PVS does not say anything about them or suggest what it is that we might do to or for them; it just excludes them from the community of those who can be thought to bear rights.

It is clear that the reasoning involved in questions of personhood are of vital importance to the study of biomedical ethics. Most of the focus of ethical thought is the person, the being who bears personal rights and responsibilities. In the past, judgments in this regard have excluded such groups as women, blacks, and American Indians. The abortion debate is the most obvious situation in which we are searching for the definition of a human being. Many in our society hold that the fetus becomes a person with all the rights and privileges of such a being at the mo-ment of conception; others hold that this status is delayed until viability. If you accept viability as the standard, then personhood is dependent on technology inasmuch as a fetus is consid-ered viable somewhere near the twenty-fourth week in the United States, but near thirty weeks in Ethiopia. With the utilization of artificial wombs in the future, personhood might be pushed back to a period near conception. Depending on where you place personhood along the scale of life, you draw very different ethical decisions. It is one thing to abort a piece of tissue (re-gardless of how remarkable) and quite another to abort a person.

ADVANCED DIRECTIVES

In 1983, at twenty-five years of age, Nancy Cruzan lost control of her car and was thrown into a ditch. Although she was resuscitated at the scene of the accident, she never regained con-sciousness. Like Karen Ann Quinlan, Nancy was diagnosed as being in PVS, and physicians es-timated that she could live for another thirty years being supported by feeding tubes. In describing her condition, her father stated that "since the accident, she has never had what we felt was a thought-produced response to anything. We feel the most humane and kind thing we can do is to help her escape this limbo between life and death."[12] Given the prognosis, the family requested that the feeding tube be removed and Nancy be allowed to die. When the Missouri Rehabilitation Center refused the request, the family took the case to the lower courts, which ruled in their favor. This affirmation was overturned by the state supreme court on the basis that the state's greater duty to preserve life outweighed any right that the parents might have to refuse treatment for their daughter.

In December 1989, the Cruzan case became the first of the right-to-die cases to be heard by the Supreme Court of the United States. In its decision, the Court upheld the Missouri Supreme Court position that not even the family should make choices for an incompetent patient in the absence of "clear and convincing evidence" of the patients' wishes. In a five–four decision, the Court ruled that states do have these rights for the following reasons:[13]

- The state has a right to assert an unqualified interest in the preservation of human life.
- A choice between life and death is an extremely personal matter and requires clear and convincing evidence of choice.
- Abuse can occur when incompetent patients don't have loved ones available to serve as surrogate decision makers.

To accommodate the **clear and convincing evidence standard** required by the court, three friends of Nancy came forward claiming to have had conversations with her prior to the accident in which she expressed the conviction that she would never want to live the life of a vegetable. As a result, the State of Missouri no longer opposed her parents in this action, and the feeding tube was removed. Nancy Cruzan died shortly after the removal.

The call for clear and convincing evidence in regard to these cases has increased the interest in **advanced directives**. Following the example set by California in 1976, most states have passed some form of living will (Figure 9-5), right-to-die, or death-with-dignity statute. There is, however, no uniformity in laws on living wills and surrogate decision makers. In some states, the advanced directives go into effect only if a patient is terminally ill and death is imminent. In others, the physician is given civil and criminal immunity from prosecution when he fails to honor the living will, when in his judgment continued treatment may be of benefit to the patient and if it is a good-faith action based on medically valid reasons. In many states the will is invalidated during pregnancy.[14]

Due to the inconsistencies and limitations found in these statutes, many authorities recommend the use of durable power of attorney over a living will. This allows you to name someone as proxy, with the authority to make medical decisions on your behalf should you become incompetent and unable to make the decisions yourself. This form of legal arrangement seems to offer the greatest flexibility in making your wishes known after you have lost competency, as the

I, _____, am of sound mind, and I voluntarily make this declaration.

I direct that life-sustaining procedures should be withheld or withdrawn if I have an illness, disease, or injury, or experience extreme mental deterioration, such that there is no reasonable expectation of recovering or regaining a meaningful life.

These life-sustaining procedures that may be withheld or withdrawn include, but are not limited to:

Cardiac resuscitation, ventilatory support, antibiotics, artificial feeding and hydration.

I further direct that treatment be limited to palliative measures only, even if they shorten my life.

Specific instructions:

A. Specific instructions regarding care I do want:

B. Specific instructions regarding care I do not want:

My family, the medical facility, any physicians, nurses, and other medical personnel involved in my care shall have no civil or criminal liability for following my wishes as expressed in this declaration.

I sign this document after careful consideration.

I understand its meaning and I accept its consequences.

Date: _____   Signed: _____

                                       Address: _____

                                       _____

This declaration was signed in our presence. The declarant appears to be of sound mind and to be making this declaration voluntarily without duress, fraud, or undue influence.

Signed by witness: _____

Signed by witness: _____

FIGURE 9-5 Living Will Statement

proxy individual is in the position to react to changes in your situation. The Society for the Right to Die suggests the following reasons for establishing a durable power of attorney:[15]

1. To give or withhold consent to specific medical or surgical measures with reference to the principal's condition, prognosis, and known wishes regarding terminal care; to authorize appropriate end-of-life, including pain-relieving, procedures.
2. To grant releases to health care providers.
3. To employ and discharge health care providers.
4. To have access to and to disclose medical records and other personal information.
5. To resort to court, if necessary, to obtain court authorization regarding medical treatment decisions.
6. To expend or withhold funds necessary to carry out medical treatments.

According to a study by the American Medical Association, only a small proportion of our citizens have any form of advanced directive in place. Young people and the poor are the least likely to request and implement these forms. As is true with many social issues, the poor and poorly informed suffer the consequences of having the least protection. The **Patient Self-Determination Act of 1990 (PSDA),** shown in Figure 9-6, mandates that all certified hospitals, nursing facilities, home health care agencies, hospices, and health maintenance organizations receiving federal reimbursement under Medicare and Medicaid provide adult clients with information on living wills and other forms of advanced directives.[16] Although nurses and other

---

PSDA was designed to support the autonomous decision-making authority of patients in regard to accepting or refusing specific medical interventions when admitted to health care facilities receiving federal reimbursements under Medicare or Medicaid. The legislation requires these facilities to:

A. Provide patients at the time of admission with information concerning their right to accept or refuse medical interventions. The facilities are charged with providing information and assistance in the preparation of advanced directives.

B. The facilities will create and maintain written institutional policies in regard to patient rights. They will provide education for the staff, patients, and community concerning advanced directives.

C. The patient's wishes in regard to refusing or executing an advanced directive will be documented in the medical record.

FIGURE 9-6   Patient Self-Determination Act of 1990

health care providers will perform a vital service in the education of patients about advanced directives, they are prohibited from serving as witnesses to durable power attorney directives that involve the patients they serve.

Although the Supreme Court held to a narrow focus in the Nancy Cruzan case, several critical aspects were reinforced by the decision. First, the Court upheld the concept that competent individuals could refuse life-sustaining treatment. Second, it made no legal distinction between tube feeding and other life-sustaining measures. Nutrition and hydration may be withheld when either of the two following conditions is met:[17]

1. The treatment is futile. In cases where all efforts to provide nutrition would be ineffective and cause pain (e.g., patients whose cardiac status is such that any IV fluids would overload the heart).

2. No possibility of benefit. While it is most often reasonable practice to provide nutrition and hydration, in those cases where the family and caregivers agree that the practice offers no benefit, such as a PVS case, there should be no barrier to discontinuance.

Decision-making processes in questions where life support is withheld or withdrawn are some of the more difficult issues in health care ethics. Even when ethicists and legal scholars have argued through the issues for decades and have come to at least an outline of what is appropriate in these difficult cases, we will often discover elements that make us question conventional judgment. Consider the case study here.

CASE STUDY

A Question of Motivation

In 1990, a twenty-six-year-old woman collapsed at home and suffered brain damage as a result of oxygen deprivation. The medical malpractice case that ensued resulted in a monetary judgment and trust fund adequate to pay for her lifetime care. Some medical and legal specialists have argued that she does not meet all the criteria of a persistent vegetative state. Nevertheless, since her initial collapse, due to her limited state of consciousness, she has been dependent on medically assisted nutrition and hydration administered by gastric tube. This level of support is necessary for her survival, as she is unable to feed herself.

(continues)

A Question of Motivation (cont.)

Although some have argued in this case that the woman's apparent eye contact, gestures, and movements indicate that rehabilitation is possible, other specialists state that these are mere reflexes. What is clear is that she did not provide written documentation of her desires prior to the event and that she is not able to speak for herself. She is not ventilator dependent, not brain dead, not in a comatose state, not terminally ill, and not in imminent danger of death given that she has had no problem assimilating the nutrition.

Unfortunately, there is disagreement in the family as to what needs to be done, and a long and exhaustive legal battle has ensued. Her husband has affirmed that he remembers his wife stating that she would not wish to be kept alive in such a condition. Her parents and siblings, on the other hand, have taken comfort in the limited responses she can give and feel that with appropriate rehabilitation, she can make some level of recovery.

The woman's parents and siblings have volunteered to take responsibility for her care, but the husband has refused this, stating that he wishes to remain true to the desires of his wife and allow her to die. The culmination of the court case came when the judiciary agreed that the feeding tube providing nutrition and hydration could be removed and the appeal to the state supreme court was refused. The tube providing nutrition and hydration was removed, which would have resulted in her death; however, in an extraordinary intervention by the governor and state legislature, the tube has been reinserted.

1. What do you think is most appropriate in this case?

2. Would it affect your judgment if you knew:

   a. The husband will gain financially when his wife dies.

   b. The husband is living with another woman and they have children.

   c. One of the nurses on staff has sworn under oath that when giving the husband an update, he said "When is that bitch going to die?"

3. To what extent do you think the motivation of participants should be taken into account in these cases?

4. In cases where there is a clear conflict of interest, should there be a mechanism to shift the decision-making burden to other individuals?

PROXY DECISION-MAKING STANDARDS

The courts have not made their decisions on the basis of personhood criteria but rather have created standards for the allowance of decisions by proxy. When an individual is not competent to refuse treatment, often the physician, hospital, or a family member may seek resolution of the problem from the courts prior to implementing a decision. Under the doctrine of **parens patriae,** the state accepts these cases on the basis of a legitimate duty, abiding in the principles of beneficence and nonmaleficence. This duty requires the protection of citizens under legal disability from harms they cannot themselves avoid. In cases in which individuals were incompetent to decide for themselves, the courts have generally used one of two proxy decision-making standards: best interest and substituted judgment.

The **best-interest standard** most often takes into account such tangible factors as harms and benefits, physical and fiscal risks. In health care, the courts might rely on such truisms as "Health is better than illness," and "Life is preferable to death." In cases in which children have been denied life-preserving care by their parents, the state has often overturned the parental decisions based on the best-interest standard.

The **substituted-judgment standard,** unlike the best-interest standard, maintains that the decision about treatment or nontreatment must remain that of the patient, based on the principle of autonomy. The fact that a patient is incompetent to make a decision for himself does not take from him the right to self-determination. A substitute is selected who is required to act in proxy for the patient—that is, to make the decision that the incompetent patient would have made if the patient had been competent. In the case of Karen Ann, her father could draw on the experiences of her previous life to determine her wants in this particular case. If patients, while competent, have clearly expressed their will through conversations or advanced directives as to their disposition in these cases, the substituted-judgment seems a rational approach.

Complicating these issues are two groups of cases—one involving competent individuals who become incompetent without expressing their wishes, and a second group, the mentally retarded, who may never have met the criterion of competence. What standard best serves these patients?

These two groups seem best served by the standard of best interest, in which the court bases its decision on the principles of beneficence and nonmaleficence rather than on patient autonomy. This appears to provide a sounder basis for decision making, especially if the individual has never been in a position to have made an autonomous decision.

The Joseph Saikewicz case is an example of the standard of best interest as it is used for patients who are incompetent to make decisions in regard to acceptance or refusal of treatment.[18] Joseph, who was profoundly retarded and had the intellectual capacity of a three year old, had lived his sixty-seven years of life in a mental institution. In 1976, he was diagnosed as having a terminal form of leukemia. Even with aggressive chemotherapy, his chances for a remission would be only 30 percent, and the remission would only extend his life for a short period of perhaps another year. Without the chemotherapy, he was expected to live for several months before succumbing to infection.

The problem with providing the chemotherapy for Joseph was that the treatment required potent drugs, which caused nausea and discomfort. Moreover, because the staff could not make the patient understand the nature of his illness or the reason for the treatment, he would probably need to be physically restrained. The institution where Joseph was treated appealed to the courts for guidance in the case. Two physicians were called to testify and spoke against the administration of the chemotherapy. The court ruled that the chemotherapy not be given, and the decision was appealed to the state supreme court, which concurred with the lower court ruling. Joseph Saikewicz had died from pneumonia prior to the time the higher court had issued its full opinion. The court ruled that a guardian could be assigned to make the judgment, but that the judgment be based on the best interest of the patient. To ensure that the patient's interests were considered, the court required that an adversarial judicial hearing be held as opposed to reliance on doctors, families, and hospital committees, as proposed in the Quinlan case.

INFORMED NONCONSENT

In the cases of Karen Ann Quinlan, Nancy Cruzan, and Joseph Saikewicz, the patients were considered incompetent to make their own decisions and needed others to determine whether treatment should be continued or withdrawn. What is to be done in cases involving competent patients who understand the nature of their conditions and the consequences of refusing care and choose informed nonconsent?

William Bartling was a seventy-five-year-old chronic pulmonary disease patient with four other terminal illnesses. There was no question as to his competence when he requested to be removed from his ventilator. The hospital refused his request due to the fact that if the device was removed, it would surely hasten his death. When the hospital refused to accept his living will as a rationale for removing the ventilator, he appealed to the courts, which affirmed the institutional decision. On several occasions Bartling attempted to remove the ventilator himself until he was placed in restraints. Although both Bartling and his wife made repeated requests in regard to his desire to refuse the care, he spent the last six months of his life on the ventilator and died before the appeals court overturned the lower court decision and ruled in his favor.[19]

Elizabeth Bouvia was a twenty-eight-year-old quadriplegic suffering from severe cerebral palsy. During her hospitalizations, she asked that her pain be controlled and that she be allowed to starve herself to death. Physicians and hospital authorities refused her request, and she was force-fed through a nasogastric tube to maintain body weight. She requested that the feeding be stopped, and the hospital refused even though her competency was not questioned. Bouvia went to court several times during the next several years, making media headlines and becoming a symbol of the right-to-die movement. The lower courts affirmed the hospital decisions, but these decisions were finally overturned by the appeals court. The court in its ruling determined that the fact that Bouvia was young and therefore had a potential for a long life was essentially irrelevant. The decision stated that the time allotted for continued life was not the issue, only the perceived quality of that life, and that "if a right exists, it matters not what motivates its exercise." Although the Bouvia case did not affirm a basic right to die, it did become a landmark decision regarding the right to informed nonconsent.[20]

These cases seem to indicate a growing consensus in regard to the allowance of personal autonomy and informed nonconsent. Several critical elements were reinforced by the court decisions:

1. The acuity of the patient is irrelevant to the allowance of treatment refusal. The patient's right to refuse care is not dependent on having a terminal illness.

2. The patient's own perceived view of her quality of life and the treatment requirements necessary to preserve it are of paramount importance. The fact that Elizabeth Bouvia could potentially live for another four decades and be a productive citizen could not overcome her autonomous choice to refuse care.

3. There is no meaningful legal distinction between mechanical life support and nasogastric feeding; both are invasive.

4. Distinctions between withholding and withdrawing care are legally irrelevant.

DNR ORDERS (DO NOT RESUSCITATE)

Cardiopulmonary resuscitation (CPR) and advanced cardiac life support (ACLS) are interventions that could theoretically be offered to all patients within the hospital. By the 1970s, it became obvious that it was not in the best interest of certain patient groups to be resuscitated, and hospitals began to initiate policies governing DNR (do not resuscitate) orders. Due to uncertainty as to appropriate criteria for selecting these patients, the late 1970s and 1980s were a period of confusion in which health care support staff were left to find their way through an ambiguous maze of verbal orders as well as DNR orders. Figure 9-7 differentiates between these various types of DNR orders. DNR policies are now required of all hospitals by the joint Commission for the Accreditation of Health Care Organizations. Figure 9-8 provides general guidelines that one might expect for the establishment of DNR policies in a health care facility.

Even given the wide use and acceptance of DNR orders, the selection of patients still raises some concern. In our age of cost containment and stretched resources, do DNR patients belong in intensive care units? Studies show that these patients in ICU are sicker, have longer stays,

Code: A call for cardiopulmonary resuscitation efforts. In the hospital setting, a code would usually contain all the elements of advanced cardiac life support, which includes oxygenation, ventilation, cardiac massage, electroshock as necessary, and emergency drugs. These are sometimes announced as "code blue" or some other designation to signal the emergency team of the need to respond.

No code: DNR (do not resuscitate). A written order placed in the medical chart to avoid the use of cardiopulmonary resuscitation efforts. In previous times, the charts were often labeled with devices such as "red tags" or "purple dots" to designate DNR status.

Slow codes: This is a practice whereby the health care team slows the process of emergency resuscitation so as to appear to be providing the care but in actual fact is only providing an illusion. The intent of the practice is more for family comfort than patient benefit.

Chemical code: Similar in intent to the slow code. In this practice, the team provides the drugs needed for resuscitation but does not provide the other services. There is a real question as to whether slow codes, chemical codes, and other forms of resuscitation that contain only partial efforts are appropriate for anything other than theatrics.

FIGURE 9-7   Language of DNR

1. DNR orders should be documented in the written medical record.
2. DNR orders should specify the exact nature of the treatments to be withheld.
3. Patients, when they are able, should participate in DNR decisions. Their involvement and wishes should be documented in the medical record.
4. Decisions to withhold CPR should be discussed with the health care team.
5. DNR status should be reviewed on a regular basis.

FIGURE 9-8   DNR Guidelines

have poorer prognosis, consume more resources (both human and fiscal), and have a higher mortality rate than do non-DNR patients.

In their *Guidelines on the Termination of Life-Sustaining Treatment and the Care of the Dying*, the Hastings Center authors concluded that the intent of DNR orders did not preclude either the use of any other treatment modalities or admission and treatment in an intensive care unit. When treatment (either curative or palliative) cannot be obtained in other units outside intensive care, the patient's rights to autonomy, beneficence, and nonmaleficence, coupled with the requirements of fidelity, make the ICU use a reasonable choice.[21]

The initiation of DNR orders is best performed after an understanding by physicians, patients, family, and staff has been reached. This is an area in which value preference will make a great deal of difference. Although patient-provider discussion in regard to DNR orders would, in theory, facilitate autonomous control by the patient, research has consistently shown that fewer than 50 percent of the patients with DNR orders discussed their resuscitative preference prior to the order being implemented.

BABY DOE

Unlike the informed nonconsent of autonomous adults or the substituted-judgment cases involving those who are irreversibly incompetent to make decisions are those situations involving withholding or withdrawing care from infants. No decisions are more filled with anguish for all involved, parents and health care providers alike. In the spring of 1982, an infant known as Baby Doe was born with an esophageal-tracheal fistula and trisomy 21, a form of mental retardation known commonly as Down syndrome. The esophageal-tracheal fistula needed immediate surgery if the infant was to be fed. The decision of whether to do the surgery would not have been questioned for a normal infant. The physicians split in their recommendations as to whether to provide the surgery in this case, the parents with court concurrence elected to refuse the surgery on behalf of their child, and the infant died. The parents based their decision on their view that it would not be in their son's best interest to survive, since he would always be severely retarded.[22]

In March 1983, in response to this case and others like it, the U.S. Department of Health and Human Services issued an Interim Final Rule, which directed that all health care facilities dealing with infants less than one year of age and who received federal funding prominently display an antidiscrimination notice protecting these infants. The notice provided a "handicapped infant hot-line" for those who might witness cases where infants were receiving less than "customary medical care."[23] Anyone in the nursery could then call and complain about care, and the federal government would send representatives to investigate the allegations. The fear of "Baby Doe squads" descending on the health care facility and involving themselves in what had previously been a rather private parent-physician arena of decision making had a serious chilling effect on deliberations having to do with infant care. The force of the notices was to place a potential conflict between the law and the moral obligations of the health care providers. Legal duties in and of themselves do not establish moral duties and vice versa.

The definition of *customary medical care* is sufficiently vague as to imply the necessity to preserve life regardless of the potential quality or value of that life to the individual. It appeared that medicine was to be forced away from any decision-making role in regard to these issues, even when infants were born with complete absence of vital parts of their brains. The national media picked up the Baby Doe issue and began to relate it to the civil rights movement and the holocaust. This feeling that something was basically wrong and that the government had a duty to protect these infants was forcefully stated by the conservative columnist Patrick Buchanan in the following interesting, although overblown, "slippery slope" argument or "wedge" line of reasoning.

> Once, however, we embrace this utilitarian ethic—that man has the sovereign right to decide who is entitled to life and who is not—we have boarded a passenger train on which there are no scheduled stops between here and Birkenau.
> Once we accept that there are certain classes, i.e., unwanted, unborn children, unwanted infants who are retarded or handicapped, etc., whose lives are unworthy of legal protection, upon what moral high ground do we stand to decry when Dr. Himmler slaps us on the back, and asks us if he can include Gypsies and Jews?[24]

As with most other important issues, responsible forces lined up on both sides. Opposing the regulations were groups such as the American Academy of Pediatrics and the American Medical Association. In support were groups such as the American Association of Retarded Citizens, who felt that the decision to provide care should be neutral in respect to handicap. In other words, if a "normal infant" would have received the surgery, then infants with handicaps should also. Of the almost 4 million infants born each year, approximately 10 percent are born prematurely or with major birth defects. Modern surgery and neonatal care has been rather miraculous; however many of these infants still face life severely handicapped. In the investigations of more than 1,500 hot-line reports following the Baby Doe case, the government found only three cases in which infants were allegedly being denied appropriate care.

In 1984, Congress passed the Child Abuse Amendment, which provided guidelines in regard to when it was appropriate to withhold medically indicated treatment from these infants. The physician is not obliged to provide care beyond that of a palliative nature when, in the treating physician's reasonable medical judgment, any of the following circumstances apply.

1. The infant is chronically and irreversibly comatose.
2. The provision of such treatment would merely
   a. prolong dying.
   b. not be effective in ameliorating or correcting all of the infant's life-threatening conditions.
   c. be futile in terms of survival.

3. The provision of such treatment would be virtually futile in terms of the survival of the infant, and the treatment itself under such circumstances would be inhumane.[25]

In 1986, following the recommendations of the President's Commission on Medical Ethics, the U.S. Supreme Court ruled that the Baby Doe regulations were not authorized under Section 504 of the Rehabilitation Act of 1973. The Court emphasized that child protection was a state responsibility and that the primary decision makers for their children should be parents, provided that these decisions were in the children's best interest. With this ruling, the federal government was out of the Baby Doe business, and parents and physicians once again could wrestle with these problems somewhat out of the public eye.

Regardless of who the primary decision makers are, the ethical problems remain. Whereas parents have a right to privacy and to be left alone in their decisions in regard to their children, this is not an absolute right and does not extend to child abuse. What is the child's best interest in these cases?

If the infant's mental and physical handicaps are overwhelming, it would be inhumane to provide life-extending care and to salvage the infant to a life whose only awareness is that of pain and suffering. On the other hand, to refuse care to a child on the whimsy of being dissatisfied with a particular model is equally distasteful. The right choice for these babies is easy to determine at the extremes, but it becomes a true problem when deciding for the infants—in which it is not clear—as to what constitutes their best interest. Perhaps these are cases that are best served by basing the judgments on the quality-of-life issue or personhood. In order to have value, life must contain some aspects of quality, such as awareness and the potential for human relationships. This view is in keeping with the writings of Richard McCormick, a Jesuit who defends a quality-of-life determination.

> It is neither inhuman nor un-Christian to say that there comes a point where an individual's condition itself represents the negation of any truly human—i.e., relational—potential. When that point is reached, is not the best treatment no treatment?[26]

Translated into the language of personhood, an infant who has no present or future potential for self-awareness or relationships can be said to have no interests at all. It then becomes incomprehensible to provide life-extending care based on the child's best interests, as it makes no difference to the child whether the equipment is maintained for five minutes or five years.

THE BORN ALIVE INFANT PROTECTION ACT

On August 2002 the Born Alive Infant Protection Act became law. The act defines being born alive as displaying any of the several specific signs of life: breathing, a heart beat, definitive movement of voluntary muscles. The law states that infants born alive, at any stage in development (and regardless of circumstances of birth), are persons and therefore entitled to equal protection under the law.

The initiative for this legislation appears to be part of the ongoing abortion controversy in which some infants who are aborted arrive outside the womb alive. The law attempts to clarify their position and to offer them protection. It is the opinion of the American Academy of Pediatrics that the new law will not affect the current approach to resuscitation of extremely premature infants and decisions regarding viability. Increased focus on the provision of palliative care offers both the families and health providers time and the tools to work through these painful decisions.[27]

ORGAN DONATION

The field of organ transplantation had its inception in the early 1950s. From the very beginning, its development has been accompanied by difficult ethical questions in regard to when it is permissible to remove organs, who should receive them, and how it is to be financed. Advances in technique and the development of powerful immunosuppressive drugs have made it possible to transplant hearts, lungs, kidneys, livers, bone marrow, skin, corneas, and pancreases from cadavers. While some of these are still rather experimental, if the past is any predictor of the future, the variety of organs suitable for transplant will increase. In all areas of transplant technology, the survival and success rate are progressively improving, with areas such as cornea transplants having a success rate in restoration of sight nearing 100 percent. Unfortunately, for the length of time that the technology has been available, there has been a huge and frustrating shortage of supply. The number of patients awaiting an organ transplant exceeded 75,000 in early 2001, while the available supply was fewer than 25,000. More than 10 percent of those awaiting transplants die each year due to a lack of available human organs.[28] This ongoing shortage has created in some cases perhaps the most challenging and basic of health care policy decisions. "Who is to live, and who is to die?"[29]

The transplantation of organs from one human to another has become somewhat commonplace. Most public opinion polls show high public support for organ donations, although not all cultural groups have shown the same level of acceptance. Some traditional cultures have strong reservations based on issues such as the need for body integrity at burial.[30]

The national policy on the procurement of tissues for transplant might be best described as volunteerism. Most donors have been young adults who were in excellent health until an unexpected and unpredictable event, such as an accident, murder, suicide, or intracranial bleed, brought on brain death. The acceptance of brain death criteria has been critical to the successful practice of organ donation. However, the need for a rapid determination of brain death creates a situation in which families are forced to deal with the horrors of sudden loss and the potential donation of a loved one's organs virtually in the same instant. To bring order to the process of organ procurement, Section 1138, Title XI of the Omnibus Budget Reconciliation Act of 1986 required hospitals to establish organ procurement protocols or face the loss of Medicare and Medicaid funding. The Uniform Anatomical Gift Act enacted in all fifty states attempts to assist in the process of increasing the availability of donor organs by recognizing the legal status of donor cards, living wills, as well as the legal authority of the next of kin, to make donations in situations in which the deceased has not indicated a preference.

The need to obtain family consent in a time of grief and stress has been a major barrier to organ procurement. Health care providers are often loath to make the request and put further stress on a family at a time of loss. Some have argued for a public policy of "required request," which would remove the decision from the health care provider and make the inquiry of the available family part of the procedures for discontinuing life support in hopeless cases. This is somewhat problematic in that it presumes that a single policy matches all situations, and it infringes on the professional autonomy and judgment of the practitioner. The required-request policies are justified by proponents as serving the greater good gained by society in general as the result of an increased supply of cadaver organs for transplants. The fact that the potential donor is often young and the family does not know what his or her views would be in the matter makes the question in a moment of stress and grief even more troubling. Even in the face of high public support for organ donations, the refusal by families in this moment of crisis is often 50 percent.

Volunteerism and public education have not provided adequate supplies of organs for donation, and the gap seems to be widening. This increasing problem has stimulated a need for the reexamination of options. Table 9-1 provides a review of potential options.[31]

Volunteerism and public education have not provided adequate supplies of organs for donations and there have been many options explored to increase the availability of the resource. Some have advocated the adoption of "presumed consent" in those cases in which neither the person nor the surrogates have rejected such use of the body. This seems a reasonable proposal given that the majority of citizens appear to favor organ transplantation, even though few complete the necessary paperwork to be a donor. Yet is this a true choice? This can be likened to the Book of the Month Club that sends you the book if you don't send back the notice rejecting the selection. Does the receiving of the book indicate consent, or is it merely that humans often do not take the trouble to reject the offer? Would a presumed consent be true consent or merely an exploitation of the all-too-human trait of failure to follow through?

Others have argued that when volunteerism fails to provide adequate scarce resources, the free market may be a better way to secure the needed organs. If organs were bought and sold on the open market, the supply would increase. For some, the very thought of selling tissue or organs is morally repellant. The National Transport Act of 1984 forbids the sale of organs in interstate commerce. Yet if we believe that the individual is the sole owner of his organs, then it would seem that he would have as much of a right to sell his property as he would in donating it.

TABLE 9-1	
Options for Increasing the Supply of Salvageable Organs	
OPTION	**DESCRIPTION**
Mandated choice	The mandated choice option would require all competent adults to decide and record whether they wish to become organ donors at their death. This might be accomplished during driver's license applications or on tax returns.
Presumed consent	Presumed consent would allow the routine salvage of organs unless the donor opts out. This shifts the responsibility of organ donation from the donor families to donors, who would be given ample opportunity during their lifetime to object or consent. In the face of no information regarding a decision, the presumption would be for consent.
Financial incentives	Although controversial and currently illegal, a commercial market in organs has been suggested. One suggestion for a nonfinancial incentive is the offering of preferred status, in which those who sign donor cards are placed ahead of others who have not signed cards, should the need arise.
Xenografting	Although there are still technical and ethical issues to work through, the ability to use animal organs as permanent replacements for failing human organs offers a solution to the acute shortage of available organs.
Altering the current meaning of death	The use of brain death as a replacement of a cardiopulmonary standard is a relatively recent concept, which has allowed the advancement of clinical transplantation. Some have argued for a modification of the brain death standard (total cessation of cortical and brain stem function) to a definition based on the loss of cortical function only. This would allow the harvesting of organs from individuals in a persistent vegetative state and from anencephalic infants.
Use of condemned prisoners	Organ donation from executed prisoners has generally been deemed to be unethical unless the individual made the decision to donate prior to conviction.

Would the placement of organs on the open market raise the price and thus disenfranchise the poor? Would the poor be exploited and coerced into selling their organs or the organs of their deceased loved ones in times of severe need? Would fiscal coercion overcome any true form of personal autonomy and consent on the part of the poor in an open market situation?

Would the placement of organs on the open market create an international trade in which organs were transferred from developing nations to rich ones? Would it be ethical to purchase organs from developing nations? In regard to matched organs such as kidneys, is the forbidding of the selling of a single kidney on moral grounds by an individual who needs the money to keep his family from starving a strange form of paternalism and self-righteousness? Which is the greater harm: the starving family or the individual with a single kidney?

Some have advocated harvesting the organs of prisoners. For prisoners who have been given the death penalty, could a nation keep such individuals alive for harvesting until a buyer needed a particular body part? Would this create too great an incentive for juries to give the death penalty? How might this affect human rights in nations that do not have strong traditions in this area? If a free market approach to selling of organs were established, it would at the very least necessitate the crafting of law that ensured that the sale was truly voluntary.

CASE STUDY

"Go Ahead and Cut Him!" Right Answer, Wrong Reason

A newly appointed transplant surgeon is called concerning a young man with fatal head trauma. The next of kin is an older brother who is in the waiting room. Before the surgeon can get beyond the first sentence about the possibility of organ donation, the brother stops him abruptly: "Go ahead and cut him. Take the organs. I hated the S.O.B.! Where do I sign?"

Altruistic counseling is designed to make an individual aware of the needs of others. In this case, the brother is filled with hatred, and there is little appreciation for the altruism of the act he is agreeing to. Should that matter now that the legal ramifications of the issue have been covered with a signed consent from the next of kin?

1. Does motivation matter in this case?

2. Is the consent valid? Does the surgeon need to seek another relative for consent?

3. How much should the concept of the greater good enter into the surgeon's decision?

There are others who argue that organs are not personal property at all but should be considered a national resource. Most authorities believe that the current system of considering organs as personal gifts, which can be freely given or withheld, is wasteful in regard to this scarce resource. What if we as a society viewed organ ownership in a communal sense, in which organ donation was considered a special social duty that was expected of any of us who die in circumstances that would allow the harvesting of our organs? In order to satisfy certain personal and cultural aversions to such a policy, one could set up a "conscientious objector" status much like those set up for pacifists who have a moral aversion to participation in war. Under normal circumstances, the retrieval of organs would be a routine expectation unless the newly dead had signed up for an exemption from policy. Such a communitarian stance would seem to have great utility in that it would increase the number of available organs and would be a great symbol of commitment to the lives of others within the community. Even the allowance of the conscientious objector status would speak to the respect that the community had for individual differences and would protect the system from authoritarian abuse.

CONCLUSION

Medical science can now save biological life so effectively that we have been forced away from using a cardiopulmonary definition of death to the certification of death by brain function. We have also as a product of our technology and therapeutics moved into a time of being able to fend off brain death, only to expose the patient to continued misery and suffering. Health care providers have reached a quandary in which the duty to respect and preserve life comes into direct conflict with the duty to prevent and relieve pain.

In this chapter we have examined several classes of patients for whom decisions of withdrawing and withholding care have been reasoned through. These decisions have gained some cultural, legal, and ethical acceptance. Reasoning will be different for the profoundly handicapped infant, the PVS patient, those who chose informed nonconsent, and the mentally retarded. In some areas such as the abortion controversy, no consensus exists within our society. In some instances, the framework of what is to be done has been postponed, and the issue has become instead who is to decide.

Some instances of nontreatment seem to have gained acceptance and are rather noncontroversial. The ninety-eight year old with severe dementia and no relatives who contracts pneumonia might be allowed to die quietly. The real questions in regard to health provider duty do not lie in the extremes, such as an infant born with no brain inside its skull, but in the middle ground where there will be a potential for personhood and meaningful life. In the extreme cases in which no potential exists, or in which the best interests of the individual seem best served by withholding or withdrawing treatment, a form of passive euthanasia has been allowed. **Euthanasia**, which literally means a gentle or easy death, has been divided into two major groupings, passive and active. This chapter has been involved in the issues of passive euthanasia—the process of doing nothing to prolong life or fend off death. Active euthanasia, as defined by the active participation of ending life, is currently forbidden by most codes of ethical conduct. Active euthanasia will form the basis of the discussion in Chapter 10.

KEY CONCEPTS

- The difference between biological and biographical life forms the basis of much of the discussion in situations in which withholding and withdrawing life support becomes necessary.

- The acceptance of the concept of brain death has allowed the rapid clinical development of organ transplantation.

- Many clinicians and scholars have begun to argue in favor of a neocortical definition of death.

- Best interest and substituted judgment are two legal standards used to assist in proxy decision making for those incapable of deciding for themselves.

- Following the Nancy Cruzan decision, the courts moved to a "clear and convincing evidence" standard for withdrawing and withholding care. The call for clearance and convincing evidence of choice have stimulated renewed interest in advanced directives.

- The courts have consistently held that competent adults have the right to informed nonconsent to care.

- The current voluntary process of securing organs for transplant has so far proved unable to meet societal demands for these tissues.

- Several modifications to the current process of securing organs for transplant are currently under consideration.

REVIEW EXERCISES

A. The case involves a young, ventilator-dependent quadriplegic patient who, after being shunted about to various facilities, sought to have his ventilator unhooked. The court recognized him as a competent adult and allowed the withdrawal of his life support.

In this case, neither the court, the health care providers, the right-to-life movement, nor the churches came forward to argue that the ventilator should be continued. After he had gained permission to withdraw from life support, the patient decided against the action and still remains on the ventilator.

The question that this case brings forward is whether the young man's demand to have the "right to die" was real or just another way of saying, "Do you care about me?" A secondary question that is equally problematic is whether the acceptance of his request was based on a respect for his personal autonomy, or was it just an answer to the, "Do you care about me?" question with a "no!"

Respond to the idea that our current acceptance of "a right to die," especially for those who are unconscious and need a proxy decision maker, is a rather slippery slope that may in the future be used not to protect individual autonomy or privacy but rather as a facade to rid us of individuals whose lives we do not value.

B. Differentiate between the various lines of reasoning and arguments needed to decide the following types of cases in regard to withdrawing or withholding care:

1. Persistent vegetative state cases

2. Profoundly retarded patient cases

3. Baby Doe cases

4. Informed nonconsent cases

Which of the above case types is best served by proxy judgments, and if so, what form: best interest or substituted judgment?

C. The philosopher Joseph Fletcher[32] issued a paper listing the characteristics of a person. The following are taken from his positive criteria:

1. Minimal IQ: Mere biological life, before minimal intelligence is achieved or after it is irreversibly lost, is without person status.

2. Self-awareness: The development of self-awareness in babies is what we watch and take such joy in. In psychotherapy, the lack of self-awareness would represent grave pathology.

3. Self control: An individual not only not controllable by others (without restraint), but also not in his own control.

4. A sense of time: Memories, a feeling of now, and expectations for the future.

5. The capability to relate to others: Interpersonal relationships seem essential to being a person in any meaningful sense.

6. Concern for others: Extra-ego orientation is a vital characteristic of a "real person."

7. Curiosity: A person is a learner; total indifference is inhuman.

8. Communication: Utter alienation or disconnection from others is not a characteristic of humanity.

9. Neocortical function: Personal reality is dependent upon cerebral function; it forms the basis between life in a biographical and biological sense.

10. Idiosyncrasy: Humans are distinct; to be a person is to have identity, to be recognizable or callable by name.

Rank-order the list from most important to least important in your view of what makes up a person. Check those that you would consider to be essential in regard to personhood. If you feel that a particular characteristic is essential, you must be willing to deny those who do not possess it the rights and privileges of person status.

In regard to the personhood criteria that you have selected, state how this would affect your decisions in the following cases.

Nancy Cruzan

Joseph Saikewicz

Elizabeth Bouvia

Baby Doe

In regard to KoKo the Gorilla, who uses sign language to communicate with humans and appears to have a kitten that she cares about and misses when it is gone, what is her level of personhood?

If an angel or alien appeared out of the sky and had all the elements that you said were essential to being a person, would the alien have all the rights and privileges of a person?

D. Assuming that Baby Doe would have grown up to know himself, know those around him, walk, talk and play, and perhaps even go to school, was the decision not to provide the surgery ethical? Regardless of how you answer, justify your decision using ethical criteria. Also note that legal decisions are ethics neutral, and vice versa: Something truly can be legally correct, medically correct, socially correct, and morally reprehensible. Ask Dr. Mengele (Nazi war criminal who performed ghoulish experiments in the death camps), for he surely felt that relative to his society, what he was doing was socially, medically, and legally correct.

E. Mr. Martinez was a seventy-five-year-old chronic obstructive pulmonary disease patient. He was in the hospital because of an upper respiratory tract infection. He and his wife had requested that CPR not be performed should he require it. A DNR order was written in the charts. In his room on the third floor, he was being maintained with antibiotics, fluids, and oxygen and seemed to be doing better. However, Mr. Martinez's oxygen was inadvertently turned up, and this caused him to go into respiratory failure. When found by the therapist, he was in terrible distress and lay gasping in his bed.

Should Mr. Martinez be transferred to intensive care, where his respiratory failure can be treated by a ventilator and his oxygen level can be monitored? Whatever your answer, provide an ethical rationale.

NOTES

1. Ruth Macklin, *Mortal Choices* (Boston: Houghton Mifflin, 1987), pp. 7–8.

2. Nancy Cruzan gravestone.

3. Ad Hoc Committee of the Harvard Medical School to Examine the Definition of Death, "A Definition of Irreversible Coma," *Journal of the American Medical Association,* November 13, 1981.

4. Thomas Furlow, "Tyranny of Technology; A Physician Looks at Euthanasia," *Humanist* 34, no. 4 (1974): pp. 6–8.

5. John Sorenson, *Determination of Death: The Need for a Higher Brain Concept in Medical Ethics,* ed. John Monagle and David Thomasma (Rockville, MD: Aspen Publishers, 1988).

6. *In re Quinlan,* 70 New Jersey 10, 355 A.2d 647, 79 A.L.R.3d 205 (1976).

7. 1957 Encyclical "Prolongation of Life" as quoted in Brody Howard, *Ethical Decisions in Modern Medicine* (Boston: Little, Brown, 1981), p. 91.

8. Gerald Kelly, *Medico-moral Problems* (St. Louis: Catholic Hospital Association, 1957), p. 129.

9. G. Meilaender, "On Removing Food and Water: Against the Stream," *Hastings Center Report* 14 (1984): pp. 11–13.

10. Joseph Fletcher, "Indicators of Personhood," *Hastings Center Report* (1972): 1–4.

11. Joel Feinberg, "The Problem of Personhood," in T. Beauchamp, and L. Walters, *Contemporary Issues in Bioethics* (Belmont, CA: Wadsworth, 1982), pp. 108–115.

12. Nancy's Father's statement.

13. *Cruzan* v. *Director, Missouri Department of Health,* 110 U.S. S.Ct., 2841 (1990).

14. Agile Freedman, "Right-to-Die Guidelines Murky in Most States," *Health Week Briefing Paper,* Phillips Medical Systems (March 1990): pp. 30–33

15. Society for the Right to Die, *Handbook of Living Will Laws* (New York: Society for the Right to Die, 1987).

16. Anne Allen, "Advanced Directives Provide Answers for Tough Questions," *Journal of Post Anesthesia Nursing* 7, no 3 (June 1992): pp. 183–185.

17. George Annas, "Transferring the Ethical Hot Potato," *Hastings Center Report* (November 1987): pp. 20–23.

18. *Superintendent of Belchertown State School* v. *Saikewicz,* 373 Mass. 728, 370 N.E.2d 417 (1977).

19. *Bartling* v. *Superior Court,* 163 Cal. App.3d 186, 195 (1984).

20. *Bouvia* v. *Superior Court,* 179 Cal. App.3d 1127 (1986).

21. Council on Ethical and Judicial Affairs, "Guidelines for the Appropriate Use of Do-Not-Resuscitate Orders," *Journal of the American Medical Association,* April 10, 1991, pp. 1868–1871.

22. Mary Rhoden, "Treating Baby Doe: The Ethics of Uncertainty," *Hastings Center Report* (August 1986): pp. 34–42.

23. J. C. Moscop and R. L. Saldanha, "The Baby Doe Rule: Still a Threat," *Hastings Center Report* (April 1986): pp. 8–12.

24. Patrick Buchanan, "The Dividing Line," *New York Times,* November 15, 1983.

25. Macklin, *Mortal Choices,* p. 123.

26. Richard McCormick, "To Save or Let Die: The Dilemma of Modern Medicine," *Journal of the American Medical Association* 229 (1979): pp. 172–176.

27. Tricia Romesberg, "Futile Care and the Neonate," *Advanced Neonatal Care,* 3, no. 5 (2003): pp. 213–219.

28. Roman Espejo, ed., *Biomedical Ethics* (New York: Greenhaven Press, 2003).

29. Arthur Caplan, ed., *Organ Transplants* (Amherst, NY: Prometheus Books, 1998).

30. Ruth Macklin, *Against Relativism* (New York: Oxford University Press, 1999).

31. Arthur Caplan, ed., *Organ Transplants* (1998).

32. Joseph Fletcher, *Humanhood: Essays in Biomedical Ethics,* (Buffalo, NY: Prometheus Books, 1979).

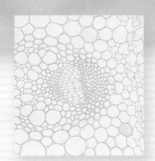

CHAPTER 10

Euthanasia:
Practice and Principles

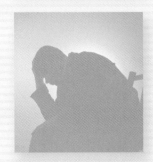

GOAL

To gain an understanding of the national debate in regard to euthanasia. The chapter will differentiate between the variety of forms that this practice takes and look at the various arguments for and against the adoption of the practice in modern health care.

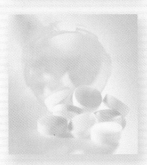

OBJECTIVES

Upon completion of this chapter, the reader should be able to:

1. Define and differentiate between active and passive euthanasia.

2. Discuss the two major arguments for the adoption of a "right to die."

3. Discuss the religious and nonreligious arguments against the adoption of active euthanasia as a practice of modern health care.

4. Outline the current position taken by the health care community in regard to the practice of both active and passive euthanasia.

5. Outline the nature of the Hospice Movement in the United States and discuss how this may impact on the debate regarding euthanasia.

6. Discuss the current ambiguity between the law and court decisions regarding mercy killing in the United States.

7. Outline the general position taken by the Supreme Court in regard to a "right to die."

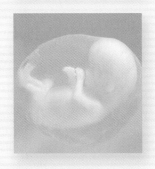

KEY TERMS

Active euthanasia	**Mercy killing**	**Voluntary euthanasia**
Hospice movement	**Palliative care**	
Involuntary euthanasia	**Passive euthanasia**	

LEGAL AND SOCIAL STANDING OF EUTHANASIA

I cannot emphasize strongly enough that people should only help each other to die if there is a bonding of love or friendship, and mutual respect. If the association is anything less, stand aside.

Derek Humphry, cofounder, Hemlock Society

Derek:

There. You got what you wanted. Ever since I was diagnosed as having cancer, you have done everything conceivable to precipitate my death. I was not alone in recognizing what you were doing. What you did—desertion and abandonment and subsequent harassment of a dying woman—is so unspeakable there are no words to describe the horror of it.

Last words of Ann Humphry, cofounder, Hemlock Society

Between these two rather remarkable quotes by the cofounders of the Hemlock Society lies the great unspoken debate over assisted suicide and self-deliverance. Within the first quote is the concern and respect for the autonomy of others, which appears to drive the right to die movement. Within the second is the great fear. What is our societal motive as we move to embrace a right to die? Are we doing so out of love and compassion—or because we have ceased to value the lives of those who are old, weak, sick, and vulnerable? Do individuals seek euthanasia because they want to control this part of their lives, or do they do so because as a society, we have made the dying more frightening than death itself?

In June 1990, Janet Adkins ended her life in a secluded county park with the assistance of the now famous, Dr. Jack Kevorkian. By the end of June 1998, Kevorkian had participated in over fifty similar events using his suicide machines (Thanatron, Mercitron). Among the deaths he has assisted with have been individuals with emphysema, Alzheimer's, rheumatoid arthritis, multiple sclerosis, as well as those declared terminally ill by their physicians. Adkins, the first, is also perhaps the most troubling. At the time of her death, Adkin's memory loss from Alzheimer's disease was still at the stage of forgetting to take her purse or missing a tennis lesson. The last evening of her life was spent among friends in cogent conversation regarding the music of Bach. Prior to her death, she had arranged with a therapist to assist her family through the bereavement period. These are not the activities of someone who normally is thought of as the classic candidate for assisted suicide. While common wisdom teaches, "It is better too early than too late." it would seem that her death was a bit premature.

Although Kevorkian, his death machine, his attendant legal problems, and incarceration has recently assumed center stage in the controversy, euthanasia is by no means a recent issue in the United States. Figure 10-1 outlines the criteria for euthanasia found in a bill brought before the New York State General Assembly and defeated in 1947. Since the early legislation and the approval of the Oregon bill states as diverse as Hawaii, Washington, and Maine have attempted similar legislation, however, although popular among segments of the public, there is no clear consensus for legalizing euthanasia.[1]

The ethical and legal issues of withholding or withdrawing life support have been reasonably worked out in cases such as those of Karen Ann Quinlan and Nancy Cruzan, and there appears to be some consensus for allowing health care providers to participate under these circumstances in **passive euthanasia**. The allowance of a deadly process to proceed without intervention is generally acceptable in the United States when the treatment is futile, and no possibility of patient benefit exists. Every day, in a hundred hospital settings, do-not-resuscitate (DNR) orders are written in charts, respirators are disconnected, IV lines are removed, and proposed surgeries are canceled. Most states today have legislation covering advanced directives, and many specifically provide that a patient or proxy can authorize the withholding or withdrawal of life-support systems. Although still somewhat controversial, the issue today does not revolve around passive euthanasia, that is, standing aside and allowing the terminal patient to die. Figure 10-2 is the anonymously written "Time to Go," which elegantly states the socially agreed upon case for passive euthanasia.

---

1. Any sane person over twenty years old, suffering from an incurably painful and fatal disease, may petition a court of record for euthanasia, in a signed and attested document with an affidavit from the attending physician that in his opinion the disease is incurable;

2. The court may appoint a commission of three, of whom at least two shall be physicians, to investigate all aspects of the case and to report back to the courts whether the patient understands the purpose of his petition and comes under the provisions of the act;

3. Upon a favorable report by the commission the court shall grant the petition, and, if it is still wanted by the patient, euthanasia may be administered by a physician or any other person chosen by the patient or by the commission.

FIGURE 10-1   Criteria for Euthanasia in Defeated Legislation

TIME TO GO

Pardon me, doctor, but may I die?
I know your oath requires you try
As long as there's a spark of life
To keep it there with tube and knife;

To do cut-downs and heart massages,
Tracheotomies and gavages.
But here I am, well past four-score.
I've lived my lifetime (and a little more)

I've raised my children, buried my wife.
My friends are gone, so spare the knife.
This is the way it seems to me
I deserve a little dignity . . .

Of slipping gently off to sleep
And no one has the right to keep
Me from my God: when the call's this clear
No mortal man should keep me here.

Your motive's noble, but now I pray
You'll read my eyes, what my lips can't say
Listen to my heart! You'll hear it cry;
"Pardon me, Doctor, but may I die?"

FIGURE 10-2   Time to Go

However, our system currently holds that there is an important distinction between assisting the death of patients and letting them die, even though the outcome seems the same. The American Medical Association (AMA) Code of Ethics states that except in special circumstances, it is illegal to deliberately cause the death of another person. The AMA does not, however, have the same admonition (special circumstances) against allowing a person to die. In the one case, you are initiating the process that brings about the death; in the other, you are just allowing a deadly process, which you did not initiate, to continue. The one case is viewed as morally wrong and the other as morally permissible. Critics of this view feel the difference is a matter of sophistry, for inherent in the decision to do nothing is the decision for death. Is the removal of the ventilator, IV lines, and feeding tubes from a patient who cannot breathe or eat for himself any less a complicity in the resulting death than if you provided a bolus of morphine to hasten the process? If there is no difference, is the bolus the more humane act?[2]

The term euthanasia comes from the Greek for *good death* and in English has taken the meaning of easy death or the *painless inducement of quick death*. The concept of easy death is further divided into two categories: passive euthanasia, which involves doing nothing to preserve life, and **active euthanasia**, which requires actions that speed the process of dying. Euthanasia is further divided, depending on whether the process is initiated by patient request, and is therefore voluntary or involuntarily implemented without patient permission.

Involuntary euthanasia, which ignores the individual's autonomous rights and could potentially bring about the death of an unwilling victim, is not easily distinguished from murder. There is very little disagreement in our society that involuntary euthanasia is morally indefensible. The focus of the current controversy that rages through our health care system is whether there is a moral difference between active and passive **voluntary euthanasia**. Several states have put statutes before the citizens in regard to legalizing voluntary active euthanasia.

It is perhaps important to differentiate between killing (involuntary euthanasia) and suicide, although neither provides the focus of this chapter, which is centered on the question of allowing voluntary active euthanasia. Tom Beauchamp offers a precise definition of suicide that separates it from the process of passive or active voluntary euthanasia. A person has committed suicide when:

1. That person brings about his or her own death;

2. Others do not coerce him or her to do the action; and

3. Death is caused by conditions arranged by the person for the purpose of bringing about his or her death.[3]

Although the frequency of occurrence is unknown, it is not a rare event for physicians to prescribe sleeping and pain medications for hopelessly ill patients who request them, knowing full well that their intended use is suicide. Some physicians see this as the last act in a continuum of care. As noted above, suicide differs from euthanasia in that the health care provider does not participate in the act of bringing about death. Any physician who becomes involved in the suicide of a patient must first be assured that the patient is indeed in a hopeless situation and not just suffering from treatable depression, common in individuals with terminal illnesses.

Prior to his conviction, one of the real problems with Dr. Kevorkian and his death machine (the Mercitron) was determining whether his patients committed suicide, whether he was practicing voluntary euthanasia, or perhaps murdering these unfortunates. When he builds his machines, advertises in newspapers (see Figure 10-3), videotapes the events, purchases the lethal dosages, arranges for undisturbed sites, puts in IV lines, and finally arranges for postmortem

> Is someone in your family
> terminally ill?
> Does he or she wish to die—
> and with dignity?
> **CALL PHYSICIAN CONSULTANT**
> (Telephone number)

FIGURE 10-3   Kevorkian Newspaper Ad

press conferences, has he stepped beyond being a mere observer when the patients push the button to release the drugs?"[4]

Some would find the acts of Dr. Kevorkian similar to the political terrorist who bombs buildings and buses in order to bring about political change. These seeming criminal acts have at times brought about positive political change. Kevorkian may be the harbinger of change and usher in a new specialty known as obiatry, practitioners of which would legally perform euthanasia in our society. Perhaps in the future there will be obiatry clinics in every major city. However, just as some terrorist acts usher in positive developments, others do nothing more than murder innocents and leave no permanent positive effects for their efforts. In a news article, the ethicist Arthur Caplan argued that Kevorkian's campaign of mercy took its heaviest toll on the poor, the disabled, and women and that his clients were more victims than beneficiaries.[5] Perhaps Kevorkian was nothing more than a serial killer with a gimmick. History has yet to determine whether Kevorkian was in the forefront of change or was just a wild, uncontrolled eccentric who captured headlines and eventually faded from the attention of the media.

A health care practitioner who deliberately hastens the death of a patient under the guise of "mercy killing" has entered into a practice prohibited under the homicide laws. Common and criminal law regard life as sacred and inalienable and look at any premeditated killing as homicide. "Consent and humanitarian motive" is never a defense under the law for murder. "He nonetheless acts with malice if he is able to comprehend that society prohibits his act regardless of his personal beliefs."[6]

The Netherlands is the only modern industrialized nation to fully sanction physician-assisted euthanasia. The full approval of the process came on January 1, 2002. This law means that physicians no longer face prosecution for carrying out mercy killings if they are performed with due care and within the established guidelines. The nation had spent nearly a decade reviewing the process before making the decision.

The process used by the Dutch is worthy of consideration. In order for the physician to assist with the euthanasia, the following must occur:[7]

- The patient must request the assistance freely and frequently, after careful consideration.
- The physician may act on the request only if the patient is terminally ill, with no hope of improvement and in severe pain.
- The physician must consult with another physician and file a report with the coroner.

During the review period, the police and prosecutor's office were charged with reviewing these cases to ensure compliance with the outlined procedures.

In the Netherlands it is usually a family physician who received the request to assist in the patient's death. The standard process was to give a large dose of barbiturates to produce a coma and then an injection of curare, which stops respiration and heart rate. It is interesting to note what types of patients availed themselves of the euthanasia option.

- Women and men are equal in requesting euthanasia.
- The average age for men is sixty-three and for women sixty-six.
- Requests are rare in people over age seventy-five and even rarer for those over age eighty-five.
- Most requests come from cancer patients, who state that they feared becoming dependent and suffering a loss of dignity, humiliation, and pain.

Almost immediately following the Dutch government's decision to fully legalize physician-assisted euthanasia, the issue was inflamed by a court finding that a doctor was guilty of malpractice for helping an eighty-six-year-old former senator die because he was tired of living. Although the court found him guilty, the doctor was neither sentenced nor fined for the offense. Many in the Netherlands feel that the protective guidelines developed during the review period are too strict. The debate now seems to be moving toward whether elderly people should be prescribed a suicide pill when they feel the time is right.

In response to the courts allowing the physician to ignore the guidelines, the Dutch Patient's Association, a disability-rights group, has begun to distribute a wallet card to its members instructing doctors that "no treatment be administered with the intention of terminating life."[8] Members of this group in a letter to the Parliamentary Committees for Health Care and Justice wrote:

> We feel our lives are threatened. We realize that we cost the community a lot. Many people think we are useless, often we notice that we are being talked into desiring death. We will find it extremely dangerous and frightening if the new medical legislation includes euthanasia.[9]

Some opponents to the legalization of active euthanasia oppose the practice on the basis of the principle of beneficence and the fear of beginning a slippery slope. Under this scenario the practice would first be limited only to voluntary patients. In that those lacking capacity must be provided the same rights as the competent, the practice could then be extended to include the noncompetent patient if the surrogate agreed. Finally, the process could be extended to include others based on a perceived need of society such as rationing.[10]

Often those opposed to the legalization of euthanasia point to Nazi-style genocide as the final point on the slippery slope. The problem with an analysis that includes Nazi Germany is that this government did not go from mercy killing to the final solution. They began with a flawed system that sought to bring about the ends of the state through the involuntary control of its citizens. There is a wide chasm between the grossness of the actions of certain totalitarian states and the perceived need for voluntary euthanasia in the context of an American medical-moral-legal framework.

In recent years, polls have indicated that a majority of American citizens favor some form of physician-assisted suicide, and in November 1995, Oregon voters approved a ballot initiative (Measure 16) that would allow a terminally ill patient to obtain a physician's prescription for a fatal drug for the expressed purpose of ending their life.[11] This decision was challenged in court with plaintiffs claiming Measure 16 violated the Equal Protection and Due Process clauses of the Fourteenth Amendment to the Constitution.[12]

Like the law in the Netherlands, the Oregon Death with Dignity Act attempts to provide protections to ensure that abuses do not occur. The law requires that the patient:

- Be a capable adult
- Is an Oregon resident
- Have a terminal illness, with less than six months to live
- Voluntarily request a prescription for lethal drugs

The request must be made both orally and in writing. The written request must be signed and dated by the patient and witnessed by at least two individuals (not to include the attending physician). The witnesses must attest that the patient is capable and acting voluntarily. At least one of the witnesses must not be a relative, heir of the patient, or someone associated with the health care facility where the patient is receiving care. The patient must reiterate the oral request at least fifteen days following the initial request.

Under the act, the attending physician has the following responsibilities:

- Determine that the patient has a terminal illness, is capable, and has made the request voluntarily
- Provide information to the patient regarding the diagnosis, prognosis, risks, and probable results of taking the prescribed medication as well as other feasible alternatives such as palliative care, hospice care, and pain control
- Refer the patient to a consulting physician to confirm diagnosis, prognosis, and for a secondary confirmation that the patient is capable and acting voluntarily

- Refer the patient to counseling if there is any indication of mental disorder

- Request that the patient notify the next of kin of his decision (compliance not required)

- Offer to the patient the opportunity to rescind the request at any time

- Complete all appropriate documentation and reports as required by law

In 1997, the Supreme Court ruled that the Constitution does not guarantee Americans a right to physician-assisted suicide and returned the issue to the state legislatures for continued debate. In its decision, the Court placed emphasis on the American tradition of condemning suicide and valuing human life. In its ruling, the Court made it clear that the states have a legitimate interest in banning physician-assisted suicide, but it also left it open to them to legalize the practice. As a result, the practice has been legalized in Oregon.[13] Figure 10-4 provides a listing of the seminal events of the right-to-die movement.

1976—Karen Ann Quinlan case: New Jersey Supreme Court ruled that the state has no right to order respiratory support to be continued. U.S. Supreme Court refused to intervene, setting no legal precedent.

1990—Nancy Beth Cruzan case: U.S. Supreme Court rules that an individual has a "right to die" grounded in the Fourteenth Amendment's guarantee of personal liberty. In its ruling, the Court called for a clear and convincing evidence standard, which spurred the interest in and development of living wills and durable power of attorney documents to provide evidence of the patient's previously expressed wish to die.

1990—Michigan pathologist Jack Kevorkian, known as Dr. Death, assists Janet Adkins in ending her life. This will be the first of over 50 similar events using his suicide machine. His activities sparked a nationwide debate regarding assisted suicide. Following many efforts to charge him with murder and other crimes, he was convicted and incarcerated.

1995—Oregon voters approved a ballot initiative (Measure 16) that would allow a terminally ill patient to obtain a physician's prescription for a fatal drug for the expressed purpose of ending his life.

1997—The U.S. Supreme Court rules that the Constitution does not guarantee Americans a right to commit suicide with the help of a physician. The issue has been left to state legislatures to decide.

FIGURE 10-4   Milestones in the Right-to-Die Movement

CASE STUDY

Extending the Right to Die: A Slippery Slope?

One of the fears of opponents regarding a "right to die" is that in the future, the courts will extend the "right" to other vulnerable populations. Under the Oregon legislation, the patient is prescribed a lethal medication but in the end must take it himself. This then is a form of physician-assisted suicide. Could it be argued that the incapacitated patient who could not take the medication without assistance has an equal right? Would this then expand the right not only to physician-assisted suicide but to physician euthanasia?

In the *Vacco* v. *Quill* case, it was argued that if a right to die could be found under the Fourteenth Amendment to the Constitution, then a law that allowed a patient who wanted to be disconnected from artificial life support to do so, but barred others who wanted to take lethal drugs to similarly hasten their death, would violate the amendment's equal protection guarantee because it treated the two groups differently.

1. Are the two groups—patients refusing care and an individual wishing a lethal prescription—the same?

2. The U.S. Supreme Court did not find a right to die under the Constitution. Do you think this was the right decision?

The result of the Supreme Court's decision was to leave to the individual states the chore of working out their legislation. It is interesting to note that the Court resisted the path it took in the 1973 landmark abortion case, when it usurped state action by finding a fundamental constitutional right to end a pregnancy. With the matter returned to the states, advocates on both sides of the issue are predicting more controversy and debate.

MERCY KILLING

An elderly woman with Alzheimer's disease that had progressed to the point that she could no longer do simple chores and whose vocabulary had shrunk to two words (*fire* and *pain*), which she screamed in German, was shot by her husband of thirty-three years. Hans Florian claimed that he shot his wife because he was seventeen years her senior and he feared that he might die first and leave her alone.[14] Under American law, he had no legal right to harm his wife and could have been brought up on the charge of murder. After considering the issues involved, the Florida grand jury refused to indict him.

In Michigan, seventy-three-year-old Bertram Harper was acquitted of murdering his terminally ill wife even though he admitted placing a plastic bag over her head. He and his wife had checked into a motel with the intention of her committing suicide. When her efforts failed, he placed a plastic bag over her head to smother her.[15]

In both the Florian and Harper cases, the facts were clear that the men had participated in ending their wives' lives, yet in both cases, they were not held accountable for the actions. What these cases indicate is a reservoir of public sentiment for **mercy killing** under certain circumstances. The practice of mercy killing is on the rise in the United States, with more cases being reported between 1980 and 2000 than in the previous half-century. Yet in almost all instances, similar to the Harper and Florian cases, the defendants have not been imprisoned for the offense. Instead the courts have found the individuals not guilty on the grounds of temporary insanity or have mandated long periods of probation.

Although the law is rather unequivocal in regard to the practice of active euthanasia, the court decisions have been quite ambiguous. This may be a proper stance for the law in that its adamant negative position provides a deterrent to all considerations of the practice and forces deliberation of the merits on a case-by-case basis. But under what circumstances is euthanasia justifiable? Is it permissible to kill the terminally ill? How about those who are not terminally ill but have only lost their appetite for life? Even if society decides that citizens have a right not only to life, liberty, and property but also to death, what part do health care practitioners play in this right? Would the role of public euthanizer have a chilling effect on the healing arts?

One highly publicized account of practitioner mercy killing, known as "It's Over, Debbie," involved a gynecology resident rotating through a large private hospital. The physician was awakened by the nurse on duty and told that a patient dying of ovarian cancer was having difficulty getting rest. When the physician entered the patient's room, he found her sitting in bed, emaciated and in severe air hunger. The patient's only words to the physician were, "Let's get this over with." The physician left the room and instructed the nurse to draw up 20 milligrams of morphine sulfate into a syringe, which he then injected intravenously into the patient after telling her and a woman visitor that "it would let her rest," and "to say good-bye." The woman died of respiratory failure within a few minutes.[16]

In that the reporting of this incident was in a "letters" format to a medical journal, there is some doubt that the case actually occurred. On the other hand, if it occurred, it poses several grave problems. First, the practitioner had not seen the patient previously, so no real patient-physician relationship had been established. Second, the physician chose to interpret the words of the patient to constitute a request for assisted euthanasia, which may or may not have been her intent. Third, the physician was morally obligated to discuss other clinical options, such as hospice, which assigns a high priority to the relief of pain and suffering. Fourth, other medications might have been used that avoided the suppression of respiration, while allowing the patient pain relief and rest. Fifth, a decision of such a devastatingly permanent nature is not one that should be taken without consultation. Given all these problems, the physician's actions could not have held up under the legal standard of basic common sense, and it is unlikely that if the physician had gone to court for this incident he would have been treated as lightly as Hans Florian or Bertram Harper.

Unfortunately there has been a cluster of cases involving allied health and nursing personnel and mercy killing. Cases in California, Michigan, Texas, Florida, Maryland, Georgia, New York, and North Carolina have all made national headlines.[17] Most of these cases came to the attention of authorities as clusters of patient deaths and were detected in quality-assurance and risk-management studies. The impact on the communities, the patients' families, and the nursing profession have been profound and negative. The intensity of the negative public reaction is perhaps a measure of how comfortable the average citizen is with the allied health practitioner or nurse as a patient advocate. When that trust is betrayed, there is a natural sense of outrage, as the "good (nurse, therapist, clinician) couldn't possibly act this way."

Mercy killing as an accepted practice is not something that can be entered into lightly, inasmuch as the act of putting someone to death—regardless of motive—involves the closure of all future options. It rules out any possibility of unanticipated discovery of wrong diagnosis, new treatments, spontaneous remission, or improvement as a result of continued treatment. There seems some right reasoning in the caution for prudence, "When in doubt—don't!"

ARGUMENTS FOR AND AGAINST EUTHANASIA

The arguments for the practice of euthanasia can be expressed in both utilitarian and duty-oriented terms. In the first case, it can be argued as a concern and compassion for those who are painfully and/or terminally ill. This view is strongly put forward by the noted ethicist and theologian Joseph Fletcher, who feels that

> it is harder morally to justify letting someone die a slow and ugly death, dehumanized, than it is to justify helping him to escape from such misery. This is a case at least in any code of ethics which is humanistic or personalistic, i.e., in any code of ethics which has a value system that puts humanness and personal integrity above biological life and function.[18]

The duty-oriented arguments are centered on an extension of personal autonomy—the rights accorded us in Western societies to live our life according to our own vision, unrestricted by the views of others. If we can live our lives according to a personal inner vision, then should this aspect of human dignity based on free choice also be extended to the termination of our lives? In Figure 10-5, the ethicist Arthur Dyck proposes a set of beliefs and propositions suitable as an ethic for euthanasia.[19]

1. An individual's life belongs to that individual to dispose of entirely as he or she wishes;

2. The dignity that attaches to personhood by reason of the freedom to make choices demands also the freedom to take one's own life;

3. There is such a thing as life not worth living whether the cause be distress, illness, physical/mental handicaps, or even sheer despair for whatever reason;

4. What is supreme in value is the human dignity that resides in the human's rational capacity to choose and control life and death.

FIGURE 10-5   The Ethic of Euthanasia

For those who oppose active euthanasia on religious grounds, the basic concern seems to be the view that our lives are not ours but gifts from God. In this view, humans hold their lives as a trust. If this is true, then we are bound to hold not only the lives of others inviolate but also our own, since to take our life is to destroy what belongs to God. In Exodus 34:7 and Daniel 13:53, scriptures taken from the Old Testament, the doctrine of the sanctity of life principle is upheld, except in rare instances of self defense. Judeo-Christian precepts generally condemn active euthanasia in any form, but allow some forms of passive euthanasia. The difference is that of omission and commission: While the Judeo-Christian philosophy might tolerate the allowance of death, acts that permit death, it draws the line in regard to acts that cause death.

Nonreligious arguments against active euthanasia usually follow a slippery slope or wedge line of reasoning. In some ways the arguments recall the parable of the camel who pleaded with his owner to be allowed to put his nose into the tent to keep it warm against the cold desert night. Once the nose was allowed, other adjustments were requested, and the owner found himself sleeping with his camel. Is there something so persuasive about putting others to death that, if allowed, would become gross and commonplace? The Nazi "final solution," which brought about the death of millions of Jews, gypsies, and other eastern Europeans, could be traced to compulsory euthanasia legislation that, at the time of its enactment, included only mental cases, monstrosities, and incurables who were a burden of the state. Using the Nazi experience as a guide, critics of active euthanasia do see some seductiveness to killing that humans do not seem able to handle. Perhaps Sigmund Freud was right as he wrote:[20]

> What no human soul desires there is no need to prohibit; it is automatically excluded. The very emphasis of the commandment "Thou shalt not kill" makes it certain that we spring from an endless ancestry of murderers, with whom the lust for killing was in the blood, as possibly it is to this day with ourselves.

The ethicist Joseph Fletcher feels that the use of the Nazi experience to show that a people can be taken down a primrose path, from a position of voluntary active euthanasia based on compassion and concern for human dignity to the grossness of the final solution, is too great a reach and is based on a false premise. He feels that what occurred in regard to the Nazi experience is not a slippery slope or wedge situation at all but rather an extension of the cruelty and lack of compassion built into the system at its very beginning. The Nazis did not go from mercy killing to the final solution; rather they started with merciless killing and proceeded from there. The Nazis did not fall into their practices on the basis of some fundamental seductiveness of killing. They began their practice through an acceptance of their bringing about the ends of the state through the involuntary control of its citizens.

Clearly, there is a wide chasm between the grossness of the actions of certain totalitarian states and the perceived need for voluntary euthanasia in the context of an American medical-moral-legal framework. The chasm is so wide that the use of the Nazi, Soviet, and Cambodian experiences is perhaps not suitable at all.

Yet, how does one decide that euthanasia is appropriate for another? Does our subjective view taken from a position of health, in regard to the quality of another's life, or how a family is suffering, justify the ending of a patient's life without his consent? Does the authority to kill an innocent individual provide the wedge that breaks down the barriers needed to protect the severely handicapped, unwanted newborns, the frail elderly, the "useless" members of our society? Once euthanasia is allowed and accepted, where is the rational ground on which to stand and declare, "This far and no more!" Perhaps the rational ground is clear and convincing evidence of the will of the individual patient, and where that is not provided or possible, there can be no allowance for outside interference with life.

It would seem that perhaps the debate involving active euthanasia in the United States is premature. Prior to deciding whether individuals have a right to self-determination regarding this issue, it would be wise to consider why the concept is so popular. Modern death often involves overwhelming fiscal costs, pain, isolation among strangers, and the invasion of one's body by technology. Perhaps even more terrifying is the chance that one will not be allowed to die at all but continue in an elongated state of unconsciousness. Is it any wonder that a now-rather-than-later mentality has infected the population?

THE HOSPICE ALTERNATIVE

It is unlikely that the increased public acceptance of active euthanasia is based on any perceived need for an extension of personal autonomy to a "right to die." It is more likely that the genesis for the support is the fear of a lingering and painful death, surrounded by impersonal technicians, in a cold and unfamiliar environment.

If this is true, then the resurgent **hospice movement** may make some arguments in regard to active euthanasia moot. The word *hospice* has been used since medieval times to indicate a place of rest for the weary traveler. In the modern use of the term, the journey is different, but the concepts of rest and comfort are retained. The best-known hospice is St. Christopher's, in Great Britain, founded by Dr. Cicely Saunders in 1967. There are none of the usual trappings of a modern hospital. The rooms are cheerful, flowers are abundant, and the patients receive personalized care designed to virtually eliminate pain and suffering. Great effort is devoted to keeping the patient clean, caring for the skin, preventing bed sores, controlling nausea and vomiting, and treating neuropsychiatric symptoms. For the patient who is terminally ill, the balance between minimizing pain and suffering and the potential for hastening death is clearly struck in favor of relief of pain and suffering. Families are encouraged to stay all day and take their meals with the patients. Dying persons, when possible, are encouraged to take home visits whenever their stamina allows for them. The physicians and staff do not make rounds in white coats, ordering this and that, but rather there is a lot of touching, hand holding, and listening. The emphasis is on honest communication with both the patients and their family. The dying patient is freed from as much pain as possible and encouraged to face the situation of death with dignity. For dying patients, the need for **palliative care** to relieve pain and suffering may rival the intensity of curative efforts found in the acute hospital setting.

Hospice programs are set up to provide palliative care, abatement of pain, and an environment that encourages dignity, but they do not cure or treat intensively. Pain suppression at this moment in medical practice is not absolute. There is no sure way to guarantee absolute freedom from pain or the side effects of modern medication. A final problem with the programs is their current lack of availability; there are many more patients who need the services than local facilities to support them. Since its inception, the hospice has ceased to be a place and has become a concept. Individual hospices now come in a variety of forms: community volunteer programs, home services, free-standing units, in-hospital palliative care units, in-hospital hospice teams, or combinations of each. In these cases, it is important for all health care providers to set a tone of caring and support. It is not the technology found in the hospital setting that dehumanizes; it is the human component or lack thereof. The basic philosophy of hospice is that dying is a natural part of life. The first two National Hospice Organization standards are: "Appropriate therapy is the goal of hospice care," and "palliative care is the most appropriate care when cure is no longer possible."[21]

The hospice concept has been very effective in dealing with the terminally ill. These are specialized units designed to reduce suffering and provide humane care for the dying. The hospice movement, while developed in England, has blossomed in the United States.

CONCLUSION

In the United States, the practice of passive euthanasia for the terminally ill and in limited cases for those who persist in a chronic vegetative state has generally been accepted by the courts and health care practitioners. Under special circumstances, health care providers have found it ethically permissible to omit further life-extending technology and to allow patients to die. Given that the end results appear to be the same for passive and active euthanasia, many advocates of euthanasia have petitioned for the broadening of the practice to include the more active forms, wherein health care practitioners could assist in hastening the dying process. Active euthanasia, which includes mercy killing, is currently forbidden under law and by all professional codes of health care ethics in the United States.

The practice of active euthanasia has been legalized in the Netherlands. Although it is illegal in most United States jurisdictions, polls indicate a shift of public opinion to favor the practice of active euthanasia. The highly publicized Quinlan, Cruzan, and Bouvia cases coupled with the activities of such groups as the Hemlock Society have brought the issue to a level of public awareness that makes its legalization a distinct possibility in the next decade. The major concerns of those favoring the adoption of active euthanasia appear to be the fear of a painful lingering death as well as the desire to further the principle of personal autonomy to include a right to die.

It is clear that modern health care delivery as it addresses the end of life is a frightening consideration for many Americans. The thought of cold, sterile rooms, filled with cold professionals, invasive tubes and instruments, lingering unconsciousness, and great financial burden all seem part of this new way of dying. Our health care policies often make the elderly spend down to poverty in order to access the care they need, in the end leaving a surviving spouse destitute. If these are the factors that have led to the great interest in euthanasia, then would it be as appealing if the dying process were less cold and terrible? The answer may lie in reforming a broken system rather than ushering in the obiatrist.

The increased availability of hospice centers may offer some relief for terminally ill patients who fear a painful lingering death, isolated from loved ones, and surrounded by cold technology and technocrats. These centers specialize in palliative care in which patients are allowed to come to grips with their mortality, and to prepare themselves for death.

Those who oppose the acceptance of active euthanasia within health care do so generally using two lines of reasoning. First, there are those who oppose active euthanasia on the basis of the principle of sanctity of life. All life in this sense has infinite value, and therefore any portion of life also has infinite value, whether that be ten minutes or ten years. Others base their opposition on the feeling that allowing assisted euthanasia for the terminally ill might be the start of a slippery slope or a beginning wedge philosophy that, once begun, could lead to extermination of the elderly or the malformed.

The argument that allowing one kind of justifiable action could conceivably increase the tendency to allow another kind of unjustified action seems somewhat spurious, unless there is a natural tendency toward the second type of action. If adopted, the slippery slope argument could easily be used to avoid any new thinking and defend the status quo in all areas of our lives.

Whatever the convictions of health care providers, they should follow the current arguments in regard to euthanasia closely. Currently, in most jurisdictions within the United States, active euthanasia is illegal and considered homicide. Given the popular support for physician assisted suicide, the legal status may change, at which time our current codes of ethics will need to be rethought and modified if assisted death becomes legal, as in the Netherlands.

KEY CONCEPTS

- The withholding or withdrawing of life support in certain types of cases and allowing a deadly process to proceed without intervention is the basis of passive euthanasia. Passive euthanasia is a generally accepted practice in cases of futility and where no possibility of patient benefit exists.

- Active euthanasia, in which the health care provider takes actions that speed the process of dying, does not have ethical or legal support in the United States.

- Involuntary euthanasia, in which the patient had not indicated a desire to be assisted in death, is not easily differentiated from murder.

- The Netherlands is the only modern industrial nation that has legalized voluntary active euthanasia.

- The current U.S. Supreme Court position on a right to die is that it is not a right that can be construed from the U.S. Constitution. The position of the Court is that this matter should be determined through individual state legislation.

- The law in regard to mercy killing is unequivocal: personal motivation is not a defense in murder. The public has been particularly outraged when this practice involves those entrusted with health care.

- The hospice movement may offer relief for the terminally ill patient and lessen the need for legislating physician-assisted suicide or euthanasia.

REVIEW EXERCISES

A. In Shakespeare's *Julius Caesar,* Brutus asks his friend Volumnius to assist him in death, after he has suffered defeat in battle.

> Thou seest the world, Volumnius, how it goes;
> Our enemies have beat us to the pit:
> It is more worthy to leap in ourselves,
> Than tarry till they push us, Good Volumnius,
> Thou know'st that we two went to school together;
> Even for that our love of old, I prithee,
> Hold thou my sword-hilts whilst I run on it.
> Volumnius replies, "That's not an office for a friend,
> My Lord."[22]

One reason often given not to continue further down the path of active euthanasia and to adopt it as a practice by health care workers is similar to that offered by Volumnius. "Putting individuals to death is not an office of a health care provider." In her article, "Where Do You Stand on Euthanasia?" Amy Haddad[23] argues that active euthanasia would harm the nursing profession, as patients currently see nurses as nurturing, compassionate patient advocates. Would their participation in death inducement place their role as nurses at risk?

B. In 1921, George Minot, at the age of thirty-six, was found to have diabetes. Following the current medical practice of his time, he attempted to control his disease by diet; however, it was obvious that he was fighting a losing battle. In 1923, insulin became available, reversed his disease, and saved his life. Minot went on with his research, and in 1927, reported that the ingestion of large amounts of liver could bring about regeneration of red cells in the bone marrow. This became the first effective treatment for pernicious anemia and won for Minot the 1934 Nobel prize.

This anecdote is often used by those who oppose both active and passive euthanasia on the basis, "Suppose a cure is found?" Respond to the argument of the miraculous cure.

C. Popular publications such as *Final Exit*[24] are little more than "how to" books and deal with emotions such as depression in a very light manner. One could imagine a person suffering from depression using the book as a suicide manual. Assuming that we have decided to allow active euthanasia, what rules would you put into place to protect against its improper usage? Create five such rules.

D. Due to our general acceptance of the rule of law in our society, we might hear the argument that we should not practice euthanasia because it is an illegal act. Is this an ethical argument? Defend your answer.

E. Write five value statements that fit your beliefs about active euthanasia as a medical practice.

NOTES

1. Thomas Mapes and Jane Zembaty, *Social Ethics: Morality and Social Policy* (New York: McGraw Hill, Inc., 2001).

2. Ronald Munson, *Intervention and Reflection: Basic Issues in Medical Ethics* (Belmont, CA: Wadsworth, 1999), p. 142.

3. Tom Beauchamp, "What Is Suicide?" in *Ethical Issues in Death and Dying*, eds. T. Beauchamp and P. Seymour (Englewood Cliffs, NJ: Prentice Hall, 1978), pp. 97–102.

4. Jack Kevorkian, *Prescription: Medicide* (Buffalo: Prometheus Books, 1991). p. 196.

5. Arthur Caplan, "Disabled Women Are Victimized by Kevorkian," *Detroit Free Press,* June 9,1992, p. 2C.

6. *Notre Dame Lawyer* 48 (1973): pp. 1202–1260.

7. Edward Tivnan, *The Moral Imagination* (New York: Simon & Schuster, 1996).

8. W. J. Smith, "Going Dutch?" *National Review* 46, no. 19 (1994).

9. R. Fenigan, "A Case Against Dutch Euthanasia," *Hastings Center Report* 19 (1989).

10. D. Brock, "Voluntary Active Euthanasia," in *Ethical Issues in Modern Medicine*, eds. S. Arras and B. Steinbock (Mountain View, CA: Mayfield, 1995).

11. Arthur Caplan, "Sledding in Oregon," *Hastings Center Report,* June 2, 1992.

12. *Lee* v. *Oregon,* B69 F. Supp. 1491 (D. Or. 1991).

13. Joan Biskupic, "Unanimous Decision Points to Tradition of Valuing Life," *Washington Post,* June 27, 1997, PAO1.

14. James Rachels, *The End of Life* (Oxford: Oxford University Press, 1987).

15. Betty DeRamus, "Without a Clear Law, We Can't Point Fingers at Assisted Suicide," *Detroit News,* October 1991.

16. Name Withheld. "It's Over, Debbie," *Journal of the American Medical Association* 259, no. 2 (1988): p. 272.

17. Beatrice Yorker, "Nurses Accused of Murder," *American Journal of Nursing* (October 1988): pp. 1327–1332.

18. Joseph Fletcher, "The Right to Live and the Right to Die." *Humanist* 34, no. 4 (1974).

19. Arthur Dyck, "An Alternative to the Ethic of Euthanasia," in *To Live and Die, When, Why and How,* ed. R. Williams (New York: Springer-Verlag, 1974).

20. Sigmund Freud, "Thoughts for the Times on War and Death, 1915, in *Collected Papers,* Vol. IV (London: Hogarth Press, 1925).

21. National Hospice Organization, Standards and Accreditation Committee, *Standards of a Hospice Program*, McLean, VA, 1979.

22. William Shakespeare, *Julius Caesar* (New York: Dover Publications, Inc., 1991).

23. Amy Haddad, "Where Do You Stand on Euthanasia" *RN* (April 1991): p. 43.

24. Humphry, *Final Exit*.

CHAPTER 11

Reproductive Issues

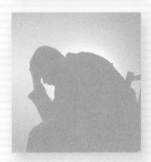

GOAL

To outline the nature of a variety of ethical issues surrounding human reproduction, including the conflict between the pro-life (anti-abortion) position and the pro-choice position (not necessarily pro-abortion, but against legislation outlawing abortion).

OBJECTIVES

Upon completion of this chapter, the reader should be able to:

1. Outline the distinction between "human" and "person," and the dispute regarding personhood criteria.

2. Describe the distinction between the quality of life and life itself.

3. List the basic facts of fetal development.

4. Outline the religious arguments against abortion.

5. Argue the issue of rights from a utilitarian understanding.

6. List the difficulties with arguments based on self-defense.

7. List the elements of the doctrine of double-effect and state when it is used.

8. Outline the significance of Thomson's analogies.

9. List the freedom of religion arguments.

10. Explain the pro-choice position from a "life plan" point of view.

11. State how an environmental perspective might affect your understanding of the abortion issue.

12. Explain how issues of civil disobedience are involved in the politics of abortion.

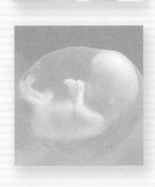

13. Explain the process of in vitro fertilization and list the ethical issues involved.

14. Provide pro and con arguments for the issue of surrogacy.

15. Outline the ethical issues surrounding in vitro fertilization.

16. Outline the ethical issues involved with the practice of surrogacy.

KEY TERMS

Conceptus (single-celled zygote)	Fetus	Speciesism
Double effect	Person	Viability
Embryo	Quickening	Zygote (multicelled zygote)

THE ABORTION ISSUE

The states are not free, under the guise of protecting maternal health or potential life, to intimidate women into continuing pregnancies.

Justice Harry A. Blackmun, Roe v. Wade, 22 January 1973

There is no difference between a first trimester, a second trimester, a third trimester abortion or infanticide. It's all the same human being in different stages of development. I finally got to the point I couldn't look at those tiny bodies anymore.

Dr. Arnold Halpern, former director of a Planned Parenthood clinic

If the anti-abortion movement took a tenth of the energy they put into noisy theatrics and devoted it to improving the lives of children who have been born into lives of poverty, violence, and neglect, they could make a world shine.

Michael Jay Tucker

The majority of women getting abortions are young. Fifty-two percent are younger than 25 years and 19 percent are teenagers. The abortion rate is highest for those women aged 18 to 19. Fifty-one percent of women who are unmarried at the time they became pregnant will elect to receive an abortion. Sixty percent of abortions are performed on woman who already have one or more children. Forty-seven percent of abortions are performed on women who have already had one or more abortions. Sixty-three percent of the abortion patients are white, however, black women are more than 3 times as likely to have an abortion, and Hispanic women are 2.5 times as likely. Forty-three percent of the women claimed they were Protestant, while 27 percent claimed they were Catholic.

For all the controversy surrounding the process, abortion is a very common experience for women. In 2001, 1.31 million abortions took place in the United States. Forty-three percent of all American women will have had at least one abortion by the time they are 45 years of age. Figure 11-1 lists the common reasons given for having an abortion. The reasons given for having an abortion are diverse and complex, ranging from concern for the health of the mother or fetus to *"I'd be looking at that dumb man's face in that child and resenting it."* For some women, the abortion came as a deep relief. Others report the experience to be devastating. Whatever the reason given, the experience of having an abortion is real, immediate, and personal. It is interesting to note that the rate of abortions has been in decline since the early 90s. According to a *USA Today*, CNN Gallup Poll in May, 1999, 16 percent of Americans believe abortions should be legal for any reason, at any time during pregnancy and 55 percent of Americans believe abortion should be legal only to save the life of the mother or in cases of rape or incest. In a Gallup Poll in January 2001, people who considered themselves to be pro-life rose from 33 percent to 43 percent in the past five years, and people who considered themselves to be pro-choice declined from 56 percent to 48 percent.[1] However, even this statistic raises a dispute as to whether the decline is a result of demographic forces, a drop in facilities performing the procedure, or changing social values.

Recently, there has been a heated debate in regard to a form of late-term abortion. As with many of these arguments, the advocates have not even managed to decide what to name the procedure in question. Pro-choice advocates favor *intact dilation and evacuation,* and pro-life advocates use the term *partial birth abortion.* It is estimated that perhaps 600 third-trimester abortions are performed each year. Most of these have involved lethal anomalies or danger to the health of the mother. The American Medical Association has supported limiting this form of abortion as it is a procedure that is never the only appropriate procedure and has no history in peer-reviewed medical literature or in accepted medical practice development.[2]

- 26.6%—want to postpone childbearing
- 21.3%—cannot afford a baby
- 14.1%—have a relationship issue or partner does not want child
- 12.2%—too young (parents or others object)
- 10.8%—child will disrupt education or career
- 7.9%—do not want more children
- 3.3%—risk to fetal health
- 2.8%—risk to maternal health

FIGURE 11-1   Reasons for Abortion

THE LEGAL DEBATE

Until 1973, except in cases where the mother's life was in danger, abortion was a statutory crime in every state of the nation. In *Roe* v. *Wade*, the Supreme Court, relying on the constitutional right of privacy emanating from the word *liberty* in the due process clause of the Fourteenth Amendment, legalized a woman's right to have an abortion. However, this right was not considered to be unrestricted, and the Court recognized the state's legitimate interest in protecting health, prenatal life, and the standard of medical practice.

The Court's decision balanced the interests of the woman and the state, allowing the woman greater freedom of action in the beginning of the pregnancy and the state a greater right to regulate the process as the fetus developed. In the decision, the court divided pregnancy into three trimesters of twelve weeks each. In the first trimester, the state has little right to regulate the process, and the decision is that of the woman and her physician. During the second trimester, the state's interest increases, at least in the area of protecting the health of the woman. Only those regulations that are directed toward this concern will be upheld as legitimate. This is somewhat problematic to those who feel that human life begins with **quickening**, as this usually occurs within the second trimester. One of the arguments against abortion was that fetuses, especially after quickening, are persons and deserved the protection under the Fourteenth Amendment. However, the Court ruled that the term *person* was used historically only postnatally. The third trimester, which begins at the twenty-eighth week of gestation, is where the Court allowed the state to shift its interest to the protection of the fetus. The fetus has reached a point of potential viability outside the womb, and the dominant interest of the state after the twenty-eighth week becomes the protection of this potential life. The Court held that once viable, the fetus cannot be aborted except in those cases where the procedure is essential for the protection of the woman's life.[3]

With the *Roe* v. *Wade* decision, the Court set off a firestorm of public debate as citizens and state legislatures attempted to gain an understanding of the dimensions of the ruling and either resist or embrace its potential outcomes.[4] One important case that made clear the primacy of the woman's rights in the first trimester, was the 1976 *Danforth* v. *Planned Parenthood of Central Missouri* case. In this case, the Supreme Court examined a statutory provision that required a woman to receive her husband's, or if a minor, her parent's or guardian's, permission prior to having an abortion. The Court held that these requirements were unconstitutional given that they imposed restrictions within the first trimester, a time when the decision was left in the hands of the woman and her physician. In regard to the issue of minors, the Court held that, like adults, minors had a constitutional right to privacy, although the scope of that protection might differ.[5]

The *Roe* v. *Wade* decision that provided women with a right to have an abortion is essentially a negative right in that it provides liberty only from interference. This liberty is somewhat like having an equal right with all others to determine what shall or shall not be done to or with one's body. The right to noninterference does not in itself create the reciprocal obligations for others to provide the means for an abortion. This has been an important battleground between pro-life and pro-choice advocates. In 1976, Congress enacted the Hyde amendment, which restricted the availability of Medicare funding for abortions. Under challenge, the amendment was modified to allow funding for abortions in those cases in which the mother's life was threatened by carrying the fetus full term or in cases of incest or rape when the incidents had been reported to appropriate governmental agencies.[6]

Pro-life forces took encouragement from the Hyde amendment. They continued to mobilize campaigns in order to defeat politicians who supported legalized abortion. Critics of the amendment objected that while abortion was still legal, it had become the privilege of the rich. They asked what a "right" to an abortion meant if you are too poor to afford the necessary services. When you ask this question, you are making an appeal to consideration under the principle of justice. Accordingly, they felt that it was the responsibility of a just society to ensure the value of an individual's rights by guaranteeing access to necessary resources. The reality of the question was reinforced by the tragic death in McAllen, Texas, of Rosaura Jiminez, a twenty-seven-year-old mother of a five-year-old child. Unable to access Medicaid for an abortion, she died in pain at the hands of a local abortionist. Rosaura was the first recorded death by illegal abortion following the passage of the Hyde amendment.

Decisions such as the *Webster* v. *Reproductive Health Services* case,[7] in which the Court held that a state could ban public employees and public health facilities from performing or assisting in performing nontherapeutic abortions, gave an indication that the Supreme Court was shifting toward a more conservative stance in regard to the abortion issue. This provided the pro-life advocates with hope that the Court would, in the future, further erode the 1973 *Roe* v. *Wade* decision.

The administration of George H. W. Bush, on January 29, 1988, barred most family planning clinics that received federal funding from providing abortion assistance or counseling.[8] This gag order became a major ethical concern within the health care community as it interposed the government between the patient and the provider. The community began to question what effect this artificial barrier had on the principle of informed consent and patient and provider autonomy. In response to the criticism of the policy, Congress passed a bill allowing abortion to be discussed as an option. However, this was vetoed by President Bush. One of the first actions of the Clinton presidency was to sign executive orders that partially overturned the gag rule, lifted the ban on the use of fetal tissue in federally funded research, and ordered a review of the prohibition on the French abortifacient RU 486. The Clinton administration lifted the barrier to federal aid for family planning centers, which offered abortion counseling, and ended the ban against overseas military hospitals performing abortions if they were paid for by private funds. In 1992, a panel of the U.S. Circuit Court of Appeals for the District of Columbia rejected the gag rule regulation issued by the Bush administration. The appeals court panel held that the administration had acted improperly and had issued the regulation without allowing for the traditional period of public comment.[9]

The abortion issue still continues to be hotly contested, and it is likely to become even more explosive as positions are stated and restated, and patience and tolerance for the views of others wane. Civil disobedience, harassment, and vandalism are increasingly prevalent across the nation as more traditional methods of changing laws and minds have been exhausted.

The main framework of *Roe* v. *Wade* is still in place and is the law of the land, in spite of the fears of those who thought that judges appointed by Reagan and Bush would attempt to reopen the case and rethink the issue. We are in the midst of a struggle of titanic proportions with neither side being able to gain a clear victory. Rules that are promulgated by one group when it gains political power are often overturned when the political tide turns.

The unfortunate level of violence with the death of physicians, attendants, and bystanders is an escalation that speaks poorly for all involved.[10] It is a hollow moral victory when pro-life advocates proclaim that fewer and fewer physicians are willing to perform abortions when the basis for their decision may be fear of physical harm for themselves and their families. On the other hand, there is little high ground when, on the basis of privacy, human life is trivialized by those who decide upon an abortion because they do not like the gender of the fetus. It must seem clear that after over three decades of political and legal struggle, the matter of abortion is one that cannot be decided by legal fiat or shifting political fortunes. We must in the end reason together if we are to bind our wounds. If either side is to truly "win," it should be by the force of their moral argument, not because they were able to coerce public opinion on a given day.

THE MORAL ISSUES

The abortion issue involves many of the same concepts that underlie the issues of euthanasia and impaired infants. In each of these issues, there are disputes concerning personhood, sanctity of life, quality of life, autonomy, and mercy—as well as larger concepts such as freedom and social stability. The health care professional is often placed in situations that involve adjudicating among these concepts, and more often is placed in situations in which others make decisions using these concepts. The fact that others make these decisions does not mean the health care professional can ignore them, for he or she is often put in the position of carrying out the decisions. So even if one has no role in the decision-making process, one may need to come to terms with actions that may be morally controversial and emotionally heartrending.

The Two Positions

The pro-life position: Anti-abortion, believes abortion is murder and should be stopped.

The pro-choice position: Believes that the decision to abort is one of personal liberty and thus should be legal.

There are two possible subpositions:

1. One may believe that abortion is wrong but, for whatever reason, is something that should be up to every individual to decide. The issue becomes an individual or personal decision.
2. One may believe there is nothing wrong with abortion or that, while abortion is wrong, it can be outweighed by other considerations.

Sanctity of Life Argument

At its most basic level, the argument for a sanctity of life position would be that the fetus is a live human and, therefore, killing him or her is wrong. Even sanctity of life positions generally allow for a few exceptions. Self-defense is a widely accepted exception to the "thou shalt not kill" proscription. Generally, it is held that if someone is trying to kill you, and the only way in which you can save yourself is by killing the other person first, that action of defense is justifiable. Some have used the self-defense argument as a reason to allow abortions in cases where the mother's life is endangered by the pregnancy. Others refute this by pointing out that self-defense is permissible only when the attacker is intending to kill you. If a hungry lion was attacking you, it would not be permissible to throw others in its path so as to satiate its hunger and escape being eaten.

Human life is thought to be sacred, or at least inviolable, on the basis of divine mandate, unalienable natural or human rights, or common collective decision. It seems a strange question, but what do we mean when we say *human*? Some argue that having a genetic code of a human being is what is essential. Others argue against this position, stating that the genetic code is not sufficient to establish humanity (acorns have the genetic code of the oak tree, yet we do not confuse the two). This dispute raises the question, Does the potential for becoming a human give an entity the same rights as a human being? Even if we accept that the fetus is a human, we often distinguish the rights of humans based on their age. A twelve year old does not have a right to drive, although he certainly has the potential to do so. Nor do minors have the right to drink, smoke cigarettes, or see X-rated movies. We do not generally provide for our children the rights and privileges that we allow the president of the United States, even though we teach them that they can potentially grow up to attain that position.

There are other problems with the genetic code argument. Down syndrome babies do not have the same genetic structure as other human beings; in fact, it is the cause of their condition. Does this mean that they do not have a right to life? The pro-life advocate would respond that a human genetic code is a sufficient but not a necessary condition of beings with a right to life. Thus, other entities may also have a right to life, but one with a human genetic code, in all its varieties, definitely has such a right.

Another question is, When does the right to life exert itself? When does it come into existence? Does the right to life come into existence with conception, with the establishment of measurable brain waves, at quickening, at viability, or upon entrance to the outside world? Figure 11-2 provides the stages of fetal development.

The Facts of Fetal Development

The next set of issues requires some discussion of the facts of fetal development. The union of the sperm and egg gives us what is called a **conceptus**. At that point, the **zygote** has a full genetic code that will determine the sex, hair color, skin color, and a variety of other attributes. At about two or three weeks, the zygote settles into the uterine wall and enters the stage in which it is described as an **embryo**. Pro-choice advocates often point out that the embryo at this stage of development is very dissimilar to what we consider human, having what appears to be a tail and gills. Pro-life advocates would quickly point out that it is a morally dangerous position taken when we base moral judgment on appearance and that whatever is there is human.

At about eight weeks, we call the entity a **fetus**, a term that will extend until birth. By the second trimester, the fetus will normally have begun to move, and the mother will be able to sense the movement at a point that is known as *quickening*. It was once believed that the fetus gained a soul at the point of quickening, but given that the event does not correspond to any major

- **Conception**—The penetration of the egg by the sperm is usually followed twenty-two hours later by syngamy, the alignment of maternal and paternal chromosomes to form a new genotype.

- **Implantation Complete**—In about fourteen days the zygote settles into the uterine wall and enters a stage when it is described as an embryo.

- **Fetus**—At about eight weeks the first neural cells start differentiating. The entity is known as a fetus; it will continue with this description until birth.

- **Distinct human form**—This occurs at about weeks 12 to 16. The fetus in this period responds to stimulation and may feel pain.

- **Quickening**—Occurs at about weeks 17 to 20.

- **Viability**—With modern technology, viability is reached by weeks 22 to 24.

- **Birth**—Normally occurs at 9 months.

FIGURE 11-2   Stages of Human Embryo Development

medical changes, most have disregarded the moment of being able to sense the motion of the fetus as important to the abortion issue. By the fifth month, neurologically, the fetus can feel pain, and therefore at least enters into a status that we afford all creatures that feel pain. In the sixth month, the fetus enters a period of potential viability, where it could possibly survive apart from the mother. Neurologically, the fetus also develops minimal consciousness during this last trimester.

Birth generally occurs after nine months, but the infant at this point is still completely dependent on the mother, or at least some mother. Pro-life theorists argue that there is very little difference between the fetus prior to birth and the infant at the moment of birth. It is left up to the pro-choice advocates to come up with an argument that would explain how the newborn has a right to life that somehow was not present in a fetus five minutes prior to birth. Since the changes are so gradual throughout development of the fetus, it is difficult to point to a stage that clearly separates a human from a pre-human.

Killing and Self-Defense

Up to this point we have assumed that killing is always wrong. But it is not true that all killing of human beings is impermissible, for there is a widely accepted exception: self-defense. If someone is about to kill you, and the only way to save yourself is to kill the other person first, then killing is permissible, at least for most people. Some believe that this means we should allow abortions when the mother's life is in danger. Others point out that killing in self-defense is permissible only when your attacker is intentionally trying to kill you. You may not, for example, kill an innocent person who threatens your life by accident. You cannot shove an innocent person in front of a speeding car in order to save yourself.

The problem with the moral assessment of such actions arises from what we may call the "multiple character" of most actions. When I turn on a light, I am not only providing illumination to a room; I may also be signaling an accomplice, testing the electricity, or any number of things. One attempt to come to terms with such complex actions—actions that have more than one meaning or consequence—focuses on the multiple character of human action. The doctrine of **double effect** comes to us from the philosopher St. Thomas Aquinas. The doctrine asks us to distinguish the intended effect of an action from other, unintended effects. This doctrine has been used to justify the death of fetuses under certain circumstances that threaten the life of the mother. Ovarian cancer sometimes must be treated with a full hysterectomy, and such an operation results in the death of the fetus. Note that the intention here is to save the mother, not to kill the fetus. Note also that it would be impermissible, according to this doctrine, to perform an abortion to save a mother from death if the procedure involved the direct killing of the fetus. It is permissible only if the death of the fetus is an indirect cause of the death of the fetus. Figure 11-3 provides the criteria for the doctrine of double effect.

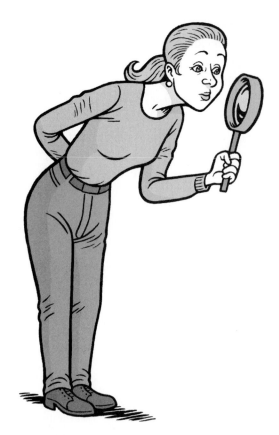

- The course chosen must be good or at least morally neutral.
- The good must not follow as a consequence of the secondary harmful effects.
- The harm must never be intended but merely tolerated as causally connected with the good intended.
- The good must outweigh the harm.

FIGURE 11-3 Doctrine of Double Effect

"Human" or "Person"?

Mary Anne Warren has argued for a distinction between "human" and "person."[11] While one is human by virtue of one's genetic code, a **person** is a member of the moral community. One becomes a member of the moral community by having certain characteristics recognized by the community as grounded in moral status and, in particular, rights. There are various characteristics that might qualify one for personhood. The following list of traits central to personhood is worth consideration:

1. Consciousness of objects and events
2. The ability to feel pain
3. Reasoning
4. Self-motivated activity

The Violinist Analogy. Thomson asks us to imagine a famous violinist whose kidneys are failing (Figure 11-4). The Society of Music Lovers, we are also asked to imagine, decides to kidnap you in the middle of the night and hook you up to the violinist for nine months or so until a kidney donor can be found. Thomson asks us whether we would feel obligated to remain hooked to the violinist for nine months or whether we would consider it morally permissible to unhook ourselves from the violinist. She anticipates that our answer will be that it is permissible to unhook ourselves because of our rights over our own bodies. The application to the abortion issue is clear. If it is morally permissible to unhook ourselves from the violinist, then, by the same reasoning, it must also be permissible to have an abortion, and this is true even if we regard the fetus as a person.

One might argue that there is a disanalogy involved, for pregnancy is not like a kidnapping. Rather, it is voluntary. Fair enough. However, what about the case of rape? Rape is, by definition, involuntary, yet many regard abortion in rape cases to be just as wrong as in voluntary pregnancies, since it is not the baby's fault it was brought about involuntarily. Such people

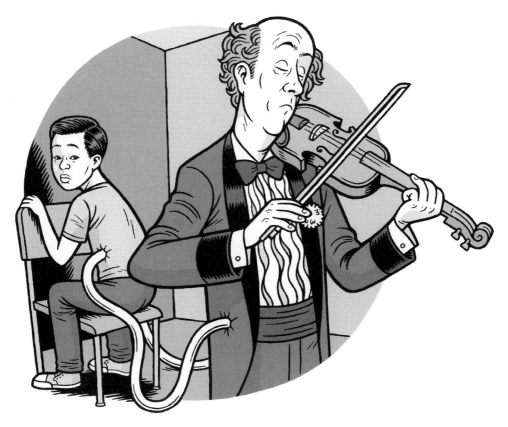

FIGURE 11-4

must therefore agree to staying hooked to the violinist for nine months. Some are willing to "bite this bullet," but many others will find themselves in a contradictory position. Notice, though, that if we are not willing to bite the bullet, we are then obligated to agree that there is at least one case when personhood may be overridden for other reasons. This is crucial, since it provides a wedge for the pro-choice person to slip an exception into the otherwise impregnable right to life of innocent persons. Once we accept this exception, so the reasoning goes, we will also be forced to accept others.

The Rapidly Growing Child Analogy. This analogy attempts to call attention to the case of abortion when the mother's life is in danger. Imagine yourself in a house with a rapidly growing child. In fact, the child is growing so rapidly that you find your exits blocked by the baby and on the verge of suffocation. The only way for you to survive is for you to kill the baby. Again, Thomson believes we will agree that killing an innocent is permissible in this case. Hence, we have another exception to the right to life of innocent persons. This case, like the one we have just considered, has problems. Is it true that it is acceptable to kill innocent people in order to save ourselves? Consider another case. You find yourself caught in a flooding tunnel and the only exit is blocked by a fat man who is lodged in the exit. The water will eventually force him out, but you will have drowned by that time. Would you be within your rights if you used dynamite to dislodge and therefore kill the fat man? Many, if not most, would say that doing so is not permissible. The argument would be that it is only right to kill in self-defense, when the other person is intentionally trying to kill you. But this does not work either, for most would regard it as permissible to kill a deranged man in self-defense even though the person is not responsible for his insanity. The only thing clear here is that self-defense cases are far from morally unambiguous. What is interesting, in spite of the ambiguity of the reasoning behind self-defense, is that the vast majority of people regard saving the life of the mother a clear case of permissible abortion. There is a vocal minority, however, who would make distinctions between cases of danger to the mother's life, namely those enamored with the doctrine of double effect.

The Carpet-Seed Children Analogy. The final analogy we will borrow from Thomson is meant to call attention to the case of failed contraception. Imagine that instead of the reproductive process being as we understand it, children are the result of airborne seeds that germinate in carpeting. We can imagine that people will be rather concerned to make sure their screens are in good working order. But we can also imagine that in spite of such diligence, holes develop in one of our screens and some seeds germinate in our carpet. Are we obligated to bring these children to term, or would we be permitted to get the vacuum cleaner from the closet (Figure 11-5)? Thomson thinks that vacuuming should be permitted. The analogy, as we have indicated, is with faulty contraception.

If one is inclined to agree to vacuuming up the carpet-seed children, one should also agree to abortion in the case of faulty contraception. The idea is that we are not responsible for unintended pregnancies if we take reasonable precautions. This brings us to the rather large topic of women's choice, on which pro-choice theorists rest so much of their case.

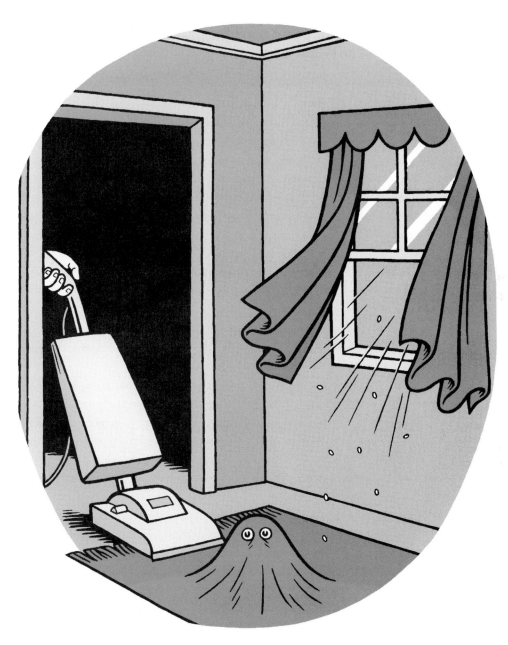

FIGURE 11-5

The Argument from Women's Liberty and the Priority of the Lifeplan

For many women, it is unthinkable to imagine a woman not having the decision of whether to continue a pregnancy. They argue that if a woman is to be free, she must have control over her reproduction, and that, given the immense responsibility of raising children, it is crucial that women be allowed to determine when it happens. Others counter that adoption is always another option, which brings the obligation down to nine months, much of which does not really interfere with a person's life. (However, it is important to note that adoption does not really work as an alternative to abortion since there are roughly 1 million abortions every year but only 50,000 couples waiting to adopt.) But the pro-choice person will respond that even this asks too much of a woman. If a woman is to compete in the marketplace with men, she cannot have pregnancy interrupting her career. To regard a woman's career—or more generally her life plan—as having so little importance that it must be set aside by the contingency of unwanted pregnancy is to regard women as less important than men. This is true whether the woman works at home or in the marketplace. What is crucial is that a woman have control over her life plan in the way a man has control. If your plan is to raise two children, then to impose a third is to violate the woman's right to choose the course of her life. This is what leads many women to say that if men became pregnant, there would be no abortion controversy.

At this point, pro-life people argue that women can "just say no." Women do not have to engage in sex. In fact, it is argued that the root of the abortion problem is precisely the modern attitude toward sex. Notice that we are now in another area of intense and deep disagreement. What we find at this level of argument are differing ideas concerning sexuality, ideas that ultimately come down to one's religious or most deeply held moral beliefs. We will discuss this broad topic later in the chapter, for now we must point out that even married women want the choice as to the time of pregnancy.

Some might argue that we are making altogether too much of the possibility of failed contraception, and that if women were merely responsible with contraception, there would be no problem. The problem with this argument is that even the pill sometimes fails, and further, many women either cannot take the pill at all or are advised not to take the pill longer than five years. Contraception other than the pill is rather less effective, and unwanted pregnancies are bound to happen. We must also remember what it is we are asking of people. We are asking that they act perfectly rationally in situations that we all know to bring out a great deal of irrationality. This is, of course, less of a problem the older we get, but the abortion issue is not one just for adults; it is one that is most tragic for minors. According to the Alan Guttmacher Institute, more than 25 percent of abortions are performed on teenagers. More than 60 percent of the females are under twenty-five.

It is in this light that we must understand why there are so many abortions. Take, for example, the typical first sexual experience for many children. Much of the time, intercourse is not on the evening's agenda, but as the night progresses, things get too hot and heavy for many teenagers to resist. Since intercourse was not planned, it is also unlikely that the teens thought ahead to bring contraceptives. Again, we must notice what we are asking of children: to behave with complete rationality in an unfamiliar situation in which their bodies' hormones are working against rationality. Now it is true that this problem can be somewhat overcome if we supply all teenagers with contraceptives, as well as sex education before they reach the age of sexuality. But many, if not most, abortion opponents would reject such practices as encouraging promiscuity.

In any case, we should not rely on the fear of pregnancy to play much of a role in preventing promiscuity. We should also respond to the idea that "if you play, you pay." The idea here is that if you consent to sex and get pregnant, it is only just. This sort of vindictiveness has no place in moral philosophy, and it certainly makes no sense from the social point of view. Should we regard children as punishment? Some argue that the task of raising a child is too difficult and demanding to turn it over to someone who is regarded as irresponsible in the first place. No one believes that "babies should have babies"; the question is how to prevent it. Given the well-known cycle of poverty of under-age, single mothers, the overriding social problem according to pro-choice theorists is teenage pregnancy, not abortion. The crucial question concerns our overall quality of life rather than biological existence. It is pointed out, for example, that 62 percent of the families of the women who have abortions have incomes well below the poverty line. So, if these children come to term, they will end up growing up in difficult circumstances and making the job of getting out of poverty more difficult for those who will raise them.

Pro-choice advocates worry about the inevitable "backstreet abortion" if abortion is made illegal, and they also worry about the quality of women's lives if they are denied the basic autonomy of reproductive self-control. The pro-life theorist, on the other hand, will see the social problem as just another manifestation of the rampant immorality of the modern age. The pro-life theorist will argue that it is quite possible to grow up "decent" in a poor household, and that to believe otherwise is to be elitist. The pro-life advocate considers the element of autonomy in reproduction more of a matter of "convenience" than a life plan that has priority over the continued existence of the fetus. It should be clear from this radical disagreement over the value of women's reproductive autonomy that we are dealing with deep-seated moral beliefs. The one side believes that self-realization through the development of one's life plan (one's "biographical life") is all important, while the pro-life theorist points to the sanctity of human "biological life." This radical disagreement over basic beliefs makes it possible to understand the violent emotions that have been unleashed in the political battle over abortion.

POLITICAL TACTICS: CIVIL DISOBEDIENCE AT THE CLINIC

In March 1993, Michael Griffin shot and killed Dr. David Gunn, an abortion doctor, outside an abortion clinic in Pensacola, Florida. This most extreme of actions shocked the nation as well as activists on both sides of the issue but was hardly unexpected, given the intensity of the abortion debate. The ever-increasing acrimony, as well as positions unlikely to change, has set the stage for even more violent action. Whatever one thinks of individuals such as Michael Griffin, the conclusion he came to is easy enough to understand: If one is completely certain that the fetus is a person, and if millions of these people are being killed, it takes only utilitarian reasoning to arrive at the conclusion that killing one person to save hundreds is morally defensible. A proponent of this form of reasoning is Randall Terry, the leader of Operation Rescue, a militant anti-abortion group. Upon hearing what Griffin had done he remarked, "We will not be outraged over the one death and not the other 4,000 precious human beings killed today by abortion."[15]

Most people find an obvious contradiction in Griffin's actions. Killing someone because that person has killed also implicates oneself. We must also remember that utilitarian reasoning is not open to Griffin, since the basis for his action was a biblical commandment. When Time magazine entitled its story "Thou Shalt Not Kill," the editors clearly meant to elicit our sense of contradiction.[16] The biblical commandment is unambiguous; there are no exceptions for a greater good.

Although the pro-choice camp has as yet refrained from violent action to protect the right of choice, it is not hard to imagine that such a response could be forthcoming as the other side grows increasingly violent. Clearly, what is needed is a plea for tolerance and a deeper understanding of why attitudes toward abortion lead to such emotional disagreement.

Short of totally eliminating them, there have also been attempts by pro-life forces to reduce the number of abortions. The Hyde amendment of 1980 cut off government funding for Medicaid abortions. The reasoning was that since pro-life people pay taxes, they should have the right to restrict the spending of their tax money to moral purposes. There is also what has been called "the gag rule." Until Clinton became president and eliminated it, doctors were not allowed to offer abortion as an alternative to pregnant women. We are likely to see laws coming into and out of effect as pro-choice and pro-life politicians come into and out of office.

TRADITIONALISM VS. MODERNISM

The abortion issue is just the most obvious point of conflict between people with different worldviews. There have been studies of the social backgrounds of pro-life and pro-choice activists, and the results are revealing. Pro-life activists tend to be more traditional and religious.

They believe that sex should be reserved for marriage, if not merely for procreation. Pro-choice activists tend to be less traditional and religious, more career oriented with higher incomes. They also tend to believe that sex is a natural expression of oneself. What is clear is that we have the well-known conflict between conservative traditionalists and liberal modernists. The former are distrustful of deviations from tradition and see society's problems as the result of straying from the traditional mores. Pro-choice activists, on the other hand, see the social problems as a result of traditionalists' failing to realize the changing of the times. They argue that it is precisely the traditionalist rejection of sex education and contraception that is the source of the problem. In the modernists' view, there would be many fewer abortions if these reforms were allowed to be instituted without resistance. For traditionalists, it is only their own resistance to the full implementation of the liberal program that prevents wholesale chaos and immorality. But since we are already in a "chaotic" situation, pro-life advocates are relying rather heavily on the possibility of a religious revival that many would resist.

Another point of view of the traditionalism versus modernism perspective on abortion is possible. Some would argue that the pro-life position is actually the more progressive of the two. The argument tries to place the attempt to give rights to the fetus within the line of development we have seen in the civil rights and women's movements. Just as people realized that African Americans, women, and homosexuals deserve the same rights as heterosexual white males, it is argued, we must extend the liberalizing program to the fetus.

ABORTION AND THE FREEDOM OF RELIGION

Given that the abortion disagreement lies so deep in our religious and moral frameworks, we are led to ask whether abortion should be regarded as a case of religious disagreement and therefore subject to the constitutional guarantee of freedom of religion. If one's view of abortion is really a result of one's religious beliefs, it would seem that the government should play no role in restricting it. It should come as no surprise that pro-life theorists reject the idea that their views on abortion are the result of their religious views but rather maintain that they are the result of basic moral reasoning. They point to the fact that while the above characterization of pro-choice and pro-life activists is true, it is also true that many nonreligious people and members of the more liberal religious sects are also opposed to abortion. They also point out that freedom of religion is not absolute. One cannot murder or steal and then argue that it should be allowed because it is part of his or her religion. Since the issue is whether abortion is murder, the freedom of religion does not come into play.

Pro-choice theorists argue that even if disagreement on abortion cuts across the various religions, as well as atheism, it is still the case that the issue is one that lies rather deep—as deep as any other religious views one might have. Abortion views tend to reflect one's most deeply held beliefs, so even if the views are not religious in the partisan sense, they are equally profound. It is argued that the disagreement is so profound that the best solution would be the same one that resulted from the religious wars of earlier centuries: tolerance.

Many people see tolerance as the best way out of our present situation. It is unlikely that one side is going to come up with an argument that will cause the opponents to suddenly "see the light" and switch sides. One problem with this continuing controversy over abortion is the way that it skews politics. People are more and more becoming one-issue voters rather than assessing the candidates' positions on all of the issues. We may also be losing good candidates because they live in areas in which the majority has a different view on the abortion issue. On the other hand, some argue that one's abortion stance is crucial to determining whether a politician understands the changing needs of women and modern social conditions generally (pro-choice) or the decline in moral standards (pro-life).

THE ENVIRONMENTAL PERSPECTIVE

Recall Thomson's carpet-seed children, whereby we tried to imagine children being the result of airborne seeds. Such a possibility is certainly far-fetched, but it does bring up an important point: that it is a contingent result of the evolutionary process that we have as many children as we do. One can easily imagine humans reproducing like frogs and many other creatures and giving birth to thousands of offspring in order to survive as a species in a situation of high infant mortality. One can also imagine that as humans advanced, they could eventually overcome the environmental forces that make it necessary to have so many offspring. Imagine that the only way to prevent our froglike humans from developing into adults is abortion. In such a case not only would it be permissible to have abortions, it would probably be necessary since the world would otherwise be quickly overpopulated. It would be necessary, also, if we were to have anything like the family structure that we have now. The suggestion is that human life, at least in its early stages, is not as valuable as some make it out to be. What would turn out to be more important would be a strong family structure. Once a family was ready to commit to a child, the sanctity of life would come into play, but fetuses would have very little value without such commitment. This is in line with an environmental perspective that sees humans as members of a biotic community with duties to maintain a balance of numbers with other members of that community.

In the People's Republic of China today, the government restricts families in most instances to one child. Severe social sanctions are imposed upon couples who attempt to avoid this dictum, and abortion is considered patriotic. The Chinese government in this instance is attempting to control the nation's population growth to allow for a continued improvement of the quality of life for all citizens. Although the Chinese restrictions on individual reproduction are a severe example, there are many individuals throughout the world who believe that an environmental perspective requires that we maintain and perhaps even encourage the use of abortion as a tool to control world population. One cannot derive a right to an abortion directly from the need to curb population growth—contraception seems better for a number of reasons—however, an aggressive attitude toward family planning fits well with an attitude of respect for nature. Pro-choice advocates often point out that many in the pro-life movement are anti-abortion and anti-contraceptive but do not have the same level of emotional commitment to advocating against the death penalty. This has led many to see pro-life people as pro-birth rather than truly pro-life.

THE FAMILY PLANNING PERSPECTIVE

The family planning perspective also asks why we should favor accidental babies over planned babies. What gives a baby who happens to be conceived when a woman is the age of eighteen more right to life than the one she would have had at twenty-eight? Given that people have the right to choose the size of their family—something that will be necessary in the long run anyway—it makes sense that they should also have the right to choose at what point they will have their children. Optimally, people want children to come when the family is financially and emotionally stable. Marriage is difficult enough without the added strain of unwanted children. Given the social problems of poverty, single parenthood, child abuse, and so on, some argue that it may be time to reconsider what is really important to the family structure.

A pro-life perspective would regard such a point of view as absurd and maybe even horrifying. Once a baby is conceived, it is a person in their view, thus possessing a right to life. In such a frame of reference, it makes no sense to compare this baby with a possible baby ten years from now. Rights belong only to existing beings. The pro-life view would see family planning as another example of the decadent culture of permissiveness.

IN VITRO FERTILIZATION

On July 25, 1978, a few days before term, a baby described by her doctors as being "nice, healthy, normal," was born and given the name of Louise Brown. The only thing not normal was that Louise had been conceived outside the human body in a laboratory dish and then implanted in her mother. Her birth received enormous press attention as the world was alerted to the birth of the first "test tube baby." Actually the term is somewhat misleading; she should perhaps have been titled the first "test tube embryo," which was then followed by the "first embryo transfer" into the mother. The normal medical expression used for the process is *in vitro fertilization* (fertilization in glass).

In vitro fertilization is a procedure in which eggs are removed from a woman and fertilized in a laboratory dish (by either the husband or another man). The embryos are then implanted in a woman (the donor or some other woman), where the egg may be brought to term. This procedure is in itself uncontroversial. The ethical issues arise because the process typically results in extra, or "spare," embryos that may then be disposed of, frozen, or experimented on, none of which is without its detractors. The spare embryos are necessary since the procedure is not an easy one for the donor; because not all the eggs fertilize; and because the implantation process may fail and thus have to be repeated.

Currently there are about 400,000 human embryos, each the size of a pinhead, stored in cylinders filled with liquid nitrogen at more than 430 fertility clinics in the United States.[17] Some have questioned what their status should be. The process of in vitro fertilization involves the freezing of embryos, rating them for quality, discarding those that hold genetic defects, and at some future time, for those that are not needed, thawing them and disposing of them. For those who believe that human life is sacred from the moment of conception, then the processes of in vitro fertilization and what happens to excess embryos becomes a moral dilemma. Do the rationalistic and impersonal practices of the in vitro processes undermine the respect for life and the concept that life begins at conception? It would seem that those who hold this view would attempt at least to limit the number of embryos harvested to the minimum number necessary, and if the excess embryos are discarded, that some ceremony of recognition of what they are would be performed. This might be similar to the special cremation services performed at some medical schools for cadavers that have been used for anatomy classes prior to their disposal.

Two other issues arise with regard to the freezing of the embryos. First, although the 90 percent success rate with thawed embryos may be acceptable for laboratory animals, it probably is not acceptable with humans, particularly if the failure or partial failure is not detectable until later in life. Second, once frozen, the embryos may outlive the donor and thus raise the possibility of postmortem conception and birth.

On the other hand, there are great potential uses that we could make of in vitro techniques. Women could postpone pregnancy without risking either infertility or the diseases of pregnancy that afflict older women by conceiving at a young age (thus avoiding the old-age dangers like Down syndrome), but then getting pregnant through implantation at an older age. This could aid women whose career choices, maturity issues, or economic situations are such that pregnancy later in life is preferable. In vitro also offers the possibility of identifying genetic abnormalities while providing an alternative to amniocentesis during the second trimester. It could also then provide a more palatable "abortion in vitro" for embryos identified as having some disease or defect.

A more recent set of issues has arisen with the use of embryonic tissue in medical research with the aim to provide treatments for diseases like Parkinson's and treatments like transplantation. These issues typically recall the arguments raised in the abortion debate over the beginning of life or personhood. For those who hold that it is wrong to abort anytime after conception, then any procedure that leads to the loss of the embryo is also wrong. But someone who believes that abortion is permissible would not likely be troubled by the use of embryos in research.

Although we have already examined most of these issues, it may be opportune to address the embryo specifically at this point. We are dealing with a blastocyst that has around one hundred cells, is approximately the size of the end of an eyelash, and completely lacks cellular differentiation. It contains mitochondria, cytoplasm, and the DNA of the mother and father. The key element is the DNA. Some people worry about the destruction of the embryo in stem cell research, but it should be noted that while the egg wall, the cytoplasm, and the mitochondria are destroyed, the DNA is not. It is precisely what gets used to form cell lines, and it should also be noted it will therefore outlive the DNA of frozen embryos.

SURROGACY

The practice of surrogacy occurs when a woman agrees to carry a baby to term and give it up to another set of parents to raise. The contracting couple may be unable to contribute genetic material for some reason or the female may be unable to carry the baby to term. Sometimes this is done for money, sometimes as a favor. It is the practice of surrogacy for money that causes the most concern, although some dislike the practice whether or not money is exchanged. Some people believe that it is unethical for a woman to be used, even with her consent, as an incubator for others. Others believe that this is just another economic opportunity for women who often have few other economic options. But this does not allay the concerns of those opposed to the practice; indeed, it makes the whole arrangement more likely to be one that involves coercion. Others remark that given the rigors of pregnancy, one should be paid even if grave economic necessity is not involved. However, there are others who question what the payment is for. Is it for the use of the "apparatus" for the nine months, or for the baby? If it is for the baby, then we have gotten into the question of the legitimacy of selling humans.[18]

Some worry that it is too hard on a woman to carry a baby to term and give it up at birth. Pregnancy is viewed as a deeply personal experience that should never be undergone for the sake of others. On the other hand, it is for this very reason that surrogacy can be a supreme gift to another.

What if the birth mother changes her mind? This is a very difficult circumstance. If the genetic material is that of the birth mother and a partner besides the contracting parents, and if the woman agrees to return any money paid to her, then one might be willing to let the baby remain with the birth mother. Others would argue that "a deal is a deal" and that the birth mother should give up the baby. One's position in this case will depend on whether one believes biological connectivity is more important than contractual agreements.[19]

If the biological material is not solely that of the birth mother and her own partner, but is contributed in whole or part by the contracting couple, then the issue is more complex. Now the case for the birth mother rests solely on the biological connectivity that comes from pregnancy. But the contracting parents also have biological connectivity because of the genetic material. They also have the contractual agreement on their side. These reasons would tend to favor the contracting parents. But again, some are loathe to remove a baby from the birth mother against her will.

Technology has brought us face to face with new and difficult issues, and merely consulting tradition will be of little use. Kantians will probably find the whole practice of surrogacy problematic since the birth mother is clearly being used as an incubator and not regarded as a rational actor. One could give a Kantian argument in favor of surrogacy on the basis that as long as there is no overt coercion and if the woman either is paid or agrees to donate her body and time for selfless reasons, then she is acting as a rational and autonomous individual. She is simply using her body like any manual laborer. Those Kantians who disagree with the practice are more likely to compare the practice to a clinical form of prostitution without the act of sex. One might wonder how one can think of the practice as prostitution given that sex is not involved, but those who do will point to the highly personal and invasive nature of pregnancy as the key analogical factors.

Utilitarians are faced with very complicated utility calculations. The simplest calculation says that everyone benefits: the birth mother is given money and the contracting parents get a child they could not otherwise have. A ultilitarian argument against surrogacy could grant this simple calculation but then argue that the long-term consequences would be negative in one or more ways, such as commodifying what should be a noncommodifed part of life, demeaning women by regarding them as incubators, depersonalizing a very personal aspect of life, or possibly creating a lower class of women whose main function in life is to produce children for others.

Another utilitarian argument against surrogacy argues that the pain of separation to the birth mother outweighs the happiness gained by the contracting parents. This might be a difficult argument to make in general since the surrogates, at least initially, feel that the pain of separation is worth a monetary reward. Most cases of surrogacy seem to bear this out. While some birth mothers change their minds, most go through with the deal and feel as if the outcome is the best one.

Surrogacy is now a fairly well-accepted practice in spite of the misgivings of some people. As long as the practice is regulated so that no coercion is used and the practice does not create a class of "breeders," the ethics of surrogacy are unlikely to be too problematic except in cases of changes of mind. If the practice does become coercive or create a class of breeders, then surrogacy should be reconsidered.

CONCLUSION

Throughout this chapter on the ethical issues surrounding reproduction, there has been little information with regard to the health provider's role and professional autonomy. The reason is that the abortion issue is not essentially a health issue but rather a social issue that takes place in the health care arena. Abortion, in most instances where it is performed, is legal. The American Medical Association in its Code of Medical Ethics, Current Opinions document, 2.01 states:

> The Principles of Medical Ethics of the AMA do not prohibit a physician from performing an abortion in accordance with good medical practice and under circumstances that do not violate the law.[20]

One's attitude toward abortion is often very intense, close, and personal. As a matter of professional autonomy, it would seem that health care providers with deeply held beliefs with regard to this matter would not be required to participate in the process. However, this may require that the provider ascertain the philosophical view of the institution where he desires employment prior to accepting duty there. It makes very little sense to look at only the salary and fringe benefits of a hospital and then find yourself working at an institution where the daily practice of abortion creates for you severe moral distress.

Health care providers, regardless of their personal feelings concerning abortion, cannot ignore the social realities of our time, such as the liberation of women and the problems of teenage mothers. There is very little indication that the abortion controversy will end anytime soon. As a matter of role duty, we must come to understand that people of intellect and honor have come to very different decisions regarding the issue. As health care providers, we do not have the luxury of treating patients with whom we have formed a patient-provider relationship with anything but the highest level of professional concern, regardless how we may feel about their decisions on reproductive issues.

Abortion is an extremely emotional issue in that it makes us consider some very important and deep moral concepts, such as personhood and the value of human life. While it is important to understand the facts of fetal development, there is no getting around the problem of philosophical disagreement over fundamentals. Abortion also requires that we review our moral intuitions. We discussed various analogies in order to determine whether our intuitions can yield a consistent moral position on abortion.

Whatever your view on abortion, it should be clear that the issue is a difficult one that reaches to the depths of our most profound thoughts on what is important in life. Nothing indicates that the controversy will end anytime soon, so how is a sensitive person to regard opponents on the issue? If one imagines that a fetus is a baby, how much effort on its behalf is rational? An adult who rushes into the street to save a toddler who has entered the pathway of an onrushing car would be considered a hero. What, then, is so extraordinary about blocking a doorway or lying down in front of an abortion clinic, if what you see yourself doing is saving babies? If, on the other hand, your view of a fetus is that of a piece of tissue—even one with remarkable potential, but still only a piece of tissue—jumping in front of cars or blocking doorways is very strange behavior indeed.

Perhaps what is missing in the debate is a level of tolerance and civility that considers the opposing view to be wrong but perhaps rational. Following the tragic killing of Dr. Gunn, the pro-choice advocates began to call the pro-life advocates "terrorists" while the pro-life movement continued to cast the pro-choice side as "baby killers." It is not likely that "baby killers" and "terrorists" are the kinds of people who will be able to sit down and reason together. Confrontations have become increasingly violent and costly as one town after another becomes a battleground.

Is there a possibility that one day people on both sides of the issue will be able to set aside their differences and come to some agreement? Maybe there is some hope in the fact that the authors of this book disagree on the abortion issue yet were able to work together in order to write this book.

KEY CONCEPTS

- Pro-choice and pro-life advocates have debated the merits of the *Roe* v. *Wade* decision for more than three decades. While each side has honed its arguments well, they do not appear to be closer to resolution.

- In the past several years, the contest has not been directed toward the issue itself as much as toward related wedge issues such as late-term abortion, double penalties for the murder of a pregnant woman, the use of fetal tissue in research, and whether the government should provide funding for abortions in federally funded programs.

- Although the pro-choice arguments presented involve issues such as rape and incest and these issues do exist, most abortions performed are related to lifestyle issues.

- The sociological backgrounds of the debaters seem to divide the advocates along traditionalist and modernist lines. Pro-life advocates appear to be more traditional and religious, while pro-choice advocates appear to be more secular and liberal modernists.

- In vitro fertilization in and of itself appears to create few ethical problems. The ethical issues are generally involved with what to do with the extra or spare embryos that are created as part of the process.

- Surrogacy is a practice that is gaining acceptance. However, issues regarding disagreements between the participants, whether one is selling a service or a baby, and whether women providing the service stereotype and demean other women, complicate the process.

REVIEW EXERCISES

A. On March 28, 1992, the *Wall Street Journal* reported that the New Jersey Supreme Court had tossed out the appeal of a man seeking to stop his girlfriend from having an abortion. Much has been written about the woman's right over her body, but relatively little about the father's rights. Does a man have the right to veto an abortion? Does he have the right to veto a pregnancy? What duties logically follow from such rights?

Use this exercise to assess the doctrine that says that for every right you have there must be someone with a correlative duty.

B. RU 486, or mifepristone, has been used by literally thousands of women in France for early first-trimester abortions. RU 486 has been found effective and safe in 96 percent of abortions in a French study. What is the appropriate position to take on RU 486, "the abortion pill"? RU 486 is a drug that prevents the blastocyst (the zygote) from embedding in the uterine wall. It does this by blocking the naturally produced hormone, progesterone, the absence of which causes the uterine wall to shed its lining and any fertilized egg.

The Ethics of RU 486: Is the zygote a person? Review the criteria of personhood to make your decision.

How is RU 486 different from the IUD? The cervical cap? The traditional pill? Compare the different forms of contraception with regard to the abortion issue.

C. One development in contraceptive technology is the "underarm pill." It is a low-dosage, slow-release pill implanted under the arm that lasts for five years.

We have discussed the severe problems of teen pregnancy in some areas. How would you feel about mandatory implantation in teenage girls in problem areas, for example, high schools where 90 percent of all girls are pregnant before graduation?

What about a national policy of underarm pill implantation? Should we implant all girls of a certain age to avoid discrimination? We could respect the wishes of certain groups who would reject the implantation, so one could also petition not to receive the pill. But then should the state be required to help to raise a child who is the result?

Should the parents who engage in child abuse be required to wear an underarm pill?

D. Some abortion foes object to fetal tissue research on the grounds that it will lead to more abortions, or at least to a feeling that the immorality of abortion may be partially offset by the fact that the tissue will be put to good use. Is this fear justified?

E. Michigan has a parental consent law stating that minors must get permission from parents or a judge before having an abortion. Imagine a similar law that adds a provision that if the parent refuses to allow the abortion it is the parent's responsibility to raise the child, not the minor's. Which would be the better law?

F. Rule utilitarians regard rights as human creations, as merely good rules that yield the greatest happiness for the greatest number. Consider the right to life from the perspective of the rule utilitarian and determine whether such a view could support the pro-life side, the pro-choice side, or both.

G. Some states have passed what is called the "informed consent" law. Such a law would require anyone considering an abortion to wait twenty-four hours and to view pictures of fetuses at the same stage as her fetus. Would such a law be a good idea? Do we require heart patients to witness open-heart surgery before they undergo the operation themselves? Is this a good analogy?

H. Do health professionals have the duty to participate in abortions even if they find them morally repugnant?

I. Examine the following statistics: What, if anything, can we learn from them? Which side does each statistic support?

1. In 1997, there were 1,400,000 abortions reported.
2. In the same year, there were 346 abortions per 1,000 live births.
3. 80 percent of all abortions are performed on unmarried women.
4. .01 percent of all abortions take place after 24 weeks.
5. 50 percent of all pregnancies are unintended.
6. 57 percent of all teenage pregnancies were terminated by abortion.
7. 13 percent of all women having abortions have been informed the fetus has a defect.
8. 55 percent of all teenagers who have an abortion inform their parents.
9. Childbirth is eleven times more dangerous than abortion.
10. 16,000 women seek abortions each year as a result of rape or incest.
11. 2,000 copies of self-abortion videos have been sold to women's groups since 1989.
12. 500,000 women die each year from pregnancy-related problems.

Use these statistics to examine the relationship between facts and values.

NOTES

1. Allan Guttmacher Institute. Statistics drawn from Institute Publications. (New York: Allan Guttmacher Institute, 2001).

2. Letter from P. J. Seward, Executive Vice President, American Medical Association to the Honorable Rick Santorum, United States Senator, dated May 19, 1997.

3. *Roe* v. *Wade* (1973), 410 U.S. 113, 164.

4. M. Faux, *Roe* v. *Wade* (New York: New American Library, 1988).

5. *Danforth* v. *Planned Parenthood of Central Missouri* (1976), 428 U.S. 52.

6. *Harris* v. *McRae* (1980), 448, U.S. 297.

7. *Webster* v. *Reproductive Health Services,* 492 U.S. 490, 190 S.Ct. 3040 (1989).

8. *Rust* v. *Sullivan* (1991). 111 S. Ct. 1750, U.S.

9. G. Pozgar, *Legal Aspects of Health Care Administration* (Gaithersburg, MD: Aspen, 1993).

10. "One Doctor Down, How Many More?" *Time,* March 2, 1993.

11. Mary Anne Warren, "On the Moral and Legal Status of Abortion," in *The Problem of Abortion,* ed. Joel Feinberg (Belmont, CA: Wadsworth Books, 1984).

12. Warren, "On the Moral and Legal Status of Abortion."

13. Michael Tooley, "A Defense of Abortion and Infantcide," in *The Problem of Abortion,* ed. Feinberg.

14. Judith Thomson, "A Defense of Abortion," in *The Problem of Abortion,* ed. Feinberg.

15. "One Doctor Down, How Many More?" *Time,* March 22, 1993.

16. "Thou Shalt Not Kill," *Time,* March 22, 1993.

17. David Hoffman, Gail Zellman, et al. "Cryopreserved Embryos in the United States and Their Availability for Research." *Fertility and Sterility.* Vol. 79. No. 5. May 2003.

18. O'Neill, Terry (ed.) *Biomedical Ethics; Opposing Viewpoints* (San Diego, CA: Greenhaven Press, Inc., 1994).

19. Scott B. Rae, "Brave New Families?: The Ethics of the New Reproductive Technologies." *Christian Research Journal,* Spring 1993.

20. American Medical Association, *Code of Medical Ethics and Current Opinions* (Chicago: American Medical Association, 1996).

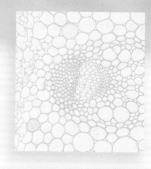

AIDS and Health Care Practice

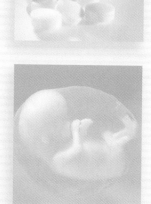

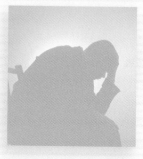

GOAL

To gain an understanding of the nature of the AIDS epidemic and to examine selected ethical problems associated with this crisis.

OBJECTIVES

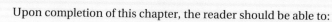

Upon completion of this chapter, the reader should be able to:

1. Discuss the nature of the disease process of AIDS and how it is acquired.

2. List the major infection control methods that have been used to bring the epidemic under control.

3. Explain how standard precautions have reduced the risk of infection for health care providers and what place they play in affirming a duty to treat.

4. List the high-risk behaviors associated with the spread of this disease.

5. List the reasons that confidentiality is perhaps more important for this patient group than for others we treat.

6. Write a rationale for the duty to treat this patient group.

7. List the conditions under which the moral duty to treat would cease to be a duty but only a moral option.

8. Write a series of guidelines that would provide the patient protection from AIDS-infected health care providers.

9. Provide rationales for the decisions both to tell and not tell health care providers the HIV status of the patients they care for.

10. Write a pro and con rationale as to whether you feel an HIV-infected practitioner should be allowed to continue practice.

11. Write a pro and con rationale as to whether you feel that providers have an obligation to patients outside of our national borders.

KEY TERMS

AIDS	**Moral duty**	**Safe sex**
High-risk behaviors	**Moral option**	**Standard precautions**

ETHICAL ISSUES OF AIDS

I remember that weekend when no patient in the intensive care unit was over the age of forty. I remember the intern who tearfully refused to come to the emergency room to see the fourth AIDS patient I had admitted to her in as many hours. She never did meet him; he died before she calmed down.

Abigail Zuger, M.D., 1986

Hundreds of thousands of lost lives later, the initial impact is over. The thunderbolts of AIDS are starting to become a fact of life. Some sense of continuity with the rest of history has become possible. AIDS continues to be a source of uniquely complex medical, legal, and social dilemmas; nonetheless, it has evolved into an entity provoking fewer immediate panicked reactions and more measured, mature analysis.

Abigail Zuger, M.D., 1993

Although this chapter focuses on the ethical issues involving AIDS (acquired immunodeficiency syndrome), it is equally instructive for other epidemic diseases. Scientists are still attempting to solve the question of where the great 1918 flu epidemic came from and when a similar epidemic will revisit. The world has grown smaller; transportation has allowed movement across the globe into areas previously isolated. Diseases such as Ebola and severe acute respiratory syndrome (SARS) could rapidly become national rather than international news. Dealing with the **AIDS** (acquired immunodeficiency syndrome) epidemic for the past quarter-century has forced American health care practitioners to rethink ethical questions regarding confidentiality, whether there is a duty to treat, the limits of a duty to warn, the meaning of distributive justice, and a host of others. The pandemic nature of AIDS is still to be dealt with and will offer lessons in regard to our duties not only to our own citizens but to the whole world. Though we have become somewhat complacent in the United States in regard to AIDS, it is instructive to remember that according to the United Nations Program on HIV/AIDS (UNAIDS) global estimates, there were still somewhere between 2.5 and 3.6 million deaths attributed to this disease in 2003. Now, a quarter-century into the epidemic, almost 22 million men, women, and children worldwide have died of AIDS and an estimated 40 million people are living with the human immunodeficiency virus (HIV), which causes AIDS. Figure 12-1 provides a chronology for the epidemic.[1]

1981 • On June 5, the Centers for Disease Control (CDC) Mortality and Morbidity Report listed an unusual outbreak of opportunistic infections such as pneumocystis carinii pneumonia among gay men.

1982 • *Acquired immunodeficiency syndrome* (AIDS) becomes the term used by the CDC to describe the unusual outbreaks of opportunistic infections.

1983 • Heterosexuals are considered at risk after two women whose sexual partners had AIDS contracted the disease.

1984 • The human immunodeficiency virus (HIV) is identified by a team of French scientists.

1985 • The Food and Drug Administration (FDA) approves the first AIDS antibody test, which is quickly used to screen the nation's blood supply.

1986 • Surgeon General C. Everett Koop issues a report calling for AIDS education and condom use.

1987 • FDA approves AZT (azidothymidine), the first antiviral agent to treat AIDS.
     • After four years in office, President Ronald Reagan publicly addresses AIDS.

1988 • The U.S. Department of Health and Human Services distributes over 107 million copies of the brochure *Understanding AIDS,* attempting to contact virtually every residential post office box in the nation.
     • The World Health Organization (WHO) declares December World AIDS Day.

1989 • The FDA approves four new drugs to treat opportunistic infections.

1990 • Congress enacts the Americans with Disabilities Act, which prohibits discrimination against persons with HIV/AIDS. The AIDS Housing Opportunity Act expands affordable housing options for people with HIV-related diseases.
     • By year's end, there are 161,073 reported cases of AIDS in the United States and 100,813 people have died of the disease.

FIGURE 12-1 Chronology of the AIDS Epidemic

1991 • An intense national debate regarding HIV-infected health professionals is sparked following reports of several patients' being infected by their dentist.
- The Occupational Safety and Health Administration (OSHA) guidelines recommend "universal precautions" for all patients.

1992 • AIDS becomes the leading cause of death among American men between ages twenty-five and forty-four and the fourth leading cause of death in women for this age group.
- The first reports of successful combination anti-retroviral therapies are reported.

1993 • President Clinton establishes the White House Office of National AIDS Policy.

1994 • AZT is shown to reduce HIV transmission from mother to infant by up to 70 percent.
- Combination therapy proves effective in battling HIV, and individualized therapy emerges as a treatment option.

1995 • The joint United Nations Program on HIV/AIDS (UNAIDS) is created.
- By year's end in the United States, there are 513,486 reported cases of AIDS, and 323,213 people have died of the disease.

1996 • The FDA approves two new protease inhibitor drugs. This new class of drugs is reported as being highly effective in controlling HIV.

1997 • For the first time in the sixteen-year history of the epidemic, the number of Americans newly diagnosed with AIDS drops, and following the introduction of protease inhibitors, AIDS deaths decline by nearly 20 percent.
- President Clinton calls for an AIDS vaccine to be developed with ten years.

1998 • CDC reports the AIDS death rate in United States dropped by 47 percent between 1996 and 1997, but the rate of new HIV infections (40,000 per year) does not decline.
- Drug-resistant HIV strains appear.

1999 • Worldwide rates of HIV/AIDS infection soar in developing nations. Due to high drug prices and poor available health care, the majority of the people with AIDS in the world go untreated.

2000 • Among gay and bisexual men in the United States, AIDS diagnosis among African Americans and Hispanics men exceeds that of whites for the first time.
- The United States and United Nations declare AIDS an issue of national security.

FIGURE 12-1   (*Continued*)

- By midyear there are 753,907 reported cases of AIDS in the United States, and 438,795 people have died of the disease.

2004
- HIV/AIDS has become an alarming international epidemic, with over 44 million infected worldwide and over 22 million deaths. The UN secretary general calls for a $7 to $10 billion program to fight AIDS in the developing world.

- Following years of decline in the incidence of new HIV infections among gay men, certain American cities are again reporting increases.

2005
- World Economic Forum's priorities include a focus on addressing HIV/AIDS in Africa.

- USDA grants tentative approval to generic AIDS Drug Regimen for potential purchase marking the first ever approval of an HIV regimen manufactured by a non-U.S. based generic pharmaceutical company.

FIGURE 12-1   (*Continued*)

Early in the 1980s, health care practitioners within major U.S. cities began to report patients with overwhelming and unusual opportunistic infections. These patients, usually young white males, presented with conditions thought to be rare and normally seen only in severely debilitated individuals or in textbooks. In June 1981, the Centers for Disease Control (CDC) reported three cases of "gay cancer," then described as gay-related immune disorder (GRID). One month later, 108 cases had been reported and 43 individuals had died. Relatively rare entities such as candidiasis of the esophagus, extrapulmonary cryptococcosis, Kaposi's sarcoma affecting a patient less than sixty years of age, progressive multifocal leukoencephalopathy, and pneumocystitis carinii became indicator diseases for what later became known as acquired immunodeficiency syndrome or AIDS. HIV is transmitted through sexual contact, exposure to infected blood or blood components, and perinatally from mothers to infants. While the HIV virus has been isolated from blood, vaginal secretions, semen, breast milk, saliva, tears, and cerebrospinal fluid, epidemiological evidence has implicated only blood, semen, vaginal secretions, and possibly breast milk in transmission. Table 12-1 lists the AIDS cases by exposure category.[2]

AIDS evidently began as a mutant virus that was picked up from a species of African monkey and transferred to humans by way of bites. It was then transmitted among the African populations via direct mucous-to-mucous contact, through semen and perhaps blood exchange. From Africa, the disease spread to Haiti, and was later carried to the United States, probably by homosexual males. The heterosexual population became infected as blood supplies became contaminated and as a result of intravenous drug use and the sharing of contaminated needles.

TABLE 12-1	
Estimated Number of Diagnosed Cases of HIV/AIDS, by Selected Characteristics, 2002	
EXPOSURE CATEGORIES	ESTIMATE
Male adult or adolescent	
Male-to-male sexual contact	11,701
Injection drug use	2,757
Male-to-male sexual contact and drug injection	943
Heterosexual contact	3,234
Other (includes hemophilia, blood transfusion, and risks not reported)	164
Total	18,798
Female adult or adolescent	
Injection drug use	1,418
Heterosexual contact	5,949
Other (includes hemophilia, blood transfusion, and risks not reported	136
Total	7,503
Child (under 13 years)	
Perinatal	144
Other (includes hemophilia, blood transfusions, and risks not reported)	18
Total	162
Race/ethnicity	
White, non-Hispanic	8,347
Black, non-Hispanic	14,398
Hispanic	3,321
Asian/Pacific Islander	140
American Indian/Alaskan Native	1,795

Female sexual partners of those infected through contaminated blood or needles contracted the disease through semen and spread the disease to other partners and perinatally to their infants.

INFECTION CONTROL METHODS

As with other epidemics, the CDC has sought to control the disease by breaking the chain of events causing the spread of the infection. This can be done in several ways, such as decreasing the susceptibility of hosts, eliminating the source of the organisms, and interrupting the mode of transmission. Although some positive reports have come from researchers seeking a vaccine to decrease the susceptibility of individuals to the HIV virus, no current vaccine exists, and most researchers believe that it will be years before a safe and effective vaccine is developed. The major efforts toward eliminating the source of the infection have been through an active educational program, legal notification requirements, and special techniques in providing barriers at the point of direct and indirect contact.

The efforts directed toward breaking the chain of infection through special techniques to reduce the spread of infection in the general public has taken many forms. These range from the rather controversial methods such as clean needle exchange programs for IV drug users and provision of free condoms for high school students, to those less controversial such as screening prospective blood donors for high-risk behaviors, increased testing of blood supplies, and the promotion of "**safe sex**" or abstinence in high-risk situations. The Health and Human Services brochure listing of both safe and **high-risk behaviors** is found in Figure 12-2.[3]

In their writings, Milliken and Greenblat have suggested several specific criteria for an ethical social policy toward control of this epidemic.[4] It was felt that only the adoption of such criteria would ensure the acceptance by the citizenry, which is a basic requisite for successful policy.

1. Methods selected must be efficacious and appropriate to the stated goals.

2. The goals selected must be ethical, and equal consideration of interest must be central to processes.

3. Implementation of the policy must avoid discrimination and be justly administered.

4. Harm to society or its subgroups that may result from the proposed policies must be identified and clearly understood.

5. The balance between harms and benefits must weigh heavily toward benefits.

RISKY BEHAVIORS

- Sharing drug needles and syringes

- Anal sex, with or without a condom

- Vaginal or oral sex with someone who shoots drugs or engages in anal sex

- Sex with someone you don't know well (a pickup or prostitute) or with someone you know has several sex partners

- Unprotected sex (without a condom) with an infected person

SAFE BEHAVIORS

- Not having sex

- Sex with one mutually faithful, uninfected partner

- Not shooting drugs

FIGURE 12-2   High-Risk and Safe Behaviors

OCCUPATIONAL RISK

In the hospital setting, efforts to protect health care workers and their patients have taken the form of adopting **standard precautions**. In that medical history and examination cannot reliably identify all patients infected with HIV or other blood-borne pathogens such as hepatitis B, standard precautions have been recommended for all patients. This is especially critical for such practitioners as nurses, respiratory care specialists, and clinical laboratory technicians, as their work brings them into medical situations in which contact with blood is common and the infection status of the patient is often unknown.

In that great numbers of health care workers did not contract the disease in the early 1980s, it has become evident that the transmission modes for HIV are rather specific. The virus is a rather fragile entity, and there is little risk for practitioners who practice standard precautions and are otherwise not involved in high-risk behaviors. One tragic exception to HIV infection being related to high-risk behaviors are the hemophiliac patients who acquired the disease in great numbers as a result of initial poor-quality testing of needed blood products used in their treatment. Of the million cases of HIV infections in the United States, only the five involved with a Florida dentist, Dr. Acer, are known to have been infected by health care providers. There appear to have been fewer than 100 health care providers who had contracted the disease from patients. Of these, most were infected through needle sticks or were caused by blood splashes into the eyes, mouth, or nose.

ETHICAL ISSUES AND THE AIDS EPIDEMIC

AIDS is a devastating epidemic with the potential for killing all who become infected. Although the risk of acquiring a hepatitis B infection is far higher, the deadly consequences of getting AIDS have made this disease a major ethical issue. In recent years, the population affected by the disease has extended to all groups, so that it is best not described by high-risk groups but rather by high-risk behaviors. The economic implications of AIDS are staggering. When one considers personal medical costs, direct costs of research, and indirect costs such as education, screening, and potential productivity losses, the disease carries a yearly price tag of over $8 billion. The economic implication of these numbers is overwhelming when you consider the already overburdened health care system. Added to these tangible costs is another set of values that defy fiscal analysis: the loss of hopes, and dreams, and potential of its victims. What is the cost of these losses, when young people are handicapped during the time of their lives when they are at the peak of their productive work and childbearing years? One real problem with solving the AIDS dilemma is that many Americans appear to be experiencing a great deal of both fear and denial concerning their own risk of acquiring AIDS, and many have rationalized the continuation of lifestyles that place them at risk.[5]

The ethical problems associated with this disease are many and cut to the very heart of what it means to be a health care practitioner. The fact that AIDS has no known cure or preventive vaccine makes it a disease that has caused the rethinking of basic fundamental issues. Do health care practitioners have a duty to treat? In a health care system already overburdened with the costs of health care, what resources should be allocated to a group of patients with a terminal disease? How much access to expensive technologies should terminal patients have? What is an acceptable risk for health care professionals? Should the patient be warned if the health care practitioner is HIV positive? Should the practitioner be warned if the patient is HIV positive? Should infected practitioners be allowed to continue practice? What is the meaning of confidentiality when it comes to AIDS, and who should be told? Examine the case involving confidentiality and the duty to warn.

CASE STUDY

A Duty to Warn?

You are a health center nurse at a local university clinic and are meeting with Mr. Green, a twenty-eight-year-old graduate student who has reported to the health center for counseling following his blood testing positive for antibodies to HIV. Although he is asymptomatic at the moment, you inform Mr. Green that while he does not currently have AIDS, there is a 5 to 35 percent probability that he will develop the disease within the next five years. You advise him that he should refrain from donating blood and should practice safe sex at all times.

During the counseling session, Mr. Jones tells you that he is bisexual and that his infection probably came from a homosexual encounter that occurred last summer. He also tells you that he is engaged to be married next month. You advise him of the need to inform his fiancé of his condition, but he tells you that it would ruin his life.

1. What are the state regulations regarding reporting HIV as a communicable condition?

2. To whom do you have duty: your real patient or the potential victim?

3. How would you handle the matter?

DUTY TO TREAT

How much risk is acceptable for health care practitioners? Although much of the media attention has been directed toward patients who have been infected with the HIV virus by health care practitioners, the truth is that it is far more likely that the practitioner will be infected by the patient than the other way around. Health care workers who have contracted the disease have included direct patient care groups such as physicians, dentists, nurses, nursing assistants, clinical laboratory technicians, and therapists, but also groups such as housekeeping and maintenance, which usually do not have direct patient contact.

Although of great concern due to the tragic consequences of infection, the risk to health care practitioners seems to be very rare. The use of standard precautions on all patients should provide an effective barrier and reduce the risk to an acceptable level. It would seem, then, that the limited risk to the practitioner would not provide a suitable rationale to refuse to treat patients

- To provide service consistent with skills

- To obtain skills if needed by patient population as consistent with scope of practice

- To provide accurate and up-to-date information

- To promote the patient's best interest regardless of personal feelings toward patient or their disease entity

FIGURE 12-3   Professional Duties in an Epidemic

with known HIV infections. In practice, it is probably not the known HIV-infected patient who is most likely to spread the disease to health care workers. Figure 12-3 lists the recommended guidelines for practice in an epidemic as provided by the Health and Public Policy Committee of the American College of Physicians and the Infectious Disease Society of America.[6] These guidelines find their basis in many health providers' code of ethics; for example, the nursing code for the care of victims of communicable disease calls for the "provision of services with respect for human dignity and the uniqueness of the client unrestricted by considerations of social or economical status, personal attributes, or the nature of the health problem." Nurses and allied health practitioners, then, have a duty to provide care commensurate with their scope of practice. Should the practitioner feel unsure about standard precautions, there is an implicit duty to obtain the needed skills and to keep up-to-date on all available information. Ignorance in this case might provide a short-term rationale for refusing to treat a patient with AIDS, but once the practitioner is trained in standard precautions, this would no longer provide a legitimate excuse. Western culture and health care practice provide historical precedence for the obligation to treat persons regardless of their social status, political affiliation, or even whether they be enemy or friend. The Good Samaritan ethic endorsed by our culture also provides strong ethical precedence for coming to the aid of those in danger or in need of help. This ethic of assistance does not, however, require that the rescuer take unacceptable risks in the process. For example, the nonswimmer is not expected to jump into the pool to save a drowning victim, for clearly this would not be in the interest of the victim or the potential rescuer.

What, then, does our culture require of us in regard to the AIDS patients? While we are not required to risk our lives in futile and perhaps dangerous gestures, under most situations that is not what we face with this patient group. While the potential for contracting AIDS within the workplace is a significant concern, it has occurred on an exceedingly infrequent basis. So this concern would not, in general, represent an acceptable rationale for refusing to treat but would create an obligation on the part of all health care workers to take appropriate protective actions.

The ANA Committee on Ethics offers some useful guidelines regarding the decision as to whether the practitioner has a **moral duty** to treat or whether the decision is left as a **moral option**. The four fundamental criteria are:[7]

1. The patient is at significant risk of harm, loss, or damage if the practitioner does not assist.

2. The practitioner's intervention or care is directly relevant to preventing harm.

3. The practitioner's care will probably prevent harm, loss, or damage to the patient.

4. The benefit the patient will gain outweighs any harm the practitioner might incur and does not present more than a minimal risk to the health care provider.

If the practitioner can answer yes to all four criteria, it would seem that a moral duty to treat would exist under the principle of beneficence. If, however, the circumstances place the practitioner in such a position that all criteria could not be answered with yes, then the decision to treat would become a moral option rather than a duty. An example of this might be an answer of no for the crucial fourth criterion, in a case in which the practitioner finds a patient bleeding from the mouth, in respiratory failure, and requiring cardiopulmonary resuscitation. Assuming that no masks or airways were in place, the decision to perform mouth-to-mouth resuscitation would not be mandated by duty.

Most health provider codes of ethics give a clear directive on the treatment of patients regardless of their disease status. These moral directives have often been ignored, and certain health care providers have refused to treat HIV-infected patients. In order to overcome this reluctance to treat this patient group, the government moved to include those infected with AIDS under the federal legislation barring discriminatory practices. This patient group is now afforded protection of Section 504 of the Rehabilitation Act of 1973 and the Americans with Disabilities Act of 1990. HIV serostatus and AIDS are now considered handicapping conditions covered under federal legislation prohibiting discriminatory practices. The failure to treat is no longer only a moral issue but also has potential legal consequences.[8] The range of concerns that can be accommodated under these acts can be seen in the *Doe* v. *Centinela Hospital* case in which an asymptomatic HIV-infected patient was refused admission to a hospital's federally funded residential drug and alcohol program.[9] The individual was refused for fear of contagion, and the hospital claimed that because the patient was asymptomatic at the time, he was not handicapped by the disease. In the decision, the court recognized that HIV-infected individuals are handicapped not only by their disease but also because others perceive them as being impaired.

CONFIDENTIALITY IN AN AGE OF AIDS

What I may see or hear in the course of the treatment or even outside of the treatment in regard to the life of men, which on no account one must spread abroad, I will keep to myself holding such things shameful to be noised about.

Hippocratic Oath

Confidentiality seems based on at least three foundations:

1. The duty-oriented acceptance of a personal right of self-determination, which requires the control over privacy and personal information

2. The utilitarian view that if confidentiality were commonly breached, the patients would be deterred in seeking medical assistance for problems with sensitive or personal aspects

3. The long-held, virtue-oriented belief among health care providers that a special relationship exists between practitioner and client that calls for the tacit agreement of confidentiality and mutual trust

It would seem that the first two of these foundations have a special importance when considering the AIDS epidemic. The nature of the illness and the recognition of its association with high-risk populations—such as homosexuals, drug users, and prostitutes—creates an enhanced danger of harm should private information be revealed beyond appropriate circles of care. Discrimination in housing, insurance, and employment and even physical harm are very real outcomes of breaches of this patient group's confidentiality. Although rarely talked about in the press or in the national call for the screening of health care workers for AIDS, these same potential results from a breach in confidentiality must be considered equally in regard to the HIV status of health care providers. Given the potential for personal harm, it is not hard to see that dedication to confidentiality is critical if this patient group is to be forthcoming in providing health care providers with the information necessary to contain the epidemic and provide adequate care. Because AIDS is still without a cure, protection of the uninfected must take precedence over other concerns, and those who are vulnerable must be warned. Unlike other infectious diseases, AIDS is also associated with a form of dementia as a result of which the infected individual may feel vindictive and intentionally try to transmit the virus.

When considering AIDS cases, the principle of confidentiality must be balanced with our obligations to provide appropriate disease control within the community and to protect vulnerable populations. Should a health care worker in the emergency department or an emergency medical technician (EMT) be notified that a patient who came into her care and whose bleeding she controlled was later confirmed to be HIV positive? In that all practitioners at this level should practice standard precautions for all patients—and understanding that, if practiced, these precautions reduce the vulnerability to a negligible risk—at first glance, the answer would seem to be no. If the risk was minimal and the practitioners were not vulnerable, confidentiality should not be broken. Stated differently, as autonomous moral agents who have accepted the role of health care provider, the practitioners have a duty to protect themselves in these cases, and if protected they would not be a particularly vulnerable population. Yet anyone who has practiced in these situations knows that they are often less controlled than one might wish. The EMT reaching into the car to remove the bleeding patient often tears the gloves that are to provide the barrier; the emergency room worker is subject to needle or sharps sticks and barrier loss. While finding out after the fact that the patient was HIV positive might not be of use in preventing the health care provider from contracting the disease, it might provide essential information in regard to the need for testing and could possibly save the family or other contacts of the health care provider. It is for these reasons that special categories of health care workers who are subject to direct body fluid contact have a right to know about the HIV status of their patients.

Surveys among practitioners show a general belief that those who are directly working with AIDS patients should be informed of their diagnosis. This information is not so much to allow practitioners to minimize personal risk as it is a fact that standard precautions are expected for all patients. The need to know has more to do with the professional tasks at hand, as it is difficult to provide adequate care without an accurate diagnosis. It is hard to imagine that a physician would feel comfortable treating a patient for whom someone else has decided that she should not be informed of the correct diagnosis. The level of professionalism of allied health practitioners and nurses would seem to make it reasonable that they also need to know the diagnosis of the patients they treat. HIV-positive status and the diagnosis of AIDS should be treated as any other disease: it should be part of the medical record. At the same time, if this were to be the policy of hospitals and clinics, it then becomes far more important that the charts be stored in a safe place so that patient confidentiality can be ensured.

AIDS is a reportable disease in every state of the union. Physicians and hospitals must report every case to the public authorities, including the names. Cases reported are also reported to the Centers for Disease Control, with the names encoded by a system known as Soundex. All CDC records fall within the protection of the Federal Privacy Act of 1974, but under statute permission are available to other federal agencies.[10]

MANDATORY TESTING

There are legitimate reasons for mandatory testing for everyone. Early diagnosis would perhaps allow for early counseling and assist in curbing the spread of the infection. Early treatment is thought to slow the progress from the HIV antibody to full-blown AIDS. Early use of antiviral drugs is thought to delay the onset of dementia and retard the later resistance to the therapeutics. If for no other reason, a mandatory system of testing would provide the types of statistics that would allow agencies to better follow the spread of the disease and allow for more reasoned allocations of resources. Public health research has shown that a majority of physicians and nurses support mandatory testing.[11]

Yet real concern exists in regard to the cost-benefit ratio of mandatory testing. The cost of these programs would not only be the cost of the individual tests but also the cost of enforcement of rules and the necessary pretest and posttest counseling. Activities would also include increased levels of segregation, education, and prevention efforts. One example of broad-based screening that may prove illustrative is the experience of testing 159,000 marriage license applicants in Illinois. Of these, twenty-three were found to be HIV positive, and the program had an estimated cost of $5.6 million, which translates as $243,000 per positive test.[12] One need ask if this money could not have been better spent in education or research. The CDC does not advocate mandatory testing. Most public health officials eschew mandatory testing and stress the importance of voluntary testing.

Another problem associated with mandatory testing is that in the absence of a cure, widespread testing could result in widespread discrimination against those that tested positive for the virus. The fact that HIV/AIDS is still commonly associated with disfavored groups—gay men, injection drug users, and prostitutes—only heightens the concern about prejudicial treatment. Although illegal, there are cases of asymptomatic individuals who have tested positive for HIV and have suddenly found themselves uninsurable, unemployable, and unable to secure housing. It is quite possible that mandatory testing would drive HIV-infected people underground, away from the counseling and health care services they desperately need. Discrimination on the basis of serological status is as wrong as discrimination on the basis of race or sex, and equally illegal. Laws at the federal, state, and local levels prohibit discrimination on the basis of a person's HIV status or disability. Health care providers must ensure that HIV testing is conducted in such a manner that respects patient autonomy and ensures patient confidentiality to the fullest degree possible.

THE INFECTED HEALTH WORKER

Although society has currently decided against mandatory testing of everyone, the issue of testing health care providers is very much alive. A Gallup poll showed a majority of the lay public (87 percent) desired mandatory testing and disclosure of HIV status by health care providers. A bill that would impose a ten-year prison sentence upon HIV-infected health care providers overwhelmingly passed in the Senate but, fortunately, failed to become law. The CDC, using statistical estimation techniques, predicted that a patient undergoing a serious invasive procedure by an HIV-infected practitioner had a 1:40,000 to 1:400,000 chance of contracting the virus. If standard precautions are used, the risk becomes essentially nonexistent. This places the risk in the same range as being hit by lightning on the way to the clinic. Indeed, HIV transmission during the course of health care provision has almost been exclusively from patient to practitioner.

However, for the six dental patients of David Acer, D.D.S., the lightning analogy gives very little comfort. These are documented cases in which an infected health care provider passed HIV on to his patients, although the mechanism for the transmission is still in question. These six

Florida cases along with the associated media coverage created an overwhelming public concern with regard to infected health care providers.

A health care provider who knows that he or she has an infectious disease, which if transmitted to patients would pose a significant threat to their health, is under an absolute obligation not to engage in any activity that creates an identifiable risk of transmission to the patient. The precautions taken to ensure patient safety must be particularly stringent in the case of a disease that is potentially fatal.

The case of *Behringer* v. *Medical Center,* at Princeton, New Jersey, dealt with an HIV-infected surgeon who was allowed to practice. Upon finding out that the staff member was infected, the hospital allowed the physician to continue practice but limited his performance to procedures that posed no risk for HIV transmission. They also required that the physician obtain a written informed consent before performing any invasive procedure. The court based this decision on the ethical principles of beneficence and nonmaleficence as well as the conviction that patients themselves should have the final decision-making role in regard to whether they are willing to be treated by an infected practitioner.[13]

One of the many problems associated with the Behringer case was the loss of personal privacy suffered by the infected practitioner as news of his infection spread rapidly across the hospital. Although we often think of confidentiality in terms of patients, we have the same responsibility to protect the personal privacy of coworkers.

The decision on how infected practitioners are to be treated in these cases seems to have been left up to the individual states, so long as their guidelines are at least equal to those promulgated by the CDC.[14] At this time, of those states that have complied with the call for guidelines, most have not required mandatory testing for health care workers nor have they required that practitioners limit their practice. The decision not to require mandatory testing seems to have been made on the basis of high cost and low effectiveness. While mandatory testing of all health care workers would seem to be a good solution, unfortunately it is ineffective because there can be a six-month lag between infection and the development of antibodies that can be identified in the test. Mandatory testing seems to offer more of an illusion of security than real substance. These tests also provide a certain level of false positives, which have the potential of destroying a practitioner's career. Most health care providers feel that rigorously enforced infection control methods would be more useful in protecting patients and providers than would mandatory testing.

Rather than requiring immediate cessation of practice or the limiting of practice to noninvasive techniques, the CDC has recommended that expert review panels be set up to decide on a case-by-case basis whether seropositive health care workers should continue to perform invasive procedures.[15] The practitioner is required to communicate the positive HIV status to the health department, which is then charged with setting up an individual review of cases and a monitoring process. The review process would call for counseling of the infected practitioner and would rate the danger to patients. If it was decided that the infected practitioner posed a threat to patients, he would be advised to notify all affiliated institutions of his status. In that certain HIV-positive patients experience a period of dementia as part of their disease process, strict practice limitations and close monitoring seem appropriate. There are indications that the Florida dentist who infected Bergalis and others may have done so on purpose, perhaps as a result of paranoia brought on by his disease.

EXPERIMENTAL TREATMENT

In the early 1960s, Americans were both horrified and mesmerized in regard to the thalidomide babies. These infants, often born with severe deformities, were the result of pregnant women taking a tranquilizer widely used in Europe, which could be purchased there without a prescription. In that this drug had not been approved for use in the United States, most often the American babies born with the thalidomide effects were from women traveling in Europe who had purchased the drug overseas. Partially in response to this tragedy, the Food and Drug Act adopted the Kefauver amendments, which required that investigational and new drugs (INDs) obtain premarket approval. This was to assure the public that drugs would not reach the market without well-controlled studies proving that they were efficacious and safe. The risks associated with human research were dramatized when five patients with hepatitis B died from liver failure, and others in the clinical group required liver transplants following clinical trials with the experimental drug fialuridine.

Although criticized by physicians, patients, and drug companies for slowing the process of pharmaceuticals reaching the market, the Food and Drug Administration guidelines maintained these standards throughout the 1960s and 1970s. Although there was a great deal of individual discomfort and frustration with the slowness of these processes, in general, the public felt that they were well served and protected.

These standards came under severe criticism in the 1980s as two rather divergent forces found common cause in speeding up the processes and began to advocate for loosening restrictions. In the Reagan era, the Council on Competitiveness, which was designed to make recommendations necessary to create a freer and more responsive business climate, advocated for accelerated approval for INDs needed to treat life-threatening conditions or for those where no alternate therapy existed.[16] This loosening of the rules would allow for drugs to reach the market still in the development stage, with some of the studies to be completed post-marketing. The second voice for change came from AIDS activists such as the AIDS Coalition to Unleash Power, which advocated for initiatives to find new drugs as well as the right of patients to have free access to new experimental therapies.[17] In response to these demands for greater and quicker access to new drugs, the National Institutes of Health and the Food and Drug Administration established a separate track to provide unproven therapies outside of clinical trials. Persons eligible to receive these drugs were those with life-threatening illnesses who could not tolerate standard treatment regimens or could not participate in the actual clinical trials.

The idea of making experimental drugs available to dying patients seems cold but rational, especially if they are part of the premarket studies. It seems a marriage made in heaven: the HIV-infected patients get experimental and perhaps useful drugs and the pharmaceutical companies get volunteers for their studies.[18]

Yet there could be no legal obligation to provide these drugs, as the law holds physicians to the standard of customary care. Customary care by definition is that which one could expect from a competent and reasonable physician. In that the drugs in question are unproved, potentially dangerous, and experimental, they could hardly be included under the umbrella of customary care.

A secondary concern in the approach of providing experimental drugs to this group of patients is that of free choice. How free is the individual in selecting to be part of the clinical study when the choice is being coerced by the lack of options? The option of a sure death as compared to a small hope is perhaps no option at all. In some way, it is similar to the burn patient who pleads to be left alone or allowed to die in the emergency room. How much of this choice is self-determination and how much is being coerced by pain?

Finally, there is a serious scientific problem associated with the use of HIV-infected patients in the clinical studies. According to published reports and television documentaries, this group of patients is desperately seeking remedies from any source. Lack of compliance with clinical research protocols has always been a minor problem in research, but what is to be done in a situation in which patients are so desperate that they will lie, cheat, or essentially do anything to gain access to what may be their only hope to personal survival? How would one do a serious study in a community that is self-medicating with whatever drugs can be found on any market? Randomized clinical trials depend on therapeutic control of the experimental clinical groups. In uncontrolled circumstances in which unauthorized drugs are being taken by either the group assigned the IND or the placebo, the possibility of nonscientific and erroneous conclusions are magnified.

In the *United States* v. *Rutherford* ruling concerning laetrile, an unsubstantiated cure for cancer, the U.S. Supreme Court ruled that the Food and Drug Administration had the legal duty to protect the terminally ill from unsafe and unproved drugs.[19] Fatally ill patients do not have a legal right on the basis of their illness to receive experimental and potentially unsafe drugs.

While the FDA processes need to be streamlined, safeguards must be maintained. The recent medications for management of acute pain in adults that were quickly taken from the market following unanticipated life-threatening side effects are an indication that we need to move cautiously in lowering the safety barriers. What is not clear is where the compromise is to be cut so as to accommodate the free market and AIDS activists and still protect the public. What is clear is that this is a decision in which social prudence is perhaps the best policy.

GLOBAL EPIDEMIC

The AIDS epidemic in the United States has seen some positive signs of becoming manageable. New therapeutic regimens are promising to turn the disease from life threatening to a chronic condition. The early dramatic rise in new cases has begun to level off and in some population groups even decline. However, even in the United States, with all the efforts toward education and treatment, the CDC survey shows that 4.4 percent of gay men in their twenties are being infected each year, about twice the incidence of infection in gay men overall. Many young men of all races have become complacent about safe sex, and if chatroom chatter is an indication, they are not only fantasizing about it but are making connections. It may become necessary in the near future for the CDC to start anew to convince a new generation of gay Americans that HIV is lethal.[20]

TABLE 12-2	
Global Estimates of the HIV/AIDS Epidemic Update, 2003	
Number of people living with HIV/AIDS	
Total	34–46 million
Adults	31–43 million
Children under 15 years	2.1–2.9 million
People newly infected	
Total	4.2–5.8 million
Adults	3.6–4.8 million
Children	590,000–810,000
AIDS deaths	
Total	2.5–3.6 million
Adults	2.1–2.9 million
Children	420,000–580,000

UNAIDS. Epidemic Update 2003

Tuskegee in Africa:
Deadly U.S. AIDS Experiments

The title for this case comes from the on-line newsletter *Revolutionary Worker*, no. 926, October 5, 1997. The newsletter likened some experiments recently held in Africa to the Tuskegee experiments in the South, in which poor African American men infected with syphilis were left untreated so that the researchers could study the natural progression of the disease.

Clinical trials in the United States have demonstrated that AZT treatment during and after pregnancy can reduce the risk of HIV transmission to the newborn to about 8 percent. Without treatment, the risk of transmission is about 30 percent.

In the African experiments, pregnant HIV-infected women were placed on lower-than-optimum dosages of the AZT protocol to assess how effective these suboptimum medication regimes were in reducing the level of transmission. Placebo control trials were matched to evaluate the risk reduction. Assume appropriate informed consent had been attained.

1. If an effective treatment is known, is it ethical to do human research using a substandard level of care? Such experiments would be ethically and politically unacceptable in the United States. Does doing them in the Third World make a difference?

2. If an effective treatment is known and the disease is fatal, should placebo trials be carried out?

Once you have thought through those questions, consider the following economic factors. The standard regime in the United States costs over $1,000 which is estimated to be about 100 times what is spent on health care for an average person in Central Africa per year. One telling quote from a journalist was, "If the cure for AIDS was a clean glass of water, Africa could not afford it."

3. If the current standard of care is so expensive as to render it literally unavailable, would it then be acceptable to do studies evaluating a lesser standard that would not afford the same level of protection but would at least be potentially affordable?

According to Peter Piot, executive director of the Joint United Nations Program on HIV/AIDS (UNAIDS), the overall epidemic is spreading faster than ever before. It is estimated that there were 5 million newly infected people with HIV in 2003, with 80 percent of these occurring in the developing world. The most vulnerable region of the world appears to be sub-Saharan Africa, where the epidemic threatens the whole health system. The recent natural disasters, social disintegration, wars, and mass population movements within the region have all worked to exacerbate the spread of HIV in the area. In many hospitals in the region, patients with AIDS occupy over 80 percent of the hospital beds. Infection rates among prostitutes in Kenya are as high as 80 percent and 55 percent in other regions. The new therapeutics that offers so much promise in the developed world are most often out of financial reach for these patients. It is estimated that the economic losses in Africa associated with AIDS may soon exceed total foreign assistance to the region.

Although the situation in sub-Saharan Africa is drastic, in regions such as Uganda prevention efforts have lowered HIV prevalence rates in certain age groups of young women. Where there is adequate funding and full government and community support, targeted prevention programs have offered some positive signs. It is not likely, however, that prevention alone will be enough to end the epidemic in the region.

Eastern Europe has also witnessed a tremendous increase of HIV infections. In that these nations are currently struggling to institute new governmental and social structure, they do not have the infrastructure of appropriate social services and prevention programs to deal with the emerging epidemic. Most new infections in the Russian Federation are occurring in people who inject drugs, and it is reported that in certain Ukrainian cities, the infection rate among injecting drug users is over 50 percent.

Southeast Asia has a rapidly developing problem in regard to HIV infections, and given its large populations, may surpass Africa in terms of absolute numbers of people infected with HIV. Asia, India, Vietnam, and Cambodia appear to have the greatest challenge in controlling the disease. The numbers of reported HIV infections in the People's Republic of China have increased over tenfold in the last five years. While the absolute numbers in China are still relatively small, the rate of increase is a major concern.

Not surprisingly, given the high infection rates, many of these nations have seen a decrease in life expectancy. The life expectancy in Thailand, Kenya, Zimbabwe, and Zambia has been reduced by at least five years. What is needed are technically and ethically sound approaches to prevention and treatment. The introduction of the female condom should help reduce the spread of the disease by sex workers. Affordable regimens to prevent mother-to-child transmission of the infection are a vital need. However, the key to control of the global AIDS epidemic appears to be a vaccine. According to Piot, "prevention will never be enough—we need a vaccine."[21]

CONCLUSION

Acquired immunodeficiency syndrome (AIDS) continues to grow as a worldwide epidemic. The disease, which at one time was centered within certain high-risk groups, has now spread to all segments of the population. The study of high-risk groups is no longer the best way to identify those at risk for the disease; rather, risk should be measured through the observance of certain high-risk behaviors.

Due to the frightening consequences of the disease and its relative newness, the public has reacted very negatively toward those infected. Victims of the disease have been stigmatized, exposed to humiliation, and have experienced loss of work, insurance, and housing. The issue of confidentiality and the attempt to sustain a level of privacy beyond that provided for other diseases often create problems for the patient and the health care provider. AIDS is the only disease about which there is any question as to whether health care providers should be told the diagnosis of their patients. In some sense, the confidentiality and privacy provided the Florida dentist were a major cause of the tragic deaths of his patients.

None of these issues has yet been satisfactorily addressed. How we finally address and resolve these problems will speak either well or ill of the ethical foundations of the American health care system. Because of the scope of the ethical problems associated with the AIDS epidemic, our actions in response to it will leave either a proud or a shameful heritage for future health care providers.

KEY CONCEPTS

- The history of dealing with AIDS has caused the rethinking and refining of our duties as health care providers during an epidemic.

- Given no current method for decreasing susceptibility to AIDS, most public health activities have been directed toward eliminating the source of the organisms and interrupting the mode of transmission.

- The adoption of standard precautions for all patients has reduced the risk of treatment of AIDS patients to an acceptable level for health care providers. Given these processes and the traditions of Western health care ethics, it would appear that health care providers have a duty to treat.

- Infected health care providers have an obligation to remove themselves from procedures that would place their patients at risk.

▪ The nature of the disease and its population groups makes confidentiality a special duty for health care providers.

▪ The AIDS epidemic is an international disaster, with some developing nations reporting over 25 percent of their populations being infected. Currently the world has not yet sufficiently addressed this growing problem.

REVIEW EXERCISES

A. In the following scenarios, determine the correct provider response. Justify your answer.

1. If the nurse attending the patient were herself immune suppressed, would this be enough to move the duty to treat an HIV-infected patient to the moral option of treating or not treating?

2. You are a respiratory therapist and have been assigned to a floor unit. You find that your department head has decided to reuse patient suction traps in order to save money. This is a breach of universal precautions. What should your response be?

3. As an EMT, you punctured your gloves while removing an auto accident victim from her car. In this case, would you have a legitimate right to know her HIV status?

4. You are a physical therapist and have been seeing Mr. Jones for months as a result of a referral from Dr. Smith. Over this time period, your relationship has grown until the patient has a better relationship with you than with his physician. One day he tells you that he is HIV positive and asks that you not tell Dr. Smith. What action do you take?

5. You are a dental hygienist and have found out that you are pregnant. Is this a rationale for refusing to treat HIV-infected patients?

6. In that Dr. Acer has caused alarm among dental patients, your clinic has decided to advertise in the local paper that all your staff is "HIV free." Is this ethical? Review your code of ethics.

B. U.S. Public Health policy has been very restrictive in accepting blood from sexually active homosexual and bisexual men with multiple partners. Some gay activists have seen this as stigmatizing the gay community, which includes both infected and noninfected individuals. This appears to be a conflict between the right to give a gift and the right of the individual who receives the blood to know that the gift of blood is pure.

State your opinion in regard to the argument. Is there a compromise position that would be satisfactory to both groups?

C. Kimberly Bergalis was a young woman apparently infected by the Florida dentist. In a letter prior to her death she wrote the following:

> I was infected by Dr. Acer in 1987. My life has been sheer hell except for the good times and closeness with my family and my enjoyment for life and nature. AIDS has slowly destroyed me. Unless a cure is found, I will be another one of your statistics soon.
>
> Who do I blame? Do I blame myself? I sure don't. I never used IV drugs, never slept with anyone, and never had a blood transfusion. I blame Dr. Acer and every single one of you bastards—anyone who knew Dr. Acer was infected—and stood by not doing a damn thing about it.

One of the assumptions that can be drawn from the above quote is that there were those who knew that Dr. Acer was infected and yet protected his privacy at Bergalis's expense. What do you think is the appropriate balance between protecting infected health care providers and protecting their patients?

D. Review the chronology of the epidemic found at the beginning of the chapter, and write a reflective response to the following questions.

1. Why do you think that it took until 1987 before President Reagan publicly addressed the issue of AIDS?

2. In 2000 the United Nations and United States declared the AIDS epidemic an issue of national security. Is it?

3. The United States has currently pledged several hundred million dollars toward the international fight against AIDS. Many in the world have criticized us for not giving more, given that the UN secretary general has estimated a need for $7 to $10 billion. What do you think is our obligation?

4. After years of decline of new infections within the gay community, some cities are reporting an increase in new HIV infections. What do you think is the cause of this, and what should be the national response?

E. Ecological analysis of social and developmental correlates of country-level HIV seroprevalence may suggest strategies for combating the HIV/AIDS epidemic.

> Countries with earlier ages at first sex, higher teenage birth rates, and higher fertility rates had higher HIV seroprevalence. Countries with high HIV seroprevalence had fewer women using contraceptives, more persons with casual sex partners, and higher herpes simplex virus 2 seroprevalence. Male circumcision and Muslim religion were collinearly associated with lower HIV seroprevalence. Countries with high HIV seroprevalence had fewer doctors, more midwives, and less access to essential medication, but health spending differences were minor.[22]

Much of the above might fall into the category of "tell me what I already know," except for the fact that we are talking about foreign lands that critically need assistance if they are to address the AIDS epidemic. Some conclusions that might be drawn from the study would call for interventions such as:

- Delaying sexual activity
- Discouraging casual sex partnerships
- Promoting male circumcision
- Promoting of the use of condoms

To what extent should U.S. assistance to a foreign land be predicated upon that nation making substantial societal change?

NOTES

1. Adapted from "The Global HIV/AIDS Epidemic: A Timeline of Key Milestones," *Kaiser Family Foundation*. www.kff.org. 2005.

2. Centers for Disease Control (CDC), *HIV/AIDS Surveillance Report*, Division of HIV/AIDS Prevention, vol. 14, 2002.

3. *Understanding AIDS*, HHS Publication no. (CDC) HHS-88-8404. 1988.

4. Nancy Milliken and Ruth Greenblatt, *Ethical Issues of the AIDS Epidemic* (Rockville, MD: Aspen Publication, 1988).

5. Ann Seidl, "HIV Testing: Patient's Rights v. Nurse's Rights," *Nursing Issues of the Nineties and Beyond* (New York: Springer, 1994).

6. Health and Public Policy Committee, American College of Physicians, and the Infectious Disease Society of America, "Acquired Immunodeficiency Syndrome," position paper, *Annals of Internal Medicine* 104 (1986).

7. American Nurses Association, *Code for Nurses with Interpretative Statements* (Kansas City, MO: American Nurses Association, 1985).

8. Robert Jarvis, Michael Closen, et al. *AIDS Law* (St. Paul, MN: West Publishing Company, 1996).

9. *Doe* v. *Centinela Hospital*, No. CV 87-2154, 1988 WL8177b (C.D. Cal. June 30, 1988).

10. George Pozgar, *Legal Aspects of Health Administration* (Rockville, MD: Aspen Publication, 2004).

11. C. H. Fox, "AIDS Transmission: Hazardous Health Care?" *Harvard Health Letter* 17 (1991).

12. M. Field, "Testing for AIDS," *Journal of Law and Medicine* 16 (1990).

13. *Estate of Behringer* v. *Medical Center at Princeton,* 592A.2d 1251 (N.J. Super. Ct. Law Div. 1991).

14. Larissa Kuntz, "CDC Shifts Control," *RT Image,* July 20, 1992.

15. Donise Grady, "Infected Healers," *American Health* (April 1991).

16. "Commission on the Federal Drug Approval Process, Final Report" (Washington, DC: Institutes of Medicine. Aug. 15, 1990).

17. AIDS Coalition to Unleash Power (ACT UP), "A National AIDS Treatment, Research Agenda" (distributed at the Fifth International Conference on AIDS, 1989).

18. Udo Schuklenk, *Access to Experimental Drugs in Terminal Illness* (New York: Pharmaceutical Products Press, 1998).

19. *United States* v. *Rutherford,* 442 U.S. 544 (1979).

20. Cathy Thomas, "A New Scarlet Letter," *Time Magazine,* June 11, 2001, pp. 82–83.

21. *UNAIDS Report* 2003.

22. *Journal of Acquired Immune Deficiency Syndrome,* 35, no. 4 (2004): pp. 410–420.

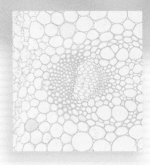

Ethical Issues and Genetic Manipulation

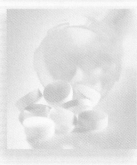

GOAL

To understand the various areas of genetic research and the moral problems that are associated with them.

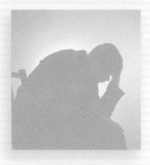

OBJECTIVES

Upon completion of this chapter, the reader should be able to:

1. Understand the purpose, practice, benefits, and dangers of genetic screening.

2. Understand the benefits of prenatal genetic testing and how it leads to the moral issues that surround abortion.

3. Describe the dangers of utilizing genetic research for the purpose of eugenics.

4. Explain the promise of the human genome project.

5. Understand the scientific advances possible with recombinant DNA as well as the dangers that unregulated research can create.

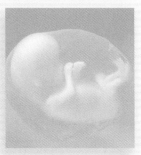

6. Put all the issues that are raised in this chapter in the context of the Faust legend.

7. Explain how ethical problems with genetics make necessary a new virtue of family planning with guidelines that help us utilize genetic counseling in an ethical manner.

8. Explain the promise and ethical pitfalls associated with gene therapy.

9. Create a policy statement that provides an ethically suitable direction in regard to cloning technology.

10. Explain the posthumanist position regarding genetic science and the discussion of ethics.

11. Explain the current state of stem cell research and provide a pro and con argument for its continuance.

KEY TERMS

Allele	**Genetic disease**	**Posthumanism**
Dominant gene	**Genetic predisposition**	**Recessive gene**
Eugenics	**Genetic screening**	**Recombinant DNA**
Gene therapy	**Genome**	**Regenerative medicine**
Genetic carriers	**Heterozygous**	**Stem cells**

I'd like to believe you can't do science if you're a really evil person, but it's probably a romantic view.

Peter Goodfellow, geneticist

The development of biology is going to destroy to some extent our traditional grounds for ethical beliefs, and it is not easy to see what to put in their place.

Francis Crick, biologist

Between the scientist and the application of his work stands society.

Bryan Appleyard, author

One day a woman's father comes home and starts ranting and raving. She has never quite seen him like this. His limbs begin moving in strange ways, and later, he begins to have seizures. Finally, the doctors have the diagnosis: Huntington's disease. Now she finds out that, because her father's disease is the result of a dominant gene, she has a fifty-fifty chance of getting it herself. This is the story of Frances.[1] It is not a happy story, but it is true, and it is repeated all too often. There is no cure for Huntington's disease, and it develops between a person's thirties and fifties, so one often finds out only after having passed the disease to one's own children. If the damage has been done, is it better not to know? After all, fifty years is a lifetime, even if it does not match our average life expectancy. Still, there is great hope, for researchers have moved fast in first finding a marker for the gene that causes Huntington's disease, and now in finding the actual gene that causes it.[2] However, the great hope that we have is associated with potential danger, for knowledge is power, and the knowledge gained in finding the Huntington's gene is the same

CASE STUDY

The Future Is Almost Now

In the not-too-distant future, given our developing knowledge and statistical abilities, medical science may allow health care providers to take a DNA sample from a fetus and create a vast probability chart—a type of medical horoscope for the infant. From this, one could fashion a lifestyle precisely tuned to our genetic predispositions.

- We may find that we can smoke without fear of cancer.
- We may need to avoid red meat to avoid a stroke in our mid-forties.
- We may be able to not worry about using sunscreen on the beach.
- We should avoid living near or working at manufacturing plants that create plastics.

Our knowledge of genetics may free us from a whole range of fears that health care professionals feel obliged to warn the whole population against. Instead of following every "good for you" health rule, we can be more precise and personal in our health care efforts. On the other hand, the probability chart may warn us of a future horrific illness.

1. How do you think that a yet-to-come diagnosis would affect you today?
2. Are you ill if you have the diagnosis of a horrific condition in the future?
3. Should your health care insurance costs be targeted to account for the horrific condition?
4. Should future employers be provided with your probability chart?
5. What if the predisposition is for a horrific disease without a current cure? Could the personal probability chart become the basis for the ultimate preventive medicine, abortion?

as that used in bioengineering—potentially one of the greatest but also most dangerous developments of human intelligence. But the stakes are high. Twenty percent of the 250,000 birth defects in children are due to known genetic causes. Should we just let **genetic disease** continue if we have the power to stop it or at least lessen its impact? The consensus so far seems to be that we should move forward, but we should be clear regarding what it means to move forward in this area.

> After thousands of years of engineering the cold remains of the earth into utilities, human beings are now setting out to engineer the internal biology of living organisms. . . . The transition is indeed staggering.[3]

THE HUMAN GENOME PROJECT AND MEDICAL PROGRESS

It is the vastness of the genetics enterprise that is so overwhelming. We may be approaching that moment in history when we can choose not only how we are going to live but who we are going to be. We are perhaps at a watershed moment, bigger in impact than the grand ideas of capitalism, socialism, or Darwinian evolution combined. The impact may be larger than the technological advances of dynamite and computers, and more significant (assuming that it did not kill us) than a meteor strike. In the end, how we answer the basic questions thrust on us by this revolution in biology will shape our philosophy, our science, our technology, and the very way we think about humans and humanity.

The human **genome** project which provides a complete list of the chemical letters that compose the map of the human genome has been completed. The promise of this information and its potential application is remarkable and may change the nature of health care itself. The psychologist Thomas Bouchard has said, "For almost every behavioral trait so far investigated, from reaction time to religiosity, an important fraction of the variation among people turns out to be associated with genetic variation."[4] Does this mean that all of the small idiosyncrasies that make us unique humans (both lovable and frustrating) are within our grasp to change? What we have not seen yet in regard to the information gained from the project is the application, but it is likely that we will shortly see a number of specific medical treatments based on the information. What is perhaps missing is the overarching vision that provides the way forward beyond the initial steps.

In our time, we will resolve what we think about cloning humans. Some have made claims that they have already cloned humans, and if it is not so, it is only a matter of time. We are a global community now, even if human cloning were forbidden here in the United States that would not stop the process from being developed. It is possible that as a species, we may back away from cloning full humans, but cloning as a technology will proceed. It is quite likely that we will master our control of the genes enough to enable us to clone distinct body parts for transplantation. In that these parts will be genetically identical to the rest of the patient's body, the problem with rejection will be resolved.

In the interim, it appears that animals will be more radically altered in our quest for body parts to assist in the human organ shortage. There are still technical problems with the transfer of animal viruses to humans and the refining of immune response suppression, but both problems can be resolved. It is not a great leap in expectation to believe that in the next several decades, xenotransplantation will become commonplace.

The alteration of agricultural products and animals for human benefit will surely be a key part of our future. It is likely that we will reengineer various types of pharmaceutical foodstuffs like corn and bananas to replace some medicines. Whole new farm factories may develop that produce high-quality proteins. We now have created monkeys that glow in the dark and placed human genes in pigs.[5] Could we in the future create a potato that tastes like pork and has human genes, giving us the option of being both a vegetarian and cannibal at the same time? For many Americans, the European ban on genetically altered foodstuffs seems both self-serving and irrational. However, when one contemplates what we could do, who knows?

Over the past hundred years, we have doubled our life expectancy, at least in the developed world. Will our biological road map let us do that again? Some hold that aging itself may be entirely a genetic process, which could be manipulated. Is immortality an option? Would that even be beneficial? Perhaps the better and more ecologically acceptable route would be to live disease free and well for eighty-five years and die quickly in our sleep after a day in which we made a hole in one on the golf course. For most of us, the option of a longer life is not acceptable if it means a longer period of helpless dependency.

The human genome project maps the whole human genome, the complete genetic makeup of the human being. Given that this is pure research, the only question to ask is whether such knowledge is proper for humans to possess. Critics of the human genome project could point to the character of Faust (or Dr. Faustus) in order to show how one can be led astray by the unquenchable thirst for knowledge. Dr. Faustus is a scholar so determined to possess more and more knowledge—especially concerning the deepest subjects such as the secret of life and afterlife—that he is willing to trade his soul to the devil for it. Faust makes the bargain and is happy with the bargain until the devil comes for his payment. In the same way, we will be happy with what our knowledge will bring us, but we will be devastated when we are called upon to pay the fee. Like Icarus, we will fly too high, and our wings will melt. This is, in fact, how Marlowe understood the character of Dr. Faustus.

> Till swoll'n with cunning, of a self-conceit,
> His waxen wings did mount above his reach
> And melting, heavens conspired his overthrow![6]

The point of the Faust and Icarus stories is generally that humankind should recognize its limitations; the failure to do so is to commit the sin of excessive pride or hubris. In secular terms, we say that humankind is in danger of overreaching its proper boundaries.

The key worry behind overreaching is that there is inevitably some disaster that comes as a result. The question is whether there will be any such fee, for no one has made any pacts with the devil in setting up the human genome project.

Some argue that there are no limits to human knowledge and that there shouldn't be. Such fears, it could be argued, are the result of theological beliefs that are no longer held. The theological basis for the Faustian view is that humans have a predetermined place in the scheme of things, and to move beyond this predetermined place is sacrilegious. Religious people do tend to believe that humankind has a place in God's plan, but most are not terribly sure that the quest for knowledge interferes with that plan; indeed, one can easily imagine that our place is to seek knowledge as a way of better knowing God's plan. For those who are not religious at all, there is no problem with God's plans in the first place. Environmentalists sometimes think of humankind as occupying a certain place in the natural order, but doing so is quite consistent with an unending quest for knowledge. There are dangers, to be sure, but they arise only when knowledge is applied.

There is a worry on the other side of the question—worry that we will put up artificial barriers to our knowledge and stop short of great discoveries that will radically increase the quality of life. Imagine if we had refrained from discovering the causes of various diseases that we have learned to cure or prevent. The fear is that we would be doing something similar if we stopped now in our quest for knowledge. Fears of the improper extension of human knowledge therefore seem to be unfounded unless one believes that the application of knowledge inevitably follows its acquisition. The question ultimately comes down to whether mankind can be trusted to use (or not use) the knowledge in question.

Modern science has achieved more than we could have dreamed possible. There is no denying the good that science has done for us. On the other hand, there is no doubt that the dangers are just as great as the benefits we have gained. Can we go too far in our attempts to understand nature? Have we gone beyond the limits of human responsibility? These are questions that arise when we consider current research in genetics and attempts to use this knowledge for the improvement of human life. Genes are the basic carriers of the information that makes us what we are. If we reach the point at which we understand these biological building blocks, will the power that comes with such knowledge be too much for humanity to use responsibly? These same questions were raised with the development of atomic science and have yet to be adequately resolved. For example, antinuclear activists argue that the consequences of a nuclear accident at a power plant outweigh the possible benefits of the plants in operation, and that the problems with waste disposal have yet to be overcome. Such questions are arising more and more in all areas of science, but genetic science has possibly the greatest potential for good and ill. In this chapter, we will examine recent developments in genetic science, particularly as it applies to medicine, and attempt to determine how we should negotiate our way through the forest of ethical issues that arise when we seek to understand and employ our understanding.

GENETICS AS SOCIAL POLICY

Other ethical issues arise when we consider the possibility of turning genetic testing into social policy. Some suggest that all parents be tested for genetic diseases in order to avoid the social and personal costs of genetic impairment. Others worry that this will lead to a coercive policy of abortion or of preventing parents from having children. Such policies raise still further issues when they are directed to certain ends, as they are with eugenics. **Eugenics** is the practice of manipulating the genes of offspring through either breeding or genetic alteration. Should we attempt to eliminate some or all genetic abnormalities? Should we attempt to improve the race of human beings by increasing intelligence through genetic selection?

> *The children of the good parents they will take to a rearing pen in the care of nurses living apart in a certain section of the city; the children of inferior parents, or any child of the others born defective, they will hide, as is fitting, in a secret and unknown place.*

> **Plato,** *The Republic,* Book V, 460C (380 b.c.).[7]

It is clear that Plato is referring to the practice of infanticide for diseased or disabled newborns. It is also clear that this practice is conceived to be part of a more general practice of eugenics, for Plato goes on to say, "if the breed of guardians is to remain pure." Sometimes what we think to be new choices are really quite old. After all, stock breeding is a form of eugenics. The dairy cow of today is a far cry from the wild cow from which it is descended. Our most recent experience with eugenics came when the Nazi experiments on human beings were revealed. It is therefore understandable if people are a bit apprehensive over any renaissance of eugenic ideas. Nevertheless, we should always give proposals a hearing lest some suspect that we are avoiding discussion out of fear of the truth.

The ability to screen and prenatally test for genetic disease raises the possibility that we could eliminate genetic diseases with a policy of negative eugenics or even improve the genetic pool of humanity by selecting for positive attributes—positive eugenics. A moderate policy of eugenics that has the intention of eliminating the most serious genetic diseases seems sensible enough, but even such a moderate approach is fraught with difficulties. The number of people carrying a recessive gene is rather large, and it is difficult to justify preventing such people from reproducing merely because they have a recessive gene. Given that it is impossible to have a genetically impaired infant with only one parent contributing a recessive gene for, say, sickle cell anemia, it would be hard to justify preventing such a couple from having children. On the other hand, if we do not eliminate these recessive genes, we will never overcome genetic disease.

An extreme program of negative eugenics faces practical difficulties that make it almost, if not in fact, impossible to implement. Could we eliminate all genetic disease? Since the majority of people carry at least one recessive gene for some genetic disease, a radical policy of negative eugenics would eliminate a large portion of the human population. But there is a more important question to ask: Would we want to eliminate all genetic disease? There are dangers involved in shrinking the gene pool. Our resistance to various sorts of biological attack is dependent to a great degree on our genetic variety. Take, for example, sickle cell anemia. We know the disease only from its negative effects here in the United States, but in malarial Africa, where the disease developed, being a carrier of the disease functions to ward off the effects of malaria.

A program of positive eugenics—here understood to include not only breeding but genetic intervention—attempts to improve the gene pool by increasing the numbers of those with positive attributes. Polls have shown that if this technology were available, many parents would make use of it. It is unlikely that we could ever develop anything like a "superhuman," but parents may be able to specify specific traits they would prefer to hand down to their children. There would be pressure upon parents (and the same would be true of nations) to utilize positive eugenics in order to increase their children's chances in a competitive market. But the problem ultimately is a scientific one; it is almost impossible to imagine a successful scientific program of eugenics, positive or negative. At this stage, the conclusion seems to be that our best course of action is to use genetic testing to help individuals rather than to alter the genetic makeup of humanity.

The names *Eugene* and *Eugenia* mean "well born" and share their entomological foundation in the ideas of eugenics. While we admire the beautiful people among us who seem so well born and move gracefully through life, it is often the nerds who become the more interesting people. Would a world of Eugenes and Eugenias be as interesting?

Stem cell research is another area that both gains from and suffers from the attempts to weld together a cohesive social policy within the glare of public debate and politics. These amazing cells are the topic of heated debate.

Human embryonic **stem cells** are the building blocks of life. They are like blank slates, potentially capable of becoming any cell in the body. Early in pregnancy, they begin to differentiate into all of the body's specialized tissues and organs.[8] Imagine the possibilities if we could figure out the switching mechanisms for these cells and coax them to grow the specialized tissues we need. It does not take a great deal of imagination to see the application in regard to spinal injuries, juvenile diabetes, multiple sclerosis, cancer, and Parkinson's disease. We could even produce organs and tissues from cloned cells that would be genetically identical to the intended recipient.

The problem is that we do not know at this time how to coax stem cells into doing any of the things we imagine that they could do. So when we are told that President Bush has banned stem cell research and is cruelly delaying cures for Parkinson's disease, multiple sclerosis, Alzheimer's, spinal cord injuries, and other afflictions too numerous to mention, you may get the feeling that we are right on the brink of these applications and the president is standing in the way. It is interesting to note that the public support for stem cell research becomes much stronger when you add Alzheimer's to the list of potential cures, even though there is little evidence that this is a potential application because Alzheimer's is so complex.

In August 2001, President Bush attempted a compromise: scientists could apply for federal funding only for research utilizing seventy-eight existing stem cell lines. (A *stem cell line* is a family of constantly dividing cells, the product of a single embryo.) Since the announcement, the true number of available and suitable lines appears to be closer to twenty than the higher number. These existing lines were created using now-obsolete techniques and are considered less suitable than some of the newer lines. However, they appear adequate for research into the switching mechanisms, even if they would not be suitable for future therapeutic applications. The restrictions do not hamper the use of private funds for the other lines, only federal funds. In effect, what President Bush did was to draw a line with federal funding. In his compromise, he managed to irritate just about everyone. In that embryos are destroyed in the process, he went beyond many of the more fundamental of his political base, and by not swinging open the door to all the lines (both present and future) with federal funding, he has left himself open for criticism that he is keeping patients from getting the miraculous cures that are being promised. As Ron Reagan, the son of the late Republican president, said at the 2004 Democratic Convention, the stem cells are "magic"; imagine "your own personal biological repair kit standing by at the hospital."[9]

The president's dilemma in regard to this research is tied to the word *embryo*. Human life begins with the embryo, which grows into a fetus, then an infant, then a child, then an adult. One can stand on pretty firm moral ground and argue against the justification of killing an adult, child, or infant for research purposes, the aim of which is to provide body parts for other human beings. We then are back to whether the embryo should have the same moral protections.

The argument from this duty-oriented position is that moral tradition teaches that we must treat every living member of the human species, including embryos, as a human person with fundamental rights, including the right to life. Some have argued that if a clear line is not drawn, then other populations, such as those in persistent vegetative states, could be at risk in the future. If you draw the line at the moment of conception, then because we are all of equal dignity, we are not at each other's disposal. Does the use of human embryos as raw materials for biotechnology undermine the value of all human life?

Yet there are problems because as humans, we often want to be on both sides of an argument depending on our current desires. When confronted with personal infertility, even those who argue that the line should be drawn at the moment of conception will often rejoice in the prospect of a process that would bring them a child, even when numerous embryos are created, then frozen, rated for their quality, discarded if they hold genetic defects, or are thawed and discarded. None of these practices would be acceptable if we were dealing with adult humans. What is to be done with the 400,000 embryos, each the size of a pinhead, that are stored in cylinders filled with liquid nitrogen at more than 430 fertility clinics in the United States?[10] If being thawed and destroyed is truly the fate of these excess embryos, why not use them for biotechnological research?

This forms the basis for a second line of reasoning in regard to stem cell research, which recognizes that investing in science and technology is always a consideration of risks and benefits. Biological research has extended human life and improved its quality. Yet every step forward has exacted a toll in harms and risks. Scientists using this form of utilitarian reasoning would argue that the benefits from stem cell research are of such great magnitude that the required destruction of human embryos in the process, especially ones that are to be discarded anyway, is permissible. Again, imagine the benefits that humanity will gain from a new specialty of **regenerative medicine** that is focused on growing specialized tissues for spinal cord injuries, diabetes, cancer, multiple sclerosis, Parkinson's disease, and many other currently unthought-of applications.

President Bush has not banned stem cell research. In an attempt at compromise, he limited the use of federal funding of projects to those using already harvested stem cell lines. The number of these lines is fewer than originally stated, probably about twenty. While this limits research with federal funding, it does not limit research with private funding, and several major centers are being established to conduct research with the newer lines. While we can and should continue to debate the issue, we should recognize that we are still in the very early stages of the research, the basic research stage. The positive applications of stem cell research are probably a decade away. Basic science is a slow, expensive, painstaking process. The final application of stem cell research may in fact not be therapeutic applications at all, but rather only an increased knowledge of how the human body works. It is important to keep in mind where we are in the science of this issue, because when politics enters the process, we are confronted by those who would take complicated science and moral issues and reduce them to pro and con bumper sticker slogans.

GENETIC ENGINEERING

> The recombinant DNA process is the most dramatic technological tool to date in the growing biotechnological arsenal. The biologist is learning how to manipulate, recombine and reorganize living tissue into new forms and shapes, just as his craftsmen ancestors did by firing inanimate matter. The speed of the discoveries is truly phenomenal. It is estimated that biological knowledge is currently doubling every five years, and in the field of genetics . . . We are virtually hurling ourselves into the age of biotechnology.[11]

Research into **recombinant DNA** is indeed a marvel of modern science, but it also brings forth some of the greatest fears of all. Scientists are now genetically altering organisms for various purposes. We have heard about genetically altered fruits and vegetables, but the range of experiments is extremely varied. The fear is that experimenters will develop organisms that will endanger humans or other living beings. The possibilities are the stuff of science fiction, and such fears have led to calls for restricting this research or even banning it altogether. Such calls have increased in recent years, and many argue for a complete ban on genetically altered foods. Additional issues have arisen concerning conflict of interest among scientists who are supported by government but turn to the marketplace for additional compensation. The ethical issues that arise involve those listed in connection with the human genome project, but others worry whether scientists can be trusted with the awesome responsibilities that come with such dangerous research. Can we rely on scientists to take the necessary precautions to keep the organisms they create harmless to human beings?

GENETIC TESTING

Doctors can test couples to see if it is possible that they will give birth to a genetically impaired infant. For example, we can now test couples for sickle cell, a disease that deforms red blood cells into thin, elongated sickle-shaped forms and causes anemia, cough, and muscle cramps. Sickle cell occurs only when both parents are carriers of the **recessive gene**. If both parents are carriers, there is a 25 percent chance that the child will have the disease. Is this too much of a risk for parents to take? Depending upon how paternalistic we are, we might (1) not allow them to have children, (2) suggest strongly that they do not have children, (3) refuse to pay the medical expenses (this would be a decision for insurance companies and/or government), or (4) merely leave it up to the parents whether to take the risk. Most would leave the decision up to the parents, but some would argue that the parents should not be allowed to have a child when the risk is so high. It is argued that it is unfair to bring a child into the world knowing that it will have such a heavy burden to bear.

Sickle cell is instructive, however, in that it is a disease that primarily afflicts people of African descent. To refuse to allow people children who are members of a minority may suggest racist motives. But there are other diseases that are not so selective. Are we to restrict people afflicted with nonracially connected genetic disease? Many people believe that it is their right to bear children, however they turn out. It is further argued that there are many afflictions that are not genetically caused or cannot be tested for. Why might such people be allowed to be born but not those with a disposition to diseases we can test for? The assumption here is that existence is a good thing; for some it may not be, and then testing would be preventing injury. This raises a deep problem: Can existence be an injury?

At first glance, human existence could be understood as an injury in utilitarian terms if the prospective life would likely contain more unhappiness than happiness. But this will not do, because ordinary life is a veil of tears for many people. To be useful for our purposes in the argument that asserts that existence can be an injury, it must be the case that bodily or mental impairment must be significantly greater than that which most people must face. This is certainly true for many diseases, and this would provide us with grounds to argue that existence can be an injury; therefore it would be immoral for such a person to be brought into the world.

Some argue that the perspective employed in such an argument is not the correct one. The proper perspective is that of the person afflicted, and from such a perspective any sort of existence may be preferable to none at all. It may be that great suffering may be endurable if just a little happiness is possible, and this is almost always the case. There is also the problem of anticipating what a future person would prefer. Given the difficulties of such calculations, some argue that there can be no good argument against having children.

A middle ground may be found by referring to actual cases. Some diseases offer only a brief and painful existence, while others are so seriously painful and prolonged that the question of a worthwhile life is out of the question. On the other hand, some diseases are not as severe. Take, for example, Down syndrome. Such children are afflicted with serious problems, but the severity varies widely. It is often pointed out that Down syndrome children frequently lead happy lives.

Some argue that we must also never underestimate the human spirit and its ability to overcome adversity. As a notable example, Helen Keller is known for having overcome devastating odds to lead a fulfilling life. The response to this argument is that one case does not a policy make. We must ground any moral policy in the reality of the overwhelming majority of cases. Policy should aim at the majority, and exceptions to the rule—the hard cases—should be regarded as exceptional. It may be too much to expect that all those with Helen Keller's afflictions be able to achieve what she did.

We may be able to test for **genetic predispositions** in the future. Some people are more genetically predisposed to certain diseases (such as cancer) and to react to toxic chemicals that cause diseases. Roughly 10 percent of the population have bodies that produce enzymes that combine with hydrocarbons and produce carcinogenic substances. One can imagine companies refusing to hire potential employees who are genetically disposed to diseases caused by the toxic chemicals used in certain industries. In fact, this is already happening without the benefit of genetic testing; the mere occurrence of several instances of a disease in a family has led companies to gauge the cost and availability of insurance accordingly.[12] One can therefore assume that as actual tests become available, the possibilities for discrimination will be great. Given that we have no control over our genetic makeup, the fairness of such practices must be questioned.

THE ROLE OF PARENTS

Virtue ethics gives us a special perspective on this question. It is the role of parents to make many decisions for their children, including the decision of life and death (or nonexistence) prior to conception and birth (assuming one is pro-abortion). One can construct a virtue ethics position that puts the decision completely in the hands of the parents. Thus, if a couple wishes to take on the burden of raising a defective child, it is morally acceptable. It must also be added that having such a child would entail duties that would go beyond those that parents of normal children would be required to assume. (Society may also gain a voice in the decision if the cost of raising the child is carried by society to any great extent. Is it legitimate knowingly to bring a child into the world with serious defects when one also knows that one cannot pay the expenses?) Prior commitments to society must be made if one takes on a risk knowing that society may very well have to carry part or all of the economic burden of tending to a child's health. But this perspective also puts the decision not to have children (or to abort) completely in the hands of parents. This would mean that parents would have the right to abort a child with characteristics that many would consider acceptable. Take, for example, the case of the Down syndrome child. A couple may have a wish for a child who can share in their preference for a rather intellectual existence, an existence that is out of the question for any Down syndrome child.

Many would accept the virtue ethics perspective when it indicates that parents may bring a defective child into the world if they wish but they would not accept the alternative side of the equation that permits parents to abort children deemed unacceptable to them for less than extremely serious reasons. Clearly, one's position on the abortion issue and the concept of personhood comes into play. If one is inclined to accept abortion, then both sides of the virtue ethics perspective make sense. If one does not accept abortion as a morally acceptable practice, then one would argue that it would be acceptable to refrain from conceiving such children but that it would not be acceptable to abort such a child once conceived.

THE POLITICS OF SCREENING

Testing large populations (screening) has a checkered history. The early sickle cell anemia screening laws are instructive. The science of testing got caught up in a whirlwind of well-intentioned legislation in the early stages of the civil rights movement. It was a way of doing good for African Americans, a group of people who were becoming increasingly politically important. But legislators are not scientists. The early legislation was often poorly written and sometimes directed at the wrong target populations.

One consistent mistake was to refer to carriers of the sickle cell as diseased. To have the disease, one must have inherited the **allele** from both parents, whereas carriers have inherited the allele from only one parent. An unanticipated problem came up as paternity discrepancies arose. If a child turned out to be **heterozygous** and neither parent was heterozygous, then it became clear that someone else was involved in the reproductive process. There are many instances where this sort of revelation has led to the breakup of otherwise stable families.

Other mistakes occurred. The state of Virginia, for example, mandated that all convicts be tested for the disease, when inmates generally have few immediate plans for reproduction. Some states used testing methods that were not the most accurate available and thus achieved an unacceptably high number of incorrect positive results. Finally, there is the issue of confidentiality. Few states were prepared to protect the confidentiality of the patients. It was feared that discrimination in employment and insurance would result, or at the least that a social stigma would be attached to those identified as carriers. The lesson of the sickle cell experience shows us that **genetic screening** requires wisdom, sensitivity, and most important, good science. We must not allow well-intentioned proposals to become practice without paying close attention to the procedures and the consequences.

RECOMBINANT DNA RESEARCH

The application of the knowledge gained from the human genome project is likely to be in the field of recombinant DNA. Scientists recombine the genetic material from one organism to another for various reasons. Sometimes it is done to improve a plant in some way, for example, to make it less susceptible to spoilage and damage, to ripen it sooner, and so on. Scientists also recombine DNA to create organisms that will attack pests of one sort or another. There have been attempts to create an organism that eats oil, for use in dealing with oil slicks. And, of course, the future holds the prospect of genetic intervention in human beings, either to combat disease or to eliminate a propensity for disease. The possibilities are endless.

Our experiences with nuclear physics give many cause for concern, and the fears associated with genetic research are similar. One fear is that such knowledge will be used by the military as another way to kill people, with disastrous results for both victim and victor. If a genetically engineered virus or bacteria were used, it would be difficult to contain and could attack us as well.

But even the peaceful uses of recombinant DNA technology are worrisome. One never knows if some experimental creature will interact with the natural environment in some negative way. Will we inadvertently create a modern-day Frankenstein's monster? The most commonly used bacterium is *Escherichia coli,* which is found in the stomachs of all human beings. Most creatures created by humans do not do well in the natural environment and are likely to die outside the laboratory, but since the attempts are precisely to create creatures hardy enough to fulfill our purposes in nature the prospect does hold some dangers. Scientists do employ special protocols for dealing with altered genetic materials, so it is unlikely that something will just be flushed down the drain where it can enter the natural environment, but as the technology becomes more common, it is likely to be in the hands of people who are not so careful.

The difficult training one must go through to become a genetic scientist will naturally restrict the numbers of those involved, but it is not always the case that people trained in the sciences are also conscious of their ethical duties. There is even one case of a scientist working on an organism to combat a disease affecting trees who was so upset at the delays the regulators were putting him through that he released the organism into the environment on his own. This is the kind of behavior that worries people. Nevertheless, the benefits we may reap from genetic engineering are too great to ignore.

GENETIC PHARMACY

One positive result of genetic engineering has been the development of the genetic pharmacy. We can now produce substances by genetic alteration that are helpful to many with medical problems. Scientists have modified bacteria to produce human insulin. This is particularly helpful to diabetics who are allergic to bovine or swine insulin. Vaccines have been produced for hepatitis B and a strain of genital herpes. Genetic pharmacy is one of the most productive and promising applications of genetic engineering.

GENE THERAPY

> It is a profound truth . . . that nature does not know best; that genetic evolution, if we choose to look at it liverishly instead of with fatuous good humor, is a story of waste, makeshift, compromise, and blunder.[13]

Genetic engineering raises the possibility of direct genetic intervention into human beings. Copies of a normal gene are injected into a cell with defective or nonpresent genes. Then the DNA of the cell is induced to incorporate the new gene so that the cell may function properly. If all goes well, when the cell reproduces, it passes along the new gene rather than the original. Eventually, the patient acquires a population of good cells that will carry out the proper functions. This method is most likely to be effective when the problem is caused by a single defective gene. Huntington's and sickle cell are this type of disease (monogenic). When a disease is the result of a combination of genes (polygenic), the potential for genetic treatment is further off, and most diseases are polygenic. Although **gene therapy** is extremely difficult, researchers are pushing ahead.

Scientists at the National Institutes of Health, for example, are engaged in the attempt to treat cancer patients with gene therapy. Some have argued that we are moving too fast into human experimentation.[14]

The speed at which we proceed is always a problem at the forefront of science and medicine, but the incredible power of gene therapy cautions prudence. We must be very sure that our attempts to improve the hand that nature deals us do not end up making things worse. For example, while the modification of somatic cells (cells that do not affect the genetic makeup of one's children) raises some moral issues, the modification of germ line cells brings us back to the whole issue of eugenics, with the attendant difficulties. Even short of altering the genetic course of the human race, there are important issues to be raised.

It is likely that we will soon be able to determine the sex of our children. Currently, many parents keep having children until they have one of the sex they prefer. As minor as this consideration is, genetic engineering can help by making sure the first child is a member of the sex preferred by the parents. One obvious problem of giving parents this power is that we may experience an imbalance of males and females. Even now, there are areas of the world where having a female child is regarded negatively, so if the technique of sex determination ever became widely available, problems could result. There is also the question of whether it is right to determine the sex of one's child. What if one chooses the sex, say, male, and the child later learns of the decision? Some might not care. Others might question their whole personality.

THE GENETIC CAUSES OF BEHAVIOR

A family in the Netherlands was found to have a mutation in a gene that coded for monoamine oxidase, a neurotransmitter that metabolizes adrenaline. The end effect of the mutation was that the affected individuals were constantly caught up in an adrenaline rush that signaled a flight-or-fight situation. The defect was on the X chromosome; women in the family generally were carriers of the defect, and its expression came out in the men. Research into the family history showed that half the men were angry, hostile, and antisocial and possessed low IQs.[15]

Suppose that these men were involved in a higher incidence of violence and antisocial behavior than others in the community. In our time, we have been asked to consider a whole range of mitigating circumstances regarding criminal acts. The classic case involved the San Francisco politician Harvey Milk who was murdered. The now famous "Twinky defense" held that the murderer had consumed too many sugary pastries and that these led to his irrational act. How much should the fact that one was abused as a child, sexually molested by a religious leader, or were currently attempting to give up smoking mitigate in a criminal case? Could a person truly be guilty if he had a "criminal gene"? If we decide that it is the gene, not the criminal act, that we should focus on, what does this do to the criminal justice system?

Although we are not likely ever to be able to fine-tune the behavior of individuals, even crude genetic modification of behavior could pose risks. One can imagine that some political leaders might prefer passivity for most of their citizenry. Or a political leader might prefer extremely aggressive people to populate the armed forces. Behavior is likely to be polygenic and substantially environmental, so that genetic engineering of this sort is unlikely. Nevertheless, there are some scientists investigating the genetic basis of criminal behavior. Imagine a case in which the presence of a certain gene causes 30 percent of those with the gene to engage in criminal behavior. Also imagine that the other 70 percent turn out to be the leaders of societies. What would be the appropriate action, if any, to take under these circumstances?

Some have suggested that all behavior is mediated through our genes and may be within our reach to modify. Just as we might find the "criminal gene," which predisposes to a life of crime, or the "homosexual gene," which leads to alternate sexual choices, it is possible that we might find the "religiosity gene," which shapes our willingness to believe in God and to strive to live a moral life. How much are we willing to change?

CASE STUDY

A Matter of Justice

In the 1980s a woman was brought to trial for the murder of her mother. As a defense, her lawyer argued that her family suffered from the genetic defect that leads to Huntington's disease and that her aberrant behavior was perhaps the first sign of its onset. Given that her father had died of the disease, she had a 50 percent chance of inheriting the genetic condition. The judge deciding the case did not accept the argument, and she was convicted. However, some years later, the woman began to display the symptoms. The judge recalled the case and ordered her release.

1. What was the correct decision: the first, which sent her to prison, the second, when she was released, or were both decisions correct?

2. If our future is in our genes and her guilt was removed by the facts of her genetic makeup, what does this say about (a) individual responsibility and (b) the morality of a criminal justice system that is focused on individual acts?

CLONING

Cloning humans, which had seemed only theoretically possible, was made a real issue with the "Well, Hello Dolly!" announcement by Scottish scientist Ian Wilmut on February 23, 1997. What Dr. Wilmut and his team had accomplished by transferring the nucleus of a somatic cell from an adult sheep into an egg from which the nucleus had been removed and then bringing that egg to full term and creating an identical twin had long been held to be theoretically possible but had never before succeeded.[16] Dr. Wilmut and Dolly suddenly burst everywhere on television, radio, Internet, journals, as the fantastic became possible and it was clear that human cloning was no longer science fiction but within human reach. "To clone or not to clone?" had become the question. In Japan, researchers believe that they have created a prototype for an artificial womb, which when combined with the technology of cloning, brings Aldous Huxley's *Brave New World* to mind.[17]

Although the question of cloning had been discussed seriously since 1960, no real strategies, helpful insights, or provisional tactical decisions had been made to assist with the current reality. This seeming inability to address novel biological developments may represent a real flaw in bioethical reasoning.

The news of the scientific breakthrough was acclaimed at both ends of the spectrum. There were those who saw it as the final attack on the family and envisioned the beginning of the apocalypse, and others who shrugged and wondered what the fuss was about. It is difficult to even enumerate all the possible uses that humans might find for the technology. Should the technology be used to

- Replace a beloved child who died an untimely death?
- Provide a child following the untimely loss of a beloved spouse?
- Provide replacement parts for an individual over a lifetime?
- Provide children to infertile couples? Gay couples?
- Promote certain types of humans such as a team of Michael Jordans?
- Continue great humans such as Mother Teresa?
- Continue the individual who wants this limited form of immortality?

Should the new technology be argued as a reproductive rights issue? Is cloning so different from other forms of reproduction as to fall outside the constitutional guarantees of procreative liberty? There are very few social constraints on personal reproduction. There appears to be all sorts of unwise, unregulated, and unrestrained procreation taking place, with even the most irresponsible people being allowed to have children. If this is the correct position regarding reproductive rights, why say no to cloning? If anything goes in reproductive rights, then anything goes, and perhaps that should include cloning.

Yet some argue that we have been morally lazy in the reproductive rights area, and the cloning issue may be the catalyst that provides the impetus to focus again on the limits of procreative liberty. Is there a legitimate place in the social community for agreements in regard to the who and how of procreation and the raising of children?

Within days of the publication of the Dolly research, President Clinton ordered a ban on federal funding related to attempts to clone humans. The president also asked the National Bioethics Commission (NBAC) to address the legal and ethical issues of human cloning within ninety days. In its deliberations, the commission examined the following concerns:

- Safety
- Individuality
- Family integrity
- Treating of children as objects
- Slippery slope issues involving eugenics
- Religious positions concerning cloning

Balanced against these concerns were issues involving the protection of personal and professional autonomy, the encouragement of scientific inquiry, and encouragement of possible biomedical breakthroughs. Figure 13-1 outlines the NBAC's decision.[18]

I. In that available scientific information indicates that the technology is not safe for humans, the use of the processes by clinicians or researchers to attempt to create a child would involve unacceptable risks to the fetus or potential child and therefore would violate important ethical obligations. The Commission, therefore recommends the following:

- A continuation of the moratorium on the use of federal funding of any attempt to create a child by somatic cell nuclear transfer.

- An immediate request to all firms, clinicians, researchers and specialty groups in the private or public domain to comply voluntarily with the intent of the federal moratorium.

II. Federal legislation should be enacted to prohibit anyone from attempting either in the clinical or research setting to create a child through the use of somatic cell nuclear transfer. The legislation should contain a sunset clause that would require a review of the issue after a specific period of time (three to five years) by an appropriate oversight body.

III. The Federal legislation should be carefully crafted so as not to have a chilling effect with other important areas of scientific research. In particular, no new regulations regarding the cloning of human DNA sequences and cell lines, as neither of these activities have the same ethical implications, as does the creation of children.

IV. In that the society appears divided on many of the important issues that surround cloning of humans, the federal government and all interested parties should encourage a national dialog on these issues in order to further our understanding of the ethical and social implications of the technology. The purpose of the dialog would be to enable society to produce long-term policies regarding the appropriate use of the technology should the time come when present safety concerns have been addressed.

V. Given the need for a fully informed citizenry regarding the use of scientific knowledge, the federal government and agencies concerned with science should seek out ways and support opportunities to provide information to the public regarding technologies involving genetics and other developments in the area of biomedical science. These efforts should especially be directed toward those areas of scientific research with the potential to affect important cultural practices, values and beliefs.

FIGURE 13-1 National Bioethics Commission Recommendations

The moral conclusion regarding cloning reached by the commission was based on the ethical duty to avoid harm or serious risk to potential children or fetuses. The fact that the technique was new and the success had been achieved following literally hundreds of failures indicated that the procedure was not safe to use in humans. Although there were many other ethical issues involved in the cloning of humans, the commission felt that these required careful, thoughtful, and imaginative reflection over time before society could respond appropriately to the technique should it become safe. Prior to the expiration of the moratorium, the commission recommended a widespread national dialog on the subject. The NBAC also recommended a sunset clause in the federal legislation that would cause a review by an appropriate oversight body prior to the expiration of the moratorium period. Although correct in recommending a ban based on safety, in the end the commission failed to answer the most basic of all the questions concerning cloning: Is the cloning of humans intrinsically wrong and if not, under what circumstances is it appropriate or permissible?

POSTHUMANISM

There are some within the camp of philosophers, including Donna Haraway,[19] Judith Halberstam,[20] and Francis Fukuyama,[21] who feel that we should not view the present situation as a cautionary tale but rather as a time to embrace the technology and possibilities of genetic engineering. While it is generally believed that human evolution is largely over given that medicine undermines natural selection, posthumanists believe that evolution is far from over. Natural selection in the biological realm is probably finished, but we humans will keep changing as a result of our interaction with the world.

Human nature is not fixed. In fact, if we consider that humans are defined anthropologically as the tool-using animal, as tools evolve, so will humans. Humans in the past changed with the transitions from horse-pulled carts to trains to personal automobiles to planes to spacecraft, or farming tools to industrial machines to computers. It is not simply human-machine interaction that changes humans; human-animal interaction is equally important. We began evolving transhumanistically when we started riding horses and domesticating dogs. However, none of this was clear until the advent of modern medical technology. Genetic manipulation, heart pacemakers, surrogacy, transplants, test tube babies, human interaction with computers, artificial intelligence, transportation vehicles, and all other inventions break down the boundary of the human body.

As we become ever more intertwined with technology, we find ourselves becoming something more than human—something "posthuman." Posthumans are also likely to welcome nonhumans to the posthuman future. Artificial intelligence, robots, created species, chimeras (species mixes), and a global Internet consciousness are all possible co-inhabitants of the future.

The key to **posthumanism** is that the "cyborg" existence is not to be resisted. Posthumanists do not question the ethics of contemporary uses of technology, or at least they do not see these developments as necessarily negative. In fact, the prospect of greater interdependence is something they find exciting and appealing. Posthumanists embrace the future. They are not oblivious to the dangers that technology raises, but they regard dangerous technology as an ongoing management issue.

The posthumanist position may be naively positive toward the future, but it is a refreshing counterpoint view to luddism. The future is coming whether we like it or not. We saw with cloning that even banning a technology will not stop its development. Nevertheless, posthumanism seems too willing to overlook the ethical issues raised by new technologies. There is ample room for compromise, however, since posthumanism can easily add ethical arguments without contradicting its central premises. One could imagine that if the posthumanist view is correct, ethical considerations in the future will still rely on duty, utilitarian, and virtue models to examine problems; however, concepts such as natural rights and human rights may become obsolete. We may, for example, still seek to maximize happiness, but the being whose happiness is to be maximized may be very different from the human of John Stuart Mill's time.

The ethical worries about issues such as cloning, stem cell research, genetic engineering, and posthumanism have as much to do with the vague fear that as humans we are "playing God" and are not up to the task. Some theological viewpoints hold that the mere possession of such profound knowledge is immoral; only God should have such power. The idea is that the attempt to gain this level of knowledge is hubris, or excessive pride. It is suggested that we leave such things to God and concern ourselves with more mundane tasks.

CONCLUSION

The advances in scientific expertise bring with them moral dilemmas. Genetic research offers great promise; we may soon be able to cure many of the genetically determined diseases and predispositions to disease. We may even be able to improve upon Mother Nature. The question is whether humankind has the wisdom to utilize this knowledge for good without violating moral rules. Only time will tell. Genetic screening will allow parents to know whether their offspring will be afflicted with disease, but in some cases this does nothing more than begin the misery sooner. Prenatal genetic testing will give parents the choice to terminate pregnancies that will lead to defective infants. Genetic testing may also justify discrimination in the minds of many. Eugenics as a state policy is unlikely and will be a long time coming, if ever, but it is fraught with the possibility that charlatans will make such proposals. The human genome project will rank among humankind's greatest achievements once it is completed, and by itself it presents no real moral difficulty; but the application of the knowledge may be more than human wisdom can handle. Recombinant DNA may be the most dangerous as it puts us in the position of creators of whole species that may or may not coexist with humanity and the rest of the natural world. In spite of the dangers, we will proceed, as we should. We may not turn away from the pursuit of knowledge even if some would misuse it.

KEY CONCEPTS

- A new and vast horizon of possibilities is opening up as the result of the ongoing biological revolution. Choices will need to be made that will affect the very concept of what we mean when we say we are human.

- The opportunities afforded by issues such as cloning, and genetic engineering fit well within the legend of Faust. Shall we rush forward on all fronts, seeking new knowledge and applying new applications of that knowledge, or accept that in some areas, humans should limit the quest and application of knowledge?

- This chapter deals with issues that can be considered small ethics—issues such as the need to protect the confidentiality of genetic profiles from insurance and employers—and large ethics, such as eugenics, where we determine what and who we are going to be in the future.

- It is unclear whether the current tools for evaluating ethical problems are capable of dealing with the unique and novel dilemmas that we are beginning to face.

- Human embryonic stem cells are the building blocks of life. Early in pregnancy, they begin to differentiate into all of the body's specialized tissues and organs.

- Most scientists working with embryonic stem cells justify the destruction of human embryos in the process by using a form of utilitarian reasoning, where the potential benefit is greater than the harm.

- Embryonic stem cell research with the resulting destruction of embryos creates a moral problem for those who hold that human life begins at the moment of conception. If this is true, then destroying embryos can be likened to killing humans and using them as raw material for biotechnical research.

- We are the only extant species of the genus *Homo*. The biological revolution may provide us opportunities to expand the species at the very least; it will provide us the opportunity to prove whether we deserve the title *Homo sapiens* (man of wisdom or thinking man).

REVIEW EXERCISES

A. If it became a general practice to abort genetically impaired infants, what would be the likely effect upon genetically impaired infants who are not aborted? Is this a reason to restrict abortions done for this reason?

B. It is likely that we will soon be able not only to detect the sex of the child very early in pregnancy but also to select the sex. Assuming such a practice could be done safely, is it morally defensible? What moral difference could it make whether parents have a male or female?

Would you want to be able to choose the sex of your children? Would you have wanted your parents to have had this power?

C. There currently are efforts to investigate whether criminal behavior is genetically determined. Aside from the scientific implausibility of all criminal behavior being explained genetically, should someone be discriminated against if his genetic makeup showed him susceptible to such behavior, even prior to actually committing a crime?

D. Most work in genetic engineering has been focused on making people better than nature and chance would make them. What would you think of a eugenics policy of producing humans who were inferior to other humans for the purpose of manual labor?

E. Given that the insurance industry is in the business of assessing risks, is it unfair for it to discriminate against individuals found to have a genetic predisposition to, say, mental health problems?

F. Imagine that you have just found out that you have Huntington's disease. You have two children; do you tell them that there is a fifty-fifty chance that the offspring of someone with Huntington's will have it as well? What if you know that they are not planning to have children? What if they are?

G. Imagine that your parents could have had you genetically altered to be better looking, as athletic as a professional athlete, and with genius-level intelligence without altering your basic personality. Would you have preferred that they had done so? If the technology existed, would parents be morally bound to have you genetically altered for the better? What if all the other parents did so except for yours?

H. Can you think of a case where humankind has acquired knowledge without using that knowledge? If not, does that mean we should refrain from continuing the human genome project?

I. Compare the character of Dr. Faustus with the character of Dr. Frankenstein. Does this help us illuminate the dilemmas surrounding genetic engineering?

J. When is the appropriate time to discuss the ethical dilemmas of the future? Do we wait until we are actually faced with the problem, or do we try to anticipate it? Anticipating the problem gives us longer to try to develop solutions, but it may also be a waste of time if the future does not play out as anticipated. Compare other scientific developments that have led to moral problems, such as atomic science, to recent developments in genetic technology.

K. Should parents be obligated to use gene therapy if it were available to fix any genetic abnormalities in their children?

L. Imagine a scenario in which a headless duplicate was cloned for each person born to serve as a source for body parts as needed by the original later in life.

1. Would such a procedure be morally problematic?

2. Would it be more ethically acceptable if animals were genetically altered to provide humans with spare organs?

M. The idea that the exploration of science is its own end is interesting and challenging to bioethical reasoning. To what extent should society restrain the efforts of scientists? What place do ethical considerations have in the decisions of science?

NOTES

1. "Frances" is a pseudonym for a person interviewed by Lois Wingerson in *Mapping Our Genes* (New York: Plume, 1991).

2. "Huntington's Gene Finally Found," *Science,* April 2, 1993.

3. Jeremy Rifkin, *Algeny* (New York: Viking Press, 1983).

4. Bryan Appleyard, *Brave New Worlds* (New York: Putnam, 1998).

5. Michael Lemonic, "Monkey Business," *Time,* January 22, 2001.

6. Christopher Marlowe, *Dr. Faustus* (New York: Signet Books, 1969).

7. Plato's *Republic.*

8. Todd Ackerman, "Stem Cell Debate May Be Far Ahead of Science," *Houston Chronicle,* August 20, 2004.

9. Jim Morrell, "Reagan's Son Urges More Support for Stem Cell Research," *Miami Herald,* July 27, 2004.

10. "If You Believe Embryos Are Human," *Time,* June 25, 2001.

11. Jeremy Rifkin. Algeny. 1983.

12. "Genetic Discrimination and Health Insurance: A Case Study on Breast Cancer," Bethesda, MD, 11 July 1995, workshop sponsored by the NAPBC and the NIH-DOE working group on the ELSI of Human Genome Research.

13. Peter Medawar, *The New Genetics and the Future of Man,* ed. Michael Hamilton (Grand Rapids, MI: William Erdmans Publishing Co. 1972).

14. "A Speeding Ticket for NIH's Controversial Cancer Star," *Science,* March 5, 1993.

15. As quoted in Roman Espejo, *Biomedical Ethics* (New York: Greenhaven Press, 2003).

16. Andy Coughlan, "Cloning of Dolly," *New Scientist,* March 1, 1997, p. 4.

17. Aldous Huxley, *Brave New World* (New York: Barrons Notes, 1984).

18. Report and Recommendations of the National Bioethics Advisory Commission, "Cloning Human Beings" (Rockville, MD, June 1997).

19. Donna Haraway, *The Haraway Reader* (New York: Routledge, 2004), See especially her "Manifesto for Cyborgs: Science, Technology for Socialist Feminism in the 1980s," pp. 7–46.

20. Judith Halberstam and Ira Livingstone, eds., *Posthuman Bodies* (Bloomington: Indiana University Press, 1995).

21. Francis Fukuyama, *Our Posthuman Future: Consequences of the Biotechnology Revolution* (New York: Farrar, Straus and Giroux, 2002).

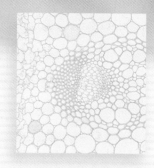

Culturally Appropriate Health Care

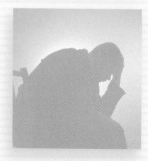

GOAL

To understand the complex nature of transcultural health through an examination of two non-Western health care traditions.

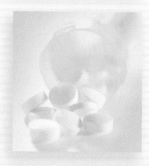

OBJECTIVES

Upon completion of this chapter, the reader should be able to:

1. Relate the concept of culture shock to modern health care provision in a multicultural nation.

2. List three ideals (principles) taken from traditional Chinese medicine (TCM) traditions and relate how they might affect the attitude of a Chinese patient seeking treatment in the American health care system.

3. List three ideals (principles) taken from Hindu healing traditions and relate how they might affect the attitude of a Hindu patient seeking treatment in the American health care system.

4. Relate how the traditions of TCM and Hindu healing beliefs relate to issues such as abortion and holistic health care.

5. List four beliefs or practices found in TCM and the Hindu healing traditions that would seem applicable to or would enhance Western health care.

6. Provide an ethical rationale for the obligation of health care providers to study the issues of transcultural health.

7. Provide a list of measures that might be useful to provide for Muslim patients.

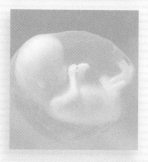

KEY TERMS

Acupuncture	Filial piety	Melting pot
Culture shock	Holistic	Moxibustion
Ethnocentric	Mass action	Xenophobic

THE E PLURIBUS IMPERATIVE

Americans have a difficult time agreeing on whether the nation should be described as a **melting pot**, where new groups are blended into the dominant culture, or a tossed salad, with each of the elements of society remaining distinct but somehow adding zest to the whole. Whatever model, whether melting pot or salad, the underlying truth is that we are a nation of immigrants, truly a multicultural society. Most Americans, even those who are not immigrants themselves, have families that came from elsewhere. Only Native Americans, the Aleuts, and the Inuit people (Eskimos) are considered native.

CASE STUDY

"Wo Bu Dong" I Don't Understand!

You are vacationing in a non-Western country. You are suddenly taken ill and admitted to the local hospital. You now wish that you had bought the travel insurance, which would have allowed you to be immediately transported home. Although the hospital appears modern and has the reputation for a reasonable standard of care, what might be your concerns?

1. What is everyone saying?

2. What is my diagnosis? Prognosis?

3. How does the system work here?

4. Will I be able to make myself understood?

5. Will I be able to get what I need?

6. Can I trust them with my life?

Since the 1950s there has been an explosion of group consciousness in the United States as many of the ethnic groups have sought to find and identify with their roots. It is the most American of all phenomena to ask yourself what it means to be a _____ American? As an example, it is hard to imagine a Chinese person in the People's Republic of China asking themselves what it means to be Chinese. They know. This rejuvenation of ethnic identity in the United States has often served to isolate and alienate individual groups. We are truly a universal nation, a pluralistic society, with competing ideas regarding basic issues such as the meaning of health and illness. This distinct feature of American culture has interesting and challenging implications for health care practice. Somehow we must not only understand that there are differences, but also confront them honestly if we are to serve the patients who make their way into our care.

As health care providers we are generally socialized into the cultures of our particular practices. This professional socialization teaches each practitioner a set of beliefs, habits, practices, likes, dislikes, and acceptable norms. This new set of learned information may or may not conform to the traditions of the individual prior to entering practice. As practitioners become more and more socialized into the provider culture, they often become further removed from the population at large in regard to its understanding of issues involving health and illness. It is this movement away from the population at large that often leads patients to complain that health care providers are speaking a foreign language. This is exacerbated when the health care provider is actually speaking a foreign language. But language is not the real issue; often the problem is that in the socialization to our particular practice, we become for all purposes a foreign culture or ethnic group to the patients we serve.

Most health care practitioners in the United States adhere rigidly to the Western system of health care delivery and often disdain any ideas of prevention and healing that fall outside the accepted scientifically proved methods. The following response from a family practice physician regarding the use of a particular herbal medicine sums up this attitude, "If it had any scientific validity, we [American physicians] would be dispensing it."

Health care providers are often not only **ethnocentric** but also **xenophobic** when it comes to practice. The only types of healers or practitioners that we tolerate are those who have been educated and certified by the provider culture. What happens to the patient with a different belief system from the practitioner in regard to illness and treatment? Are practitioners truly able to meet the needs of patients if they do not understand how the patient views health, illness, or treatment?

Individuals who find themselves in transition from one setting to another, where one fails to understand the basic cues of social intercourse, are susceptible to the high stress malady known as **culture shock**. What often happens in this situation is that a communication barrier is raised, which often is described as being either a problem patient or an uncommunicative one. Consider, for instance, the patient with a heart condition who is restricted to bed. Although he is told to remain in bed and appears to understand, he is found several times a day standing and gazing out his window. The nurses complain to each other that the patient is uncooperative.

The patient, a devout Muslim who by faith is required to pray several times a day facing in a particular direction, feels that the religious priority overcomes the requirement of bedrest. Understanding and a change in bed position might have solved what unfortunately became a breakdown in communication in which all involved, especially the patient, lost. As a nation of immigrants we have patients who face these challenges every day. Hospitals are daunting places, even for people with medical backgrounds. Often we think that our communication problems are the differences in the patient's language. Yet this is only one of the barriers, and perhaps not even the most important. The question becomes whether we as practitioners are standing in the way of their getting well. The influence of cultural factors on the response of patients and families to ill health and hospital care plans cannot be underestimated. Always remember that quality care is a lot more than diagnostics, procedures, and drug administration.

This chapter will examine two traditional systems of health care practice separate from the Western tradition. Both the traditional Chinese medicine (TCM) and Hindu healing beliefs are traditions that extend in time well before the traditions of the West and still retain hundreds of millions of adherents. The final section of this chapter examines how the Islamic faith shapes and influences the attitudes and behaviors of adherents to this religious tradition. Given that Islam is only one of the five major religions in the world and given that there are many nonmajor religions, and Chinese and Indian traditional medicine practices are just two of many that deserve examination, it should be clear that this chapter does not intend to be all inclusive. Rather, this chapter hopes to convince the reader of the need to study further and that if we as health professionals wish to serve patients in this multicultural nation and do more than just celebrate diversity, we will need to broaden our clinical horizons in regard to other cultures.

TRADITIONAL CHINESE MEDICINE

The People's Republic of China offers an interesting history of health care ethics. Unlike most other nations of the world, China has a richly recorded cultural history that extends back for over forty centuries. Medicine in China, a system of diagnosis and health care approaches, has a written history that extends back for over twenty centuries. Traditional Chinese medicine as a comprehensive profession includes internal medicine, surgery, and dietary components and evolved as early as the Zhou dynasty in eleventh century B.C.E. These practices include acupuncture and moxibustion, massage, diet, herbal remedies, meditation, and both moving and static exercises. While the practices contained within TCM appear very distinct, they all share the same underlying assumptions regarding the human body and its place in the universe.

As in the Western tradition, doctors in ancient China practiced individual medicine where health care is aggressively patient centered. It was recognized that skill was an important aspect of health care practice, and physicians were admonished to read extensively and profoundly, combine theory and practical knowledge, and write out what they learned in practice so that future generations of patients and physicians could benefit. The extensive written documentations of traditional Chinese medicine set it apart from all other folk medicine practices. According to these traditions, a physician who relied solely on skills and failed in the virtues was a poor physician. This can be clearly seen in the *Rules of Pediatrics,* one of the classic works of Chinese medicine, written by Xia Yuzhu in the Qing dynasty. It noted that many were not called to the work. Individuals who were cruel, overly aggressive, stubborn, hesitant, frivolous, impatient, or greedy were not qualified to learn medicine. What, then, were the virtues required?

TCM Virtues of Intellect

Providers were admonished to:

- Be tireless in pursuing studies
- Study geography, astronomy, ecology, and psychology as the practice of health care required a holistic understanding of the patient and his environment
- Learn from everyone: the learned, ordinary people, subordinates

An interesting application of the intellectual virtues is found in the story of the god of agriculture in Chinese legendary history. Shen NongShi reportedly tasted hundreds of plants to find beneficial herbs. In doing this he was poisoned as many as seventeen times per day and finally succumbed after eating a poisonous insect with 100 feet.

Virtues of Humanity and Justice

Providers were called upon to:

- Provide care for all without consideration of station
- Provide care without consideration of weather, contagion, filth, or odor
- Consider the health of the people and health of the nation as one

These virtues are amplified in a famous allusion found in the story of Dong Feng, a TCM physician of the Three Kingdoms' period (220–280 C.E.). Dong Feng treated the poor free of charge and would not take money from them. When they presented gifts, he would refuse but asked them to plant apricot trees around his house. Over the years, a forest of ten thousand trees grew into a great orchard. Dr. Dong then exchanged the fruit for grains, which he distributed to the poor. It is reported in this way that twenty thousand poor were relieved. In a major hospital in Beijing a mirror stands in the entry inscribed with the Chinese characters, "Warm Spring in the Apricot Garden," which speaks of the great respect for health care providers.

Personal Virtues

Practitioners were to practice the virtues of:

- Humility; physicians were encouraged to learn from ordinary people and subordinates
- Self-sacrifice
- Avoidance of self-interest, whether fame, fortune, or governmental position
- Collegial respect, where one is warned against arrogant attitudes toward colleagues
- Maintain good manners, respect for patients, and harmonious behaviors

An interesting allusion amplifying these virtues can be found in the story of Li Gao who practiced in the Yuan dynasty (1271–1368 C.E.). During this period, an acute epidemic covered the land. In order to provide care for many, Dr. Li wrote his prescriptions on a wooden board and hung it in the street to let people use it free of charge. This tradition is still honored, and in Nan Xi Hill in Guilin, one can still find an original post where prescriptions had been left.

EASTERN AND WESTERN TRADITIONAL PRINCIPLES

When we compare the ancient Chinese principles with writings such as the Hippocratic Oath, there are both similarities and interesting differences. In the Western tradition there is more of a guild mentality, especially in regard to safekeeping the information, to the group of practitioners bound within the oath. Fame and fortune are promised blessings for those practitioners who keep their oath. Principles such as confidentiality are highlighted in the Western tradition and do not appear in the Chinese counterpart. Both sets of tradition call for continued study, justice for all, and the avoidance of conflicts such as gratuities and sexual misadventures with patients.

The role of the environment and the holistic nature of care were central to TCM, while the Western tradition focused more on the disease entity and its particular cure. The principles of health care practice in Chinese traditional medicine do not need to wait until a disease appears, as the system works best in an environment where the practices become an aspect of daily life. The great TCM physicians kept their patients well rather than waiting for them to be stricken.

The early codification of traditional Chinese medicine had a tendency to freeze the traditional practices so that they remained unchanged over a period of time. Today, as in the past, TCM possesses two outstanding features: its **holistic** nature and the codified applications of treatment according to differentiation of symptom-complexes. Illness is seen as a process of disharmony that needs alleviating rather than as a machinery breakdown that needs fixing.

Perhaps the most basic principle in TCM is the concept of yin and yang. The universe is composed of mutually dependent opposites, each giving meaning to the other. Yin represents cold, stillness, passiveness, darkness, within, and potential. Yang represents warmth, activity, light, outside, and expression. Illness is an imbalance of these mutually dependent opposites.

The traditions speak of several basic substances that are important in the maintenance of health:

- Qi—Energy or life force; everything in the universe is composed of Qi.
- Blood—Nourishes, moistens, and lubricates the body. Blood is the very material manifestation of Qi. Blood is important in helping anchor the mind and in allowing clear and stable thought processes.
- Jing—Essence, the underpinning of all aspects of organic life.
- Shen—Mind or spirit of the individual.

The meridian system is the energy distribution system for the basic substances. These are often depicted as a system of channels that distribute the substances across the body. Since these channels do not fit any known anatomical structure, they are best thought of as a process rather than a structure.

According to tradition, the *zang-fu* organs (liver, heart, spleen, lung, and kidney) form the core of the organ entity in which tissues and sense organs are connected through a network of channels and collaterals. While the functions of the *zang-fu* organs are distinct, they work in coordination. Pathology within the *zang-fu* organs can be reflected on the skin surfaces through communication along the channels and collaterals, and problems at the skin surfaces may also be reflected to their related *zang* or *fu* organs.

The human body is seen as an organic whole that is unified with nature. Changes in environment, geography, seasons, and even alterations between day and night may directly or indirectly affect health. The establishment of treatment regimes is expected to be in accord with the different seasons and environments.

The practice of TCM requires the differentiation of syndromes. It is important for the physician to come to understand the causative factors, the location, and nature of the problem in order to come to a conclusion regarding the confrontation between pathogenic factors and antipathogenic factors that are in play. Within the system, similar diseases may manifest themselves differently while different disease entities may share the same syndrome complex. Treatment is focused on the syndrome rather than the particular disease. Therefore, different treatments exist for the same disease entity, and different diseases may be treated by the same methods.

Health care practice and ethics in ancient China served as a core for occupational development and motivation. To the credit of these ancient practitioners, their holistic practices focused on the health of the individual, their families, and the nation. Good physicians were treated as cultural heroes. Their emphasis on the classics and continuing study allowed for the early development of a unified set of theories. The early codification, however, did create some limitations

CASE STUDY

A Difference in Perception

In TCM clinics, there is very little technology used for diagnosis. Diagnosis is made by looking, hearing, questioning, smelling, and touching and includes an extended conversation over a whole host of seemingly irrelevant information. It is a hands-on operation where the physician examines the pulses, looks at the tongue, smells the person, and palpates the body and from this gives a diagnosis.

Think of the last time you met with your physician. Generally the conversation was brief (five minutes or less). Someone else took your pulse and blood pressure, and weighed you. The physician gave vague answers as to what the condition was until test results came in.

Now imagine that you are an elderly Chinese person who is accustomed to the traditional approach. Also imagine that you firmly believe that you possess an energy anatomy, which allows for a flow of energy (*qi*) around and through your body. Your definition of health includes the concept of balance and harmony of this *qi* as it flows about and that the physical manifestation of this *qi* is blood.

1. What must you think of the fact that your traditional doctor was able to come to a diagnosis without modern technology? Would the Western clinician seem more or less competent?

2. What would you think about the fact that your old doctor talked to you about your family and your life and the new one gave you only five minutes? Would the Western clinician seem to be as caring as the traditional physician?

3. What would you think about having to give blood? Not only does it hurt but it also affects the *qi* flow. Your old doctor understands this and does not hurt you.

Assume that you answered the above questions as (1) the doctor is less competent than the old one, (2) less caring than the traditional one, (3) and that somehow this giving of blood was interfering with your *qi* flow.

If this is what is going on in your patient's mind, would you find it hard to imagine that you will have the following happen.

1. The patient comes to you only late in the sequence of the problem and always after having tried traditional therapies.

2. The patient leaves your service as quickly as possible and fails to follow up with later clinic appointments.

in that it was steeped within the culture and therefore important elements such as **filial piety** obstructed surgical and anatomical study, and the restrictions in treating women hindered the development of areas such as gynecology.

As health care practices developed in the West, especially in the twentieth century, medicine began to purge itself of the practices of folk medicine, and practitioners began to subject the discipline to scientific reasoning. That which could not be proven and reproduced by experiment became suspect. Health care in the West was dynamic and was seen to be in ascendancy at the turn of the nineteenth century. While TCM was respected and favored by the people in China, the intellectual and national leaders began to move toward Western medicine. This shift was accelerated with the fall of the dynastic leaders and the establishment of the republic. In 1929 and again in 1933, leaders within the Nationalist Party attempted to ban traditional practices altogether. TCM physicians such as Hun Tieqiao, Sun Bohua, and Shi Jinmo led the opposition to these changes, presenting petitions to the capitol at Nanking and aided the establishment of the Hua Bei Medical School to train TCM physicians.

REVOLUTIONARY SOCIALISM AND CHINESE HEALTH CARE

Another major shift in Chinese health care and health care ethics came with the rise of communism in post–World War II China. With revolutionary socialism came the discrediting of many of the ancient philosophers whose thinking formed the basis of Chinese health care ethics. The tenants of Confucian thinking became counterrevolutionary. Modern health care ethics in Communist China were to serve the state and promote the development of communist morality. In its ideological construction, the ethics of health care were to build up revolutionary zeal, communist morality, and discipline. Health care and health care workers were to serve the people with all their hearts and souls and to guarantee the health of the laboring class. Revolutionary humanitarianism called for the rejection of old superstitions, the break down of class consciousness, the placing of service before personal interest, and cooperative efforts between practitioners.

As in ancient China, stories of People's Heroes exemplify the characteristics of the ideal practitioner within the communist state. The following three stories show the virtues expected by a physician in the new communist state:

1. Dr. Zhang Zhenyu worked as a medical professional for over forty years. On one occasion, a patient who had larynx cancer began to bleed and obstructed the tracheotomy tube. When it became apparent that the patient could not breathe and given that there was no suction device available, Dr. Zhang sucked the pus and blood from the patient's throat and opened the airway.

2. Dr. Tang Yaoqing was a surgeon in Ruijin Hospital in Shanghai. It was customary for physicians to take a fee for setting patients' and relatives' mind at ease of 200 yuan. Dr. Tang refused the fee and performed surgery for necrotic pancreatitis. A second surgery was necessary and the family again came forward with the fee. Because the physician refused the fee, the patient became concerned that perhaps the physician had no faith in the outcome of the surgery. The patient became so pessimistic over the outcome of the surgery that he removed his own oxygen and IV tubes. Hearing this, the physician took the fee and performed the surgery. Once the surgery was successful, the physician returned the fee to the family.

3. Dr. Sun Bingyan, from the Foundation of Oncology and Orthopedics in Beijing, researched herbal medicine and screened dozens of poisonous samples from the over 2,000 within the pharmacopea. These herbs were for external use and could not be taken orally. Not wanting to risk others, the physician tried each of the drugs on himself. His wife attempted to stop his efforts but he continued in his work. Although he became ill on many occasions, he persevered and was credited for finding drugs useful for the treatment of certain cancers.

Within these stories are the major themes of revolutionary humanitarianism:

- Serving the people with all your heart and soul
- Self-sacrifice for the people's health
- Humility and the avoidance of personal gain
- The need to show respect for science and seek the truth from facts

Health care providers in the People's Republic could not be as openly concerned with earning wealth as were their Western counterparts. Problems such as maldistribution of health care services were amenable to government fiat; professionals could be sent to practice where the government perceived the need. Programs such as the "barefoot doctors," in which relatively low-skilled practitioners were sent into the countryside, served the nation well.

Within communist practice, the science of medicine could be explored and advanced, at least in areas considered essential by those in power. TCM was also maintained along with Western-style health care because its less expensive holistic traditions seem adaptable to **mass action** programs of community health. Public banners with slogans admonishing the citizens to keep Beijing free of flies or to perform other sanitation measures are common fare and remarkably effective. It is the availability of social control that has allowed China to engage in difficult mass action policies such as the one-child policy designed to lower the population pressures.

One of the weaknesses of the system is that the health professionals themselves are not the keepers of their traditions. Unlike their Western counterparts, Chinese physicians are not self-regulating and have not set up their own code of ethics. Professional conferences in China focus on the skills of medicine, and the ethical aspects of practice are governed by the communist apparatus. Also, central control of health care does not always promote the effective use of health care resources. It is an unfortunate truth that even in a republic of equals, some are more equal than others. The disruption of health care services, research, and professional careers associated with the Cultural Revolution that followed the death of Mao in 1976 was a testament to the fallacy of central control that was unresponsive to the needs of the professions and the patients they serve.

FISCAL REFORM AND CHINESE HEALTH CARE

A recent critical shift that dramatically affected health care provision and ethics in China is the government movement to fiscal reform. In one of the popular stories within China, the communist leader Deng Xiao Pieng is quoted as saying that he is not bothered with whether the cat is black or white so long as it catches mice. The moral of the story is that labels are not as important as pragmatic outcomes. While no one is willing to label what is taking place as capitalism, given that the nation is communist, there appears to be a huge shift toward free market experiments. Moving from a highly controlled environment to one that is based on a free market causes social disruptions, and many of the social programs of the old regimes have been dismantled without a safety net set up to protect the weak. While senior members of the government and those involved in manufacturing seem to have guaranteed health access, those involved in agriculture (60–70 percent of the population) are in a fee-for-service position.

The acquisition of wealth is no longer considered to be a vice among the citizens. Most health care providers work in public institutions, and many feel they are being left out of the new options. The ethics of health care have been imposed from the outside for the last three quarter-century, so those in practice are somewhat adrift in how to respond to the new situation. There is a critical need for the establishment of new rules of practice that fit the current situation. In the past, slogans such as "Dedicate yourself to medical enterprise and bring benefits to mankind," "Serve the patients with heart and soul," or "Be honest in performing medical duties" could motivate and give direction; however, in the new China, while they still may inspire, they fail to give adequate direction. The traditions of Chinese health care practice are very much in keeping with virtue ethics, but, unfortunately, as in the United States the health care environment is shifting so rapidly that it is difficult to always determine what the good practitioner should do in a given situation.

There is much to be admired in the traditions of health care provision in the Chinese culture. Chinese physicians are listeners, spending far more time with their patients than is common in Western practice. They are holistic in their approach to the patient and their family. TCM, while it is a slow process, seems very effective in chronic care as the therapies appear to raise the whole immune system of the patient and are very cost-effective. It is clear that for acute conditions, Western health care is often more appropriate. Many Chinese practitioners seek to integrate the two systems and handle acute care with Western medicine and chronic care with traditional practices. Chinese patients and their families seem more participative in their health care, and it is not uncommon to have the patient and family bring a copy of the medical records to the clinic and discuss the treatment options, advising the physician as to what is most practical given their situation. Within the culture itself are facets that promote good health. A nation that cycles to work, lives in stable families, and eats vegetables and sea foods in modest quantities has much to be said for itself in regard to promoting good health.

INDIAN MEDICAL ETHICS

India is a land of many faiths. Hinduism, Islam, Sikhism, Jainism, and Christianity coexist in a spiritual conglomerate seen nowhere else in the world. Nevertheless, the dominant world view is Hindu. Hinduism is a very old and sophisticated philosophical religion. The great thinkers of India are the equal of some of the greatest philosophers of the West. India also has a venerable medical tradition going back to the Arthaveda. This means we must disabuse ourselves of any feeling of intellectual superiority from the outset if we are intent on understanding Indian medical ethics. Furthermore, while India is a predominantly poor country, it has a large, modernized medical sector that is quite Western and technological. India is thus a study in contrasts. While key attitudes toward medical practice are grounded in a worldview thousands of years old, some practices are largely the result of the application of modern technology to an overpopulated and underdeveloped society.

Understanding Hindu ethics requires that we understand something of the general Hindu worldview. Hindus have traditionally organized society into distinct castes. This is still true even though caste has lost much of its legal sanction. In spite of the government's efforts to undermine the influence of caste, one is still either a Brahmin (priest), Ksatriya (warrior), Vaisya (merchant), or Sudra (manual laborer). There are also those outside the caste system altogether, the Untouchables. Each caste is further subdivided according to one's specific occupation. Thus, there are literally thousands of castes. One's duty, or in Hindu terms, *dharma*, is linked to one's caste, sex, and stage of life. Hinduism therefore has much in common with virtue ethics in that duty is relative to the agent. Caste is not a matter of choice even though it probably originated that way. People are born into their station in life, but it is far from arbitrary. Hindu are born into the caste they deserve. But how can this be? How can we deserve anything before we have had opportunities for action? The answer lies in the doctrine of *samsara*.

Hindus believe in reincarnation or *samsara*. They believe that they have lived many times in the past and that they will live again in other bodies in the future. The assignment of bodies to reincarnated souls (the Hindu term for soul is *atman*) is dictated by one's conduct in a past life. This is called *karma*. If we act immorally in this life, it will be reflected in our assignment to a caste in a future life. Our present caste is a function of our actions in our past lives. Engaging in unsavory activities leads to the accumulation of impurity or karmic matter. Impurity can also be gained by contact with those of lower caste. In either case, it is the accumulation of karmic matter that causes rebirth. From a Western perspective, this may sound odd since the punishment for sin is getting to live again. But this merely points to a difference between the Western and Indian worldviews. For the Indian, life is suffering, and rebirth is a repetition of suffering. So the Indian prefers bringing the cycle of suffering to an end. There are three acknowledged ways to end, or at least get closer to the end of, the cycle of rebirth: the way of works, the way of loving devotion, and the way of knowledge.

The *way of works* is the most popular of the paths to salvation. One follows this path by performing the prescribed rituals: sacrificing to the gods, paying the three debts (to one's teacher, to one's ancestors, to the gods), performing the rites of birth, puberty, marriage and death, and so on. The *way of loving devotion (bhakti)* is the path for those who find the deepest expression of their religious needs in the worship of a personal deity such as Vishnu, Krishna, or Shiva. The *way of knowledge* is taken by those more intellectually inclined, those more up to the task of the deep self-reflection into the vagaries of the soul. Such adherents study the Upanishads and other key texts and meditate in order to achieve *moksha,* or release or liberation.

Moksha provides the enlightened one with a release from the cycle of rebirth. One who achieves *moksha*—and only Brahmins are in the appropriate spiritual position to do so—does so by overcoming ignorance, which in the religious sense means realizing that one's sense of oneself as a separate entity in a world of entities is false. Hindus believe in monism, the view that everything is ultimately a single reality. They believe this in spite of the well-known fact that Hindus believe in many gods. But even the gods are merely aspects of the one. The same is true of the *atman* or soul. *Atman* is really just the Brahman that is in us. Our awareness of our soul is therefore also an awareness of God, or Brahman.

Hindu ethics and metaphysics have the common aim of bringing us to the consciousness of our oneness with Brahman. This has led to a key criticism of Hindu ethics: that it focuses more on the personal than the interpersonal, which is the proper domain of ethics. It is sometimes claimed that Hindus are selfish in their single-minded concern with enlightenment. In response, however, Hindus argue that ethics are not neglected; indeed, they are the precondition of enlightenment. One cannot even begin the search for enlightenment until the baser aspects of personality are under control. The key doctrine in this regard is that of *ahimsa,* or nonviolence. Respect for life is very deep in the Hindu world view and is represented most clearly in cow worship and vegetarianism. Cows represent the gentle fullness of life, the fertility of life that generates life. Vegetarianism shows a respect for the animal world that goes far beyond anything in the West. A religious offshoot of Hinduism, Jainism, takes *ahimsa* as so important that care is taken lest one accidentally inhale or step on insects.

Another problematic aspect of Hinduism is the focus on detachment. Ethics in the Western sense is centrally a matter of regard for the other, but Hindus emphasize the precise opposite:

detachment. In fact, it is a duty of the elderly to progressively detach themselves from the things and people of this world. Only by detaching oneself from the world can one adequately prepare for union with Brahman. The Hindu has a clear sense of the stages of life. While one is first a student and then a householder with all the obligations inherent in these social roles, one also must turn away from these worldly obligations and become a forest dweller and then a *sannyasin,* one who has renounced the world. As different as this is from the Western conception of the end of life, it does have its benefits. Death is not the great horror that it is to the Westerner; rather, it is simply another stage one takes in the path toward oneness with Brahman. We will see that this attitude comes into play in our discussion of euthanasia.

Abortion and euthanasia are the core issues in medical ethics, so our treatment of these issues will be the centerpiece of our discussion of Indian ethics. Both issues raise the problem of personhood, and we have already seen that the Hindu has a very different notion of the self. The Westerner begins from the presupposition of the individuated self. Since Descartes, this has been conceived as the thinking thing that animates the body. While the Hindu agrees that the soul is an immaterial thing that animates the body, it is not properly speaking an individuated self. As we have already indicated, the Hindu idea of the soul, *atman,* is not really distinct from God or Brahman. It is mere illusion that we are distinct from each other and from God. Enlightenment largely consists of overcoming this illusion.

Abortion in India

The treatment of the abortion issue is instructive, for the debate in India mirrors the argument in the West. One can derive the positions of the opposing sides from the traditions. One tradition, for example, is based on the *Rig Samhita,* which refers to Vishnu as the protector of the unborn. And as Julius Lipner argued, it is clear that abortion was regarded by some as reprehensible. The *Maharayana Upanishad* is only one of several texts that list the abortionist as a serious offender. And it is clear in texts such as *The Law Book of Vishnu* that killing an embryo is as bad as killing a Brahmin, a serious offense indeed. Further, the evil of killing of the fetus is not necessarily derived from that of the pregnant woman; rather, the fetus is understood to be valuable in its own right.

On the other hand, evidence can be gleaned from the *Bhagavad Gita* in favor of abortion. One reason Krishna gives to Arjuna in favor of killing his relatives and friends in battle is that one can do no real harm to the *atman* or soul since it is immortal. Similarly, nothing one can do to the fetus can hurt its *atman.* This would, of course, also justify arbitrary murder if it were not restricted to cases in which one was fulfilling the duties dictated by one's social role. In the case of women, whose duty has been to provide their husbands with sons, the knowledge that one is pregnant with a girl has been one of the primary reasons for abortion and even infanticide in India. This has been such a problem that in January 1995, the Indian Parliament voted to outlaw abortions done after amniocentesis or ultrasound has shown the baby is female.

Whatever the merits of the arguments of the two sides, it is clear that Indian women have availed themselves of the practice of abortion in rapidly increasing numbers. In 1991 and 1992, there were 6.7 million abortions in India. Especially troubling is the fact that only 600,000 of these were performed legally. A large part of the problem seems to be the lack of contraceptives in use. Sixty percent of all married couples in India use no form of contraception. Of the remaining 40 percent that do use contraception, two-thirds use female sterilization.

India is an underdeveloped and overpopulated country with a shortage of medical facilities. While family planning is regarded as extremely important, the task is overwhelming. It is predicted that India's population will pass China's within twenty years. The problem is partly one of tradition, but it is greatly exacerbated by massive numbers of people with little or no access to contraception. India is at a comparative disadvantage with regard to China, because as a democracy, India can't employ the social control measures available to the People's Republic.

The abortion debate will only intensify as India modernizes. It is hard to imagine that India will forgo the practice given the severity of the population pressures. On the other hand, Indian politicians, like those in the United States, will find themselves torn between opposing viewpoints. Both sides will turn to tradition, using the arguments mentioned above, and the pro-abortion forces will argue for the necessity of the procedure given the burgeoning population. As it stands, there is little hope that India will get the problem under control anytime soon, and if that is the case, it is easy to imagine that India's democracy could be threatened by the need for drastic measures. China's success has been possible only through the heavy hand of government control of reproduction, and Indian politicians may find the totalitarian option a better alternative than social chaos.

Euthanasia in India

Euthanasia has a long history in India because it has been a part of the ascetic tradition. The history of euthanasia in India is an interesting one, for it begins by asserting the preferability of living for one hundred years. The next stage is to prefer death in battle as part of the heroic ethic of the Ksatriyas. Ksatriyas could achieve salvation by dying in battle. Also acceptable was suicide for the purpose of avoiding the shame of capture. By extension, warriors who do not die in battle are shamed. To avoid this shame, warriors developed a code in which self-willed death in old age conferred the same reward as death in battle. Later, proponents of the Jain religion, an offshoot of Hinduism, developed a religious version of the heroic self-willed death. The idea was that one could conquer the negative influence of the body by denying it food at the end of life. This view was, in turn, applied by Hindus and Buddhists as well as Jains to those near the end of life as a merciful alternative to drawn out suffering. Sometimes, however, the alternative was not self-imposed starvation, although that practice did continue; rather, one either jumped into fire or water or jumped off a cliff. The practice of *sati*, or widow burning, has been justified in a similar way. The net result of this tradition was greater sympathy for those with a debilitating disease at the end of life. This is not to say there was universal agreement with self-willed death; indeed, the opposite is true. The counter traditions in Hinduism and Buddhism have always been stronger than the pro-euthanasia position. Nevertheless, there was an important minority position in favor of euthanasia.

Westerners may be able to learn from the Indian experience with self-willed death. An important issue in Western euthanasia cases concerns the propriety of denying food and water to a dying person. One can imagine an Indian observer attempting to allay our concerns in the matter. On the other hand, it is clear that in the Indian context, such a practice had to be voluntary; otherwise, strength of will was not involved and could not lead to instant salvation and an end to the cycle of rebirth. Westerners might be justified in ignoring this qualification for the comatose since they do not base the justification on an end to rebirth but on considerations of mercy. Most important, however, is the idea that euthanasia can be understood as a matter of personal autonomy rather than as denial of the value of life. If a person wishes to end her life because autonomy is no longer possible, then we may be able to justify the action if the end of life is imminent. We are still left with the problem of cases in which autonomy is severely impaired yet bodily existence is likely to continue indefinitely. Even here, however, the Indian tradition suggests that allowing self-willed death is not clearly immoral since perfectly healthy ascetics commit suicide in an effort to end the cycle of rebirth.

The Hindu Code of Professional Ethics for Physicians

The Ayurvedic literature contains many directives concerning the physician's ethical duties. The *Atreya Anushasana,* which predates the Hippocratic Oath by two centuries, contains the following directives:

1. The physician who by his conduct allows the disease to progress or adopts hasty measures even before the right time is to be considered a sinner and stands liable for punishment.

2. Drugs and recipes should be suitable and effective; no harmful therapy should be adopted however much it has been extolled.

3. The scope of medical science is not merely to relieve suffering but to restore health; strive to maintain and promote health but do not undermine the natural strength of the patient.

4. The scope of medical science is merely to lend a helping hand to those who are sinking in the quagmire of disease; it is just an aid. Physicians should not assume too much either to themselves or their science in case of a cure.

5. It is impossible to guarantee life in all cases even by experts, even under ideal conditions, nor can death be predicted as certain when suitable conditions do not exist.

6. Treatment is to be done to the last breath, for many a hopeless patient recovers by the grace of God.

7. Medical science should not be used for selfish gains or for money, but should be for the service of all creatures.

8. Medical practice is quasi-faceted: friendship with all, sympathy and compassion for the sick, utmost care, and attention toward the manageable patient and connivance of the hopeless.

9. He who makes medicine merchandise shall only reap a heap of sand, casting away a heap of gold.

10. He who bestows health and relieves pain is worthy of every kind of worship and all the fruits of righteousness shall accrue to him.

11. Physicians, by relieving the suffering, attain heaven without performing sacrifices.

12. Practicing the profession on the principles of philosophy of life, looking after the health of the deserving and the needy, showing kindness and compassion to all beings is the *dharma* for the medical man; accepting from the rich just enough money to meet the minimum needs, his life, and his dependents is the *artha*; respecting the elders, scholars, professional brethren, and nobles and receiving honors from them, winning love and affection of all by sympathetic service is the *kama*; by practicing thus, the physician is sure to attain salvation or *moksha*.

From this selection from the Ayurvedic Code, we note a few important points. First, note the emphasis on separating medicine from profit. Western medicine, especially in the United States, is very much a profit-oriented practice. In fact, many become doctors precisely because of the high pay. Indian tradition saw a danger that is becoming increasingly obvious: the subordination of the value of health to that of profit. Second, the great respect accorded to doctors is not without merit, for doctors do perform an extremely valuable function. So our response to the first problem should not be to impoverish or lower our respect for doctors. Medicine should always be regarded as one of the noblest of callings. Third, doctors need to be sensitive to the emotional needs of the patients. The patient is not a machine that needs to be fixed. The patient is a human being with all the associated fears and misgivings over disease, death, and treatment. Fourth, in spite of the partial acceptance of the Indian tradition for euthanasia, this does not mean abandoning the severely sick or elderly to their fate. Care must continue as long as the patient requires. Fifth, it is important not to overestimate the powers of the medical community. No matter how sophisticated medical science becomes, death will always be waiting for us in the end. Thus we must come to terms with death. India is far more advanced than the West in this regard. The Indian idea of the stages of life with the final stage being a withdrawal from the world is more realistic and sober about the facts of the human life span.

MUSLIM PATIENTS

The Islamic faith is the cultural core for many immigrants from the Middle East, Bosnia, Turkey, Pakistan, Malaysia, Indonesia, and parts of Africa and Polynesia. The Muslim faith, like Christianity, is a universal religion, which finds adherents in literally every nation in the world. Just as the practice of Christianity is somewhat different in various parts of the world, the same can be said for Islam. However, there are certain foundational practices that appear the same regardless of culture. In the United States, the Islamic community is a rapidly growing segment of our population. It is safe to assume that every American health care provider will meet a Muslim patient at some stage in his career. This necessitates that each of us gains an understanding of the essentials of Islam to improve our care of this patient population. Figure 14-1 provides suggestions on how we might better serve this population.

The basic message of Islam can be summed up in the Arabic expression, *"La ilaha illa Allah: Muhammadun rasulu Allah,"* which states that there is no God but Allah and that Muhammad is his final messenger or prophet. This is the Muslim creed. Muslims are fiercely monotheistic; they believe in Allah (God Almighty). Islam literally means "submission," and the term *Muslim* means "one who has submitted to Allah." Along with their belief in a monotheistic God, Muslims believe in angels of God, prophets of God, and books of God (e.g., Torah, Bible, and the Holy Qur'an). Muslims believe that the God of Islam, Christianity, and Judaism is the same god. In the early church, Muslims had great respect for Jews and Christians as fellow "people of the book." For them, the teachings of the Torah and Bible are the works of God, which may have been misunderstood or mistranslated. According to the Islamic faith, it is this confusion that caused God to send his final prophet, Muhammad, and the last of the divine revelations, the

---

- Respect patients' modesty and privacy.
- Provide meals in accordance with Muslim traditions.
- Accommodate prayer and Qur'an reading.
- Within statutory restraints, do not insist on autopsy or organ donation.
- Always examine a female patient in the presence of another female.
- Where possible, provide a same-sex health care provider as the patient.
- Preferably no male should be in the delivery room except the husband.
- Encourage advanced directives.

FIGURE 14-1   Muslim Patients: Suggestions for Care

Holy Qur'an, to the world. Like most Jewish and Christian traditions, Muslims believe in a final day of judgment when the wicked will be punished with suffering and the faithful will be rewarded with eternal life in heaven. Fate plays a great part in Muslim faith, and according to tradition, whatever happens that is good or evil is predestined by God.

According to Muslim tradition, all people share the common parentage of Adam and Eve. In this light, every human being is a member of the same universal family. Because of this common heritage, there is no room for racial prejudice, social injustice, second-class citizenship, or concepts of ethnic or national superiority within the teachings of the Qu'ran or in the exemplary example found in the life of Muhammad.

The Islamic faith has no priesthood or clergy in the same sense as Christians think of such religious leaders. Islamic religious leaders are men with special training in Islamic law. In the community, they serve as judges in the religious courts, counselors for those with legal problems, teachers in the religious schools (*madrasahs*), and prayer leaders in the mosques. They do not however, perform ceremonies on behalf of other believers, hear confessions, or act as intermediaries between believers and God.

Five Pillars of Islamic Faith

Perhaps the most foundational of Islamic beliefs are the five basic fundamental Muslim obligations, collectively known as the Five Pillars of the Faith.

The first pillar is belief in Allah and his final prophet, Muhammad. In order to be considered a Muslim one must recite the formula of "witness": "I bear witness that there is no god but Allah. I bear witness that Muhammad is the Apostle of God."

Salaat, or prayers, the second pillar, consists of fixed sets of standing, bowing, prostration, and sitting in worship of Allah. Muslims are required to pray five times per day (at dawn, noon, midafternoon, sunset, and early evening) while facing Mecca. Before praying, they wash their hands, face, and feet as a ritual purification in worship. One prayer during the week requires attendance at the mosque. This is the Friday noon prayer. Like Sunday for Christians, Friday is a special day for Muslims, but it is not a day of rest. Muslims often work in the morning and the afternoon on Friday, leaving their work for a few hours around noon to gather at the mosque.

Cleanliness plays an important part in the Islamic faith. By tradition, it is said that cleanliness is half the faith and a Muslim cannot pray or hold a copy of the Qur'an without having first washed beforehand. There are various types of washings. One is *ghusi,* or washing the entire body in accordance with the example of Muhammad. It is necessary to have *ghusi* on embracing Islam; after sexual intercourse, menstruation, and childbirth; and before burial. Another is *wudhu:* washing the hands, mouth, nostrils, face, and forearms; wiping the head, ears, and the neck; and washing the feet with clean water, in accordance with the example of the prophet Muhammad, so as to be pure for *Salaat.* A person who has done *wudhu* remains in the appropriate state for prayer until it is nullified by any of the conditions that make it necessary for renewal (emissions of impurities from the body, such as urine, feces, or prostatic fluid) or loss of consciousness by whatever means, usually sleep or fainting.

The third pillar is *Zakaat,* or alms. Giving to the poor is a religious obligation, but it also forms the important social purpose of wealth distribution. After a Muslim has attained a certain financial level prescribed by the doctrines of the church, Islamic law prescribes that one-fortieth of his wealth is the proper amount he should give in alms. This is not considered a gift but rather a right due to those who cannot support themselves.

Fasting during the month of Ramadan, the annual religious fast that occurs during the ninth month of the Muslim lunar calendar, is the fourth pillar. By tradition, all Muslims above adolescence refrain from eating or drinking between dawn and sunset each day of that month. In that fasting is considered inward and outward purification, some Muslims may keep optional fasts beyond the requirements of Ramadan. Exempted from fasting are pregnant, lactating, or menstruating women; the ill; and travelers. Islamic doctrine puts the onus on the sick person to decide whether to fast, and the patient may wish to consult a practicing Muslim physician in making this decision.

Hajj, or pilgrimage, is the fifth pillar. The twelfth month of the Muslim year is the month of pilgrimage. All Muslims who can afford it are required to make a pilgrimage to Mecca at least once in their lives.

Guidelines for Health Providers

There are a number of areas where the Islamic faith affects the attitudes and behavior of Muslim patients. It is important that all health providers have some basic understanding of these attitudes and beliefs so that accommodations can be made where appropriate. It is also important to remember that these are guidelines only. The practice of the Islam faith may differ slightly in various parts of the world, and most traditions allow exceptions to its rules in emergency situations; however, the situation should truly be life threatening.

Food Service

Perhaps the most common of all areas where the faith can be easily accommodated is in food service. In the Qur'an, Muslims are enjoined to eat what is "good." It is common knowledge that pork and all its products (ham, bacon, lard, and sausage) are forbidden to Muslims. Equally forbidden but less known are the admonitions against the eating of wild animals that use claws or teeth to kill their victims, (all birds of prey, rodents, reptiles, worms, and the like). Muslims eat halal meat (the animal is slaughtered according to Islamic tradition and rites), which is a practice similar to the Jewish practice to make meat kosher. Many baked goods contain lard or shortening. A listing of ingredients that specifies "vegetable shortening" is the only way to be sure that the product is suitable. Gelatin, used in "Jell-O" and marshmallows, also presents a problem, as it is derived from connective tissue of vertebrate animals.

Whenever possible, halal food should be made available to Muslim patients. When this is not possible, the patient should be given the choice of having seafood, eggs, fruits, and vegetables. Care must also be taken in the general food preparation so that separate utensils are used; for example, a knife used for slicing pork must not be used to cut anything that will be given to Muslim patients.

Some traditions of the faith have taken the position that Muslims living in predominantly Christian countries may eat commercial meat (apart from pork), pronouncing God's name on it at the time of eating. Consequently the question of halal is not considered relevant by all Muslims living in Western countries.

Muslims are counseled to eat in moderation and always to leave food. It should be expected that small portions of uneaten food will be left on the plate. However, if large amounts are being left, the practitioners should try to ascertain if there is a problem of food acceptance. When serving food or drink, allow for the receipt in the right hand. Muslims consider the left hand unclean; therefore, when eating or giving or receiving food, only the right hand should be used.

Depending on the ethnic traditions of Muslim patients, they may prefer to eat from several plates with their fingers rather than from one plate with a knife and fork. Ask for guidance in this from the patient, a family member, or interpreter.

Strict adherence to fasting and diet regulations may create problems with compliance in the taking of medications and following medication schedules. Where a choice exists, medicines containing alcohol should be avoided. When the patient is fasting, the midday dose of medication may offer a problem unless the schedule can be reorganized. Doses once or twice daily would be a more practical schedule when applicable.

Hygiene

Personal hygiene plays an important role in the Islamic religion. Special care must be made for patients who are in-patients to provide them with the opportunity for cleanliness, especially associated with discharges, urine, stool, and bleeding from any orifice, bearing in mind that the patient may wish to pray in bed. The ambulatory patient may need help to the bathroom for washing. A beaker of water for washing should be made available to bedridden Muslim patients whenever they use a bedpan. A patient who is physically unable to wash up or would be hurt by washing up may instead use dry cleaning (called *tayammum*) in which he strikes his hands on a clean surface and then brushes his palms over his hands and face. Maternity nurses should note that women are excused from prayer during menstruation or postpartum bleeding.

Religious Observance

All Muslims have the obligation of daily prayer. If possible, a room should be made available as a prayer room. The hospital chapel may serve this purpose provided no icons are present. In that the patient or visitor must face toward the Ka'aba (a small square house of prayer in

Mecca), the general direction of this site should be known so as to assist the patient or visitor. If the patient is in a coma, it is preferred that the face of the patient be turned toward Mecca. For Muslims, bowing and prostrating themselves symbolically is an essential part of prayer. If necessary, this can be done sitting, lying down, or even mentally, depending on the patient's degree of incapacity.

Within most Muslim communities, it is considered a virtue to visit the sick. Sick Muslims are usually happy to receive many visitors, and often families consider it a duty to notify as many people as possible of the illness. Because of this emphasis within the faith, where possible, arrangements should be made to accommodate large numbers of visitors. It is important for Muslims to be given an opportunity to recite the Qu'ran or prayers in front of the patient or in a room nearby. Often relatives will go out of their way to conceal this practice so as not to embarrass or bother the hospital personnel. Again, when possible, the relatives should be encouraged to pray if they wish.

There are several interesting traditions associated with the birth of infants. Many parents will desire that the newborn have the call to prayer recited in each ear. Parents may request that a learned person from the Islamic community perform this service. Also some parents, following the example of Muhammad, may wish that the hair of the newborn be removed soon after birth. Circumcision is performed on all male children. The timing of this varies, but it must be done before puberty.

Modesty

By tradition, Muslims are not allowed to expose their bodies. A female is required to be covered from head to ankles. Only her face, hands, and feet are to be exposed. Men are not allowed to expose the area between the waist and knees. Medical examination techniques should be modified so that as little of the patient is exposed as possible, while not inhibiting the medical procedures. It is preferable for a female Muslim to be cared for by females and a male Muslim by males. As with all religious observance, you will find various degrees of adherence to this dress code depending on individual preference and the ethnicity of the group. Where possible and where suitable clothing can be made available, patients should be allowed to be dressed according to the requirements of their faith.

Grieving and Bereavement

For a Muslim, the whole of this life constitutes a trial and test during which his final destiny is determined. By Islamic tradition, grieving is allowed for only three days. Muslims feel that death is predestined by God and that it is the beginning of eternal life. As a result of this, more orthodox families my appear inappropriately calm and accepting of death by Western standards of expected conduct.

When a Muslim patient on service dies, it is preferable that his face be turned toward Mecca and his whole body, including face, be covered with a sheet. By tradition, the body should be handled as little as possible as Muslims believe that the body is hypersensitive to pressure and pain. The body must be handled with the utmost respect and only by a member of the same sex. The body is cleaned, scented, and covered with a clean cloth. If no relative is available, a leader within the Islamic community should be notified. Often relatives wish to pray at this time, and where possible, accommodation should be made. Cremation is prohibited, as are postmortems. However, it is understood that the statutory laws of the country must be followed.

Modifying Conditions

The Islamic faith is in many ways practical in its approach and allows adaptation for unavoidable circumstances. It is understood that in situations of life-threatening emergency, the preservation of life overrides all the guidelines previously presented. Islam allows exceptions to its rules in emergency situations, but these situations must be truly life threatening. Also, those diagnosed as having a mental illness are absolved from all the obligatory requirements of Islam. They are not required by faith to perform the obligatory prayers or fast.

Health Care Ethics: A Muslim Perspective

The rapid development of modern medicine in areas of sustaining life support, organ transplantations, gene therapy, abortion, and surrogacy have caused all communities, Muslims included, to attempt to bring order to their beliefs. For guidance on these matters, Muslims first turn to the Qur'an.

> Blessed be He in whose hands is the Dominion, and he has Power over all things. He who created life that He may test which of you are best in deed and He is exalted in might, oft forgiving (Qur'an 67: 1–2).

It is impossible to provide a detailed exploration of health care ethics from a Muslim perspective in this book; however, several issues provide insights into the thinking.

Abortion, Euthanasia, and Suicide

No soul can die except by Allah's permission.

Qur'an 3:185

The teachings make it very clear that life and death are in Allah's hands and that human beings should not play God. Suicide, euthanasia, and abortion are forbidden by the religion. The practice of euthanasia is regarded as murder by the person who is performing it, and it is considered suicide for the person ending his or her life. In the case of abortion, Islam considers abortion of a viable fetus as infanticide except when it is necessary to save the mother. Even in this situation, every attempt should be made to save both lives.

Prolongation of Life by Artificial Means

Islam teaches that everyone has been created for a particular life span. Thus, while the faith gives great importance to saving lives, it recognizes the limitations of medical science and makes it clear that dying is part of the contract with God, who has the final decision. The quality of life is equally or more important than the duration of living. Physicians and the family should recognize their limitations and not attempt heroic measures for the terminally ill patient or to prolong a life of misery artificially.

Transplants

The Islamic faith allows for the acceptance of blood products and most human organs, assuming the following conditions can be met:

1. The donor must not be put at risk while alive.
2. There must be no coercion in the obtaining of the organ (e.g., financial, social, or family pressure).
3. No vital organ can be removed for implantation while the person is alive.
4. Cadaver to living is not permitted since it involves the desecration of the dead body.
5. Xenotransplants are permissible. Because animals can be eaten and become part of the body, the use of animals for transplants would seem to fit within the guideline.

Issues in Biotechnical Reproduction

The teachings of the special place of marriage from the Prophet Muhammad are clear: "Marriage is my tradition. He who rejects marriage is not of me." Therefore, the violation of this sacred contract by a biomedical technique is problematic under Islamic law. Reproduction through biotechnical means would be sanctioned only if it is the product of an intact marriage (i.e., during the life of the marriage). Artificial insemination using the sperm from the husband, fertilized in the uterus of the wife or the test tube, would be allowed. The use of sperm or eggs from others and surrogate motherhood would not meet the test due to questions of who the mother is and questions of lineage. Cloning would also seem to be a forbidden practice.

CONCLUSION

The United States is filled with a large variety of traditions with an impact on health care practice. It is important for providers to be sensitive to these differences among our patient populations as they affect how willing the patient is to comply with our regimes or even whether the patient is willing to risk entry into our system.

In the United States we are in a period of dynamic social change in which hundreds of thousands of immigrants from around the world are flocking to our shores. Along with their hopes, aspirations, personal problems, talents, and dreams, these new immigrants bring with them their views of health, illness, and appropriate health practices. Although a review of traditional practices within the diverse homelands of these immigrants reveals the existence of meaningful health care traditions different from those practiced in the West, there is a reluctance of many health care providers to see the benefits or to be willing to accept these differences.

Health care practice in the West is based on scientific reasoning and high technology. Western health care is a system of marvels: organs can be replaced, the blind can be made to see, and the dead can be revived. On the surface it would seem that modern medicine as taught and practiced in the West should be embraced by all. What can one truly take from a health care tradition that is not built on an understanding of germ theory?

Yet some patients do not seem able to follow prescriptions given, will not show up for appointments, do not comply with treatment regimes, and are not even willing to access the system until they are in severe distress and then leave as quickly as possible. Under current practice, something is being missed in regard to these patients, and the system is failing them. Is it because the patients and practitioners have different views regarding health, illness, and appropriate practice? Can it be that the patients often believe that the care offered would make them sicker or is incompatible with their illness? In some sense, what the patient believes is not as important as whether the provider is sensitive to the facts surrounding the belief system of the patient and is willing to respect the differences. It is important to come to understand how patients understand illness and their relationship to it and also what motivates them to seek medical assistance and then to follow the advice given. There is an ethical and professional imperative to build the bridges of understanding that allows for successful practice among those with a different view of health, illness, and appropriate practice.

KEY CONCEPTS

- Often the lack of cultural cues within the health care setting is severe enough for non-Western patients as to create culture shock and interfere with the ability of the patient to benefit fully from the service.

- The health care traditions of cultures such as that of India and China have a long and valid history. However, the ideals of the health care does not spring from Hippocratic traditions; therefore, the non-Western patient and Western practitioner may have very different expectations.

- Whether one is Mormon, Methodist, Muslim, or Mennonite, the traditions of the faith will affect the patient's behavior. Health care providers, to the extent possible, should come to understand the needs of these and other patient populations and provide appropriate accommodations.

- The principles of beneficence, nonmaleficence, role duty, and justice provide an ethical and professional imperative for health care providers to build bridges of understanding that allow successful practice among those with a different view of health, illness, and appropriate practice.

REVIEW EXERCISES

A. A health care code of ethics based on the traditions of medical practice in China would be very different from the AMA code of ethics. Review the AMA code found in the appendix and review the virtues found in traditional Chinese medicine practice and revolutionary socialism as outlined in the chapter. Write a seven-rule code of ethics to fit the virtues found in ancient and modern Chinese health care practice.

B. A study regarding Navajo culture indicates that there are problems associated with the legal requirements of the Patient Self-Determination Act that requires the practitioner to discuss life-threatening conditions and seek to elicit answers regarding the patient's wishes in regard to the use of life-supporting technologies. The problem lies in the fact that within the traditional Navajo culture in times of illness, there is a need to speak and think positively and avoid the negative. The requirement that health care providers review all the adverse possibilities seems to go against the need to remain positive in the face of illness. Given that the requirements are designed to promote patient autonomy and are legally required, what is the practitioner to do?

C. Several African populations practice the tradition of female circumcism. Assume that one of the families moved to the United States and brought their young daughter in to the emergency room with severe trauma and infection caused by this process and it was clear that the young girl did not feel that she had been abused. Would it be necessary to report the family for child abuse? Would you feel differently if the young woman had come to you prior to the event and made it clear to you that she did not want to participate in this cultural ritual?

D. Several traditional populations do not donate organs at the same rate as the majority population in the United States. There are many reasons for this, including in some cases a cultural need for body integrity following death. Given that these groups have decided not to provide organs, should they receive organs on the same basis as groups that more readily donate them?

E. The World Health Organization defines health as a "state of complete physical, mental, and social well being and not merely the absence of disease." Do you think that this definition fits the definition of health that we use in the American medical model? In what ways is it the same, in what ways different?

Think about how you might define health if your model was based on a nongerm theory system in which illness was caused by some individual who wished you ill and was using some magical/religious basis to bring about your problem.

BIBLIOGRAPHY

Some of the information presented in this chapter was drawn from the following sources.

Yusuf Ali, trans., *The Holy Quran* (Washington, DC: Amana Corporation, 1990).

Shahid Athar, *Information for Health Care Providers When Dealing with a Muslim Patient* (Downers Grove, IL: Islamic Medical Association of North America, 2004).

B. Bowman, et al., eds., *World Cultures* (Needham, MA: Prentice Hall, 1999).

Hassan Gaveebo, "An Islamic Code of Medical Ethics," *Journal of Islamic Medical Association* 20 (1988).

Geng Junying and Su Zhihong, *Acupuncture and Moxibustion* (New York: New World Press, 1993).

Geng Junying and Su Zhihong, *Basic Theories and Principles* (New York: New World Press, 1993).

"Islamic Medical Ethics," special issue of *Journal of Islamic Medical Association* (January 1988).

Li Wen Peng, *Medical Ethics* (Shan Dong Province University, 1993).

Julius Lipner, "The Classical Hindu View on Abortion and the Moral Status of the Unborn," in *Hindu Ethics: Purity, Abortion and Euthanasia*, Harold Coward, Julius Lipner, and Katherine Young, eds. (Albany, NY: SUNY Press, 1989).

K.R. Srikanta Murthy, "Professional Ethics in Ancient Indian Medicine," *Cross Cultural Perspectives in Medical Ethics: Readings*, Robert Veatch, ed. (Boston: Jones and Bartlett, 2000).

Kalvero Oberg, *Culture Shock* (Indianapolis: Bobbs-Merrill, 1954).

Sheng Yi Ru and Zeng Meng Liang, ed., *Model and Style of Medical Ethics in China* (Traditional Chinese Medicine Publishing House, 1994).

Rachel Spector, *Cultural Diversity in Health and Illness* (Stamford, CT: Appleton and Lange, 1996).

Tom Williams, *Chinese Medicine* (Rockport, MA: Element Books, 1996).

Katherine K. Young, "Euthanasia: Traditional Hindu Views and the Contemporary Debate," *Hindu Ethics: Purity Abortion and Euthanasia* (Albany, NY: SUNY Press, 1989).

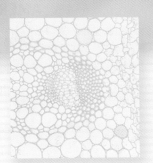

Codes of Professional Ethics: Selected Health Professions

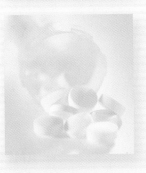

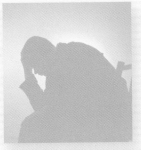

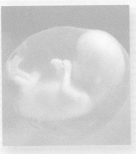

AMERICAN ACADEMY OF PHYSICIAN ASSISTANTS

Statement of Values of the Physician Assistant Profession

- Physician assistants hold as their primary responsibility the health, safety, welfare, and dignity of all human beings.
- Physician assistants uphold the tenets of patient autonomy, beneficence, nonmaleficence, and justice.
- Physician assistants recognize and promote the value of diversity.
- Physician assistants treat equally all persons who seek their care.
- Physician assistants hold in confidence the information shared in the course of practicing medicine.
- Physician assistants assess their personal capabilities and limitations, striving always to improve their medical practice.
- Physician assistants actively seek to expand their knowledge and skills, keeping abreast of advances in medicine.
- Physician assistants work with other members of the health care team to provide compassionate and effective care of patients.
- Physician assistants use their knowledge and experience to contribute to an improved community.
- Physician assistants respect their professional relationship with physicians.
- Physician assistants share and expand knowledge within the profession.

AMERICAN ASSOCIATION FOR RESPIRATORY CARE

Statement of Ethics and Professional Conduct

In the conduct of professional activities the Respiratory Therapist shall be bound by the following ethical and professional principles. Respiratory Therapists shall:

Demonstrate behavior that reflects integrity, supports objectivity, and fosters trust in the profession and its professionals. Actively maintain and continually improve their professional competence, and represent it accurately.

Perform only those procedures or functions in which they are individually competent and which are within the scope of accepted and responsible practice.

Respect and protect the legal and personal rights of patients they care for, including the right to informed consent and refusal of treatment.

Divulge no confidential information regarding any patient or family unless disclosure is required for responsible performance of duty, or required by law.

Provide care without discrimination on any basis, with respect for the rights and dignity of all individuals.

Promote disease prevention and wellness.

Refuse to participate in illegal or unethical acts, and refuse to conceal illegal, unethical or incompetent acts of others.

Follow sound scientific procedures and ethical principles in research.

Comply with state or federal laws which govern and relate to their practice.

Avoid any form of conduct that creates a conflict of interest, and shall follow the principles of ethical business behavior.

Promote health care delivery through improvement of the access, efficacy, and cost of patient care.

Refrain from indiscriminate and unnecessary use of resources.

Effective 12/94
Revised 3/00
(Reprinted with permission from the American Association for Respiratory Care)

AMERICAN ASSOCIATION OF MEDICAL ASSISTANTS
Code of Ethics and Creed

Code of Ethics

The Code of Ethics of AAMA shall set forth principles of ethical and moral conduct as they relate to the medical profession and the particular practice of medical assisting.

Members of the AAMA dedicated to the conscientious pursuit of their profession, and thus desiring to merit the high regard of the entire medical profession and the respect of the general public which they serve, do pledge themselves to strive always to:

A. render service with full respect for the dignity of humanity;

B. respect confidential information obtained through employment unless legally authorized or required by responsible performance of duty to divulge such information;

C. uphold the honor and high principles of the profession and accept its disciplines;

D. seek to continually improve the knowledge and skills of medical assistants for the benefit of patients and professional colleagues;

E. participate in additional service activities aimed toward improving the health and well-being of the community.

AAMA Creed

I believe in the principles and purposes of the profession of medical assisting.

I endeavor to be more effective.

I aspire to render greater service.

I protect the confidence entrusted to me.

I am dedicated to the care and well-being of all people.

I am loyal to my employer.

I am true to the ethics of my profession.

I am strengthened by compassion, courage and faith.

AMERICAN DENTAL ASSOCIATION

Principles of Ethics and Code of Professional Conduct

(*With official advisory opinions revised to January 2004*)

II. Preamble

The American Dental Association calls upon dentists to follow high ethical standards which have the benefit of the patient as their primary goal. Recognition of this goal, and of the education and training of a dentist, has resulted in society affording to the profession the privilege and obligation of self-government.

The Association believes that dentists should possess not only knowledge, skill, and technical competence but also those traits of character that foster adherence to ethical principles. Qualities of compassion, kindness, integrity, fairness, and charity complement the ethical practice of dentistry and help to define the true professional.

The ethical dentist strives to do that which is right and good. The *ADA Code* is an instrument to help the dentist in this quest.

III. Principles, Code of Professional Conduct, and Advisory Opinions

Section 1 PRINCIPLE: PATIENT AUTONOMY ("self-governance"). The dentist has a duty to respect the patient's rights to self-determination and confidentiality.

This principle expresses the concept that professionals have a duty to treat the patient according to the patient's desires, within the bounds of accepted treatment, and to protect the patient's confidentiality. Under this principle, the dentist's primary obligations include involving patients in treatment decisions in a meaningful way, with due consideration being given to the patient's needs, desires, and abilities, and safeguarding the patient's privacy.

Section 2 PRINCIPLE: NONMALEFICENCE ("do no harm"). The dentist has a duty to refrain from harming the patient.

This principle expresses the concept that professionals have a duty to protect the patient from harm. Under this principle, the dentist's primary obligations include keeping knowledge and skills current, knowing one's own limitations and when to refer to a specialist or other professional, and knowing when and under what circumstances delegation of patient care to auxiliaries is appropriate.

Section 3 PRINCIPLE: BENEFICENCE ("do good"). The dentist has a duty to promote the patient's welfare.

This principle expresses the concept that professionals have a duty to act for the benefit of others. Under this principle, the dentist's primary obligation is service to the patient and the public-at-large. The most important aspect of this obligation is the competent and timely delivery of dental care within the bounds of clinical circumstances presented by the patient, with due consideration being given to the needs, desires, and values of the patient. The same ethical considerations apply whether the dentist engages in fee-for-service, managed care, or some other practice arrangement. Dentists may choose to enter into contracts governing the provision of care to a group of patients; however, contract obligations do not excuse dentists from their ethical duty to put the patient's welfare first.

Section 4 PRINCIPLE: JUSTICE ("fairness"). The dentist has a duty to treat people fairly.

This principle expresses the concept that professionals have a duty to be fair in their dealings with patients, colleagues, and society. Under this principle, the dentist's primary obligations include dealing with people justly and delivering dental care without prejudice. In its broadest sense, this principle expresses the concept that the dental profession should actively seek allies throughout society on specific activities that will help improve access to care for all.

Section 5 PRINCIPLE: VERACITY ("truthfulness"). The dentist has a duty to communicate truthfully.

This principle expresses the concept that professionals have a duty to be honest and trustworthy in their dealings with people. Under this principle, the dentist's primary obligations include respecting the position of trust inherent in the dentist-patient relationship, communicating truthfully and without deception, and maintaining intellectual integrity.

AMERICAN DENTAL HYGIENISTS ASSOCIATION
Code of Ethics

1. Preamble

As dental hygienists, we are a community of professionals devoted to the prevention of disease and the promotion and improvement of the public's health. We are preventive oral health professionals who provide educational, clinical, and therapeutic services to the public. We strive to live meaningful, productive, satisfying lives that simultaneously serve us, our profession, our society, and the world. Our actions, behaviors, and attitudes are consistent with our commitment to public service. We endorse and incorporate the Code into our daily lives.

2. Purpose

The purpose of a professional code of ethics is to achieve high levels of ethical consciousness, decision making, and practice by the members of the profession. Specific objectives of the Dental Hygiene Code of Ethics are

- to increase our professional and ethical consciousness and sense of ethical responsibility.
- to lead us to recognize ethical issues and choices and to guide us in making more informed ethical decisions.
- to establish a standard for professional judgement and conduct.
- to provide a statement of the ethical behavior the public can expect from us.

The Dental Hygiene Code of Ethics is meant to influence us throughout our careers. It stimulates our continuing study of ethical issues and challenges us to explore our ethical responsibilities. The Code establishes concise standards of behavior to guide the public's expectations of our profession and supports existing dental hygiene practice, laws, and regulations. By holding ourselves accountable to meeting the standards stated in the Code, we enhance the public's trust on which our professional privilege and status are founded.

3. Key Concepts

Our beliefs, principles, values, and ethics are concepts reflected in the Code. They are the essential elements of our comprehensive and definitive code of ethics, and are interrelated and mutually dependent.

Approved and ratified by the 1995 ADHA House of Delegates.

4. Basic Beliefs

We recognize the importance of the following beliefs that guide our practice and provide context for our ethics:

- The services we provide contribute to the health and well being of society.

- Our education and licensure qualify us to serve the public by preventing and treating oral disease and helping individuals achieve and maintain optimal health.

- Individuals have intrinsic worth, are responsible for their own health, and are entitled to make choices regarding their health.

- Dental hygiene care is an essential component of overall healthcare and we function interdependently with other healthcare providers.

- All people should have access to healthcare, including oral healthcare.

- We are individually responsible for our actions and the quality of care we provide.

5. Fundamental Principles

These fundamental principles, universal concepts, and general laws of conduct provide the foundation for our ethics.

Universality The principle of universality assumes that, if one individual judges an action to be right or wrong in a given situation, other people considering the same action in the same situation would make the same judgement.

Complementarity The principle of complementarity assumes the existence of an obligation to justice and basic human rights. It requires us to act toward others in the same way they would act toward us if roles were reversed. In all relationships, it means considering the values and perspective of others before making decisions or taking actions affecting them.

Ethics Ethics are the general standards of right and wrong that guide behavior within society. As generally accepted actions, they can be judged by determining the extent to which they promote good and minimize harm. Ethics compel us to engage in health promotion/disease prevention activities.

Community This principle expresses our concern for the bond between individuals, the community, and society in general. It leads us to preserve natural resources and inspires us to show concern for the global environment.

Responsibility Responsibility is central to our ethics. We recognize that there are guidelines for making ethical choices and accept responsibility for knowing and applying them. We accept the consequences of our actions or the failure to act and are willing to make ethical choices and publicly affirm them.

6. Core Values

We acknowledge these values as general guides for our choices and actions.

Individual autonomy and respect for human beings People have the right to be treated with respect. They have the right to informed consent prior to treatment, and they have the right to full disclosure of all relevant information so that they can make informed choices about their care.

Confidentiality We respect the confidentiality of client information and relationships as a demonstration of the value we place on individual autonomy. We acknowledge our obligation to justify any violation of a confidence.

Societal Trust We value client trust and understand that public trust in our profession is based on our actions and behavior.

Nonmaleficence We accept our fundamental obligation to provide services in a manner that protects all clients and minimizes harm to them and others involved in their treatment.

Beneficence We have a primary role in promoting the well being of individuals and the public by engaging in health promotion/disease prevention activities.

Justice and Fairness We value justice and support the fair and equitable distribution of health-care resources. We believe all people should have access to high-quality, affordable oral healthcare.

Veracity We accept our obligation to tell the truth and assume that others will do the same. We value self-knowledge and seek truth and honesty in all relationships.

7. Standards of Professional Responsibility

We are obligated to practice our profession in a manner that supports our purpose, beliefs, and values in accordance with the fundamental principles that support our ethics. We acknowledge the following responsibilities:

To Ourselves as Individuals . . .

- Avoid self-deception, and continually strive for knowledge and personal growth.
- Establish and maintain a lifestyle that supports optimal health.

- Create a safe work environment.
- Assert our own interests in ways that are fair and equitable.
- Seek the advice and counsel of others when challenged with ethical dilemmas.
- Have realistic expectations of ourselves and recognize our limitations.

To Ourselves as Professionals . . .

- Enhance professional competencies through continuous learning in order to practice according to high standards of care.
- Support dental hygiene peer-review systems and quality-assurance measures.
- Develop collaborative professional relationships and exchange knowledge to enhance our own life-long professional development.

To Family and Friends . . .

- Support the efforts of others to establish and maintain healthy lifestyles and respect the rights of friends and family.

To Clients . . .

- Provide oral healthcare utilizing high levels of professional knowledge, judgement, and skill.
- Maintain a work environment that minimizes the risk of harm.
- Serve all clients without discrimination and avoid action toward any individual or group that may be interpreted as discriminatory.
- Hold professional client relationships confidential.
- Communicate with clients in a respectful manner.
- Promote ethical behavior and high standards of care by all dental hygienists.
- Serve as an advocate for the welfare of clients.
- Provide clients with the information necessary to make informed decisions about their oral health and encourage their full participation in treatment decisions and goals.
- Refer clients to other healthcare providers when their needs are beyond our ability or scope of practice.
- Educate clients about high-quality oral healthcare.

To Colleagues . . .

- Conduct professional activities and programs, and develop relationships in ways that are honest, responsible, and appropriately open and candid.

- Encourage a work environment that promotes individual professional growth and development.
- Collaborate with others to create a work environment that minimizes risk to the personal health and safety of our colleagues.
- Manage conflicts constructively.
- Support the efforts of other dental hygienists to communicate the dental hygiene philosophy of preventive oral care.
- Inform other healthcare professionals about the relationship between general and oral health.
- Promote human relationships that are mutually beneficial, including those with other healthcare professionals.

To Employees and Employers . . .

- Conduct professional activities and programs, and develop relationships in ways that are honest, responsible, open, and candid.
- Manage conflicts constructively.
- Support the right of our employees and employers to work in an environment that promotes wellness.
- Respect the employment rights of our employers and employees.

To the Dental Hygiene Profession . . .

- Participate in the development and advancement of our profession.
- Avoid conflicts of interest and declare them when they occur.
- Seek opportunities to increase public awareness and understanding of oral health practices.
- Act in ways that bring credit to our profession while demonstrating appropriate respect for colleagues in other professions.
- Contribute time, talent, and financial resources to support and promote our profession.
- Promote a positive image for our profession.
- Promote a framework for professional education that develops dental hygiene competencies to meet the oral and overall health needs of the public.

To the Community and Society . . .

- Recognize and uphold the laws and regulations governing our profession.
- Document and report inappropriate, inadequate, or substandard care and/or illegal activities by any healthcare provider, to the responsible authorities.

- Use peer review as a mechanism for identifying inappropriate, inadequate, or substandard care and for modifying and improving the care provided by dental hygienists.

- Comply with local, state, and federal statutes that promote public health and safety.

- Develop support systems and quality-assurance programs in the workplace to assist dental hygienists in providing the appropriate standard of care.

- Promote access to dental hygiene services for all, supporting justice and fairness in the distribution of healthcare resources.

- Act consistently with the ethics of the global scientific community of which our profession is a part.

- Create a healthful workplace ecosystem to support a healthy environment.

- Recognize and uphold our obligation to provide pro bono service.

To Scientific Investigation . . .

We accept responsibility for conducting research according to the fundamental principles underlying our ethical beliefs in compliance with universal codes, governmental standards, and professional guidelines for the care and management of experimental subjects. We acknowledge our ethical obligations to the scientific community:

- Conduct research that contributes knowledge that is valid and useful to our clients and society.

- Use research methods that meet accepted scientific standards.

- Use research resources appropriately.

- Systematically review and justify research in progress to insure the most favorable benefit-to-risk ratio to research subjects.

- Submit all proposals involving human subjects to an appropriate human subject review committee.

- Secure appropriate institutional committee approval for the conduct of research involving animals.

- Obtain informed consent from human subjects participating in research that is based on specifications published in Title 21 Code of Federal Regulations Part 46.

- Respect the confidentiality and privacy of data.

- Seek opportunities to advance dental hygiene knowledge through research by providing financial, human, and technical resources whenever possible.

- Report research results in a timely manner.

- Report research findings completely and honestly, drawing only those conclusions that are supported by the data presented.

- Report the names of investigators fairly and accurately.

- Interpret the research and the research of others accurately and objectively, drawing conclusions that are supported by the data presented and seeking clarity when uncertain.

- Critically evaluate research methods and results before applying new theory and technology in practice.

- Be knowledgeable concerning currently accepted preventive and therapeutic methods, products, and technology and their application to our practice.

AMERICAN HOSPITAL ASSOCIATION

The Patient Care Partnership: Understanding Expectations, Rights and Responsibilities

When you need hospital care, your doctor and the nurses and other professionals at our hospital are committed to working with you and your family to meet your health care needs. Our dedicated doctors and staff serve the community in all its ethnic, religious and economic diversity. Our goal is for you and your family to have the same care and attention we would want for our families and ourselves.

The sections explain some of the basics about how you can expect to be treated during your hospital stay. They also cover what we will need from you to care for you better. If you have questions at any time, please ask them. Unasked or unanswered questions can add to the stress of being in the hospital. Your comfort and confidence in your care are very important to us.

What to Expect During Your Hospital Stay

- **High quality hospital care.** Our first priority is to provide you the care you need, when you need it, with skill, compassion, and respect. Tell your caregivers if you have concerns about your care or if you have pain. You have the right to know the identity of doctors, nurses and others involved in your care, and you have the right to know when they are students, residents or other trainees.

- **A clean and safe environment.** Our hospital works hard to keep you safe. We use special policies and procedures to avoid mistakes in your care and keep you free from abuse or neglect. If anything unexpected and significant happens during your hospital stay, you will be told what happened, and any resulting changes in your care will be discussed with you.

Reprinted with permission of the American Hospital Association, copyright 2003.

- **Involvement in your care.** You and your doctor often make decisions about your care before you go to the hospital. Other times, especially in emergencies, those decisions are made during your hospital stay. When decision-making takes place, it should include:

  - *Discussing your medical condition and information about medically appropriate treatment choices.* To make informed decisions with your doctor, you need to understand:
    - The benefits and risks of each treatment.
    - Whether your treatment is experimental or part of a research study.
    - What you can reasonably expect from your treatment and any long-term effects it might have on your quality of life.
    - What you and your family will need to do after you leave the hospital.
    - The financial consequences of using uncovered services or out-of-network providers.

    Please tell your caregivers if you need more information about treatment choices.

  - *Discussing your treatment plan.* When you enter the hospital, you sign a general consent to treatment. In some cases, such as surgery or experimental treatment, you may be asked to confirm in writing that you understand what is planned and agree to it. This process protects your right to consent to or refuse a treatment. Your doctor will explain the medical consequences of refusing recommended treatment. It also protects your right to decide if you want to participate in a research study.

  - *Getting information from you.* Your caregivers need complete and correct information about your health and coverage so that they can make good decisions about your care. That includes:
    - Past illnesses, surgeries or hospital stays.
    - Past allergic reactions.
    - Any medicines or dietary supplements (such as vitamins and herbs) that you are taking.
    - Any network or admission requirements under your health plan.

  - *Understanding your health care goals and values.* You may have health care goals and values or spiritual beliefs that are important to your well-being. They will be taken into account as much as possible throughout your hospital stay. Make sure your doctor, your family and your care team know your wishes.

  - *Understanding who should make decisions when you cannot.* If you have signed a health care power of attorney stating who should speak for you if you become unable to make health care decisions for yourself, or a "living will" or "advance directive" that states your wishes about end-of-life care; give copies to your doctor, your family and your care team. If you or your family need help making difficult decisions, counselors, chaplains and others are available to help.

- **Protection of your privacy.** We respect the confidentiality of your relationship with your doctor and other caregivers, and the sensitive information about your health and health care that are part of that relationship. State and federal laws and hospital operating policies protect the privacy of your medical information. You will receive a Notice of Privacy Practices that describes the ways that we use, disclose and safeguard patient information and that explains how you can obtain a copy of information from our records about your care.

- **Preparing you and your family for when you leave the hospital.** Your doctor works with hospital staff and professionals in your community. You and your family also play an important role in your care. The success of your treatment often depends on your efforts to follow medication, diet and therapy plans. Your family may need to help care for you at home.

  You can expect us to help you identify sources of follow-up care and to let you know if our hospital has a financial interest in any referrals. As long as you agree that we can share information about your care with them, we will coordinate our activities with your caregivers outside the hospital. You can also expect to receive information and, where possible, training about the self-care you will need when you go home.

- **Help with your bill and filing insurance claims.** Our staff will file claims for you with health care insurers or other programs such as Medicare and Medicaid. They also will help your doctor with needed documentation. Hospital bills and insurance coverage are often confusing. If you have questions about your bill, contact our business office. If you need help understanding your insurance coverage or health plan, start with your insurance company or health benefits manager. If you do not have health coverage, we will try to help you and your family find financial help or make other arrangements. We need your help with collecting needed information and other requirements to obtain coverage or assistance.

While you are here, you will receive more detailed notices about some of the rights you have as a hospital patient and how to exercise them. We are always interested in improving. If you have questions, comments, or concerns, please contact _____.

AMERICAN MEDICAL ASSOCIATION
Principles of Medical Ethics

Preamble

The medical profession has long subscribed to a body of ethical statements developed primarily for the benefit of the patient. As a member of this profession, a physician must recognize responsibility to patients first and foremost, as well as to society, to other health professionals, and to self. The following Principles adopted by the American Medical Association are not laws, but standards of conduct which define the essentials of honorable behavior for the physician.

I. A physician shall be dedicated to providing competent medical care, with compassion and respect for human dignity and rights.

II. A physician shall uphold the standards of professionalism, be honest in all professional interactions, and strive to report physicians deficient in character or competence, or engaging in fraud or deception, to appropriate entities.

III. A physician shall respect the law and also recognize a responsibility to seek changes in those requirements which are contrary to the best interests of the patient.

IV. A physician shall respect the rights of patients, colleagues, and other health professionals, and shall safeguard patient confidences and privacy within the constraints of the law.

V. A physician shall continue to study, apply, and advance scientific knowledge, maintain a commitment to medical education, make relevant information available to patients, colleagues, and the public, obtain consultation, and use the talents of other health professionals when indicated.

VI. A physician shall, in the provision of appropriate patient care, except in emergencies, be free to choose whom to serve, with whom to associate, and the environment in which to provide medical care.

VII. A physician shall recognize a responsibility to participate in activities contributing to the improvement of the community and the betterment of public health.

VIII. A physician shall, while caring for a patient, regard responsibility to the patient as paramount.

IX. A physician shall support access to medical care for all people.

Adopted June 1957; revised June 1980; revised June 2001.

Code of Medical Ethics, copyright 2004, American Medical Association.

AMERICAN NURSES ASSOCIATION

Code of Ethics for Nurses

Provision 1. The nurse, in all professional relationships, practices with compassion and respect for the inherent dignity, worth, and uniqueness of every individual, unrestricted by considerations of social or economic status, personal attributes, or the nature of health problems.

Provision 2. The nurse's primary commitment is to the patient, whether an individual, family, group, or community.

Provision 3. The nurse promotes, advocates for, and strives to protect the health, safety, and rights of the patient.

Provision 4. The nurse is responsible and accountable for individual nursing practice and determines the appropriate delegation of tasks consistent with the nurse's obligation to provide optimum patient care.

Provision 5. The nurse owes the same duties to self as to others, including the responsibility to preserve integrity and safety, to maintain competence, and to continue personal and professional growth.

Provision 6. The nurse participates in establishing, maintaining, and improving health care environments and conditions of employment conducive to the provision of quality health care and consistent with the values of the profession through individual and collective action.

Provision 7. The nurse participates in the advancement of the profession through contributions to practice, education, administration, and knowledge development.

Provision 8. The nurse collaborates with other health professionals and the public in promoting community, national, and international efforts to meet health needs.

Provision 9. The profession of nursing, as represented by associations and their members, is responsible for articulating nursing values, for maintaining the integrity of the profession and its practice, and for shaping social policy.

Reprinted with permission from American Nurses Association, Code of Ethics for Nurses with Interpretive Statements, © 2001 nursesbooks.org, American Nurses Association, Washington, DC.

Preface

Ethics is an integral part of the foundation of nursing. Nursing has a distinguished history of concern for the welfare of the sick, injured, and vulnerable and for social justice. This concern is embodied in the provision of nursing care to individuals and the community. Nursing encompasses the prevention of illness, the alleviation of suffering, and the protection, promotion, and restoration of health in the care of individuals, families, groups, and communities. Nurses act to change those aspects of social structures that detract from health and well-being. Individuals who become nurses are expected not only to adhere to the ideals and moral norms of the profession but also to embrace them as a part of what it means to be a nurse. The ethical tradition of nursing is self-reflective, enduring, and distinctive. A code of ethics makes explicit the primary goals, values, and obligations of the profession.

The Code of Ethics for Nurses serves the following purposes:

- It is a succinct statement of the ethical obligations and duties of every individual who enters the nursing profession.

- It is the profession's nonnegotiable ethical standard.

- It is an expression of nursing's own understanding of its commitment to society.

There are numerous approaches for addressing ethics; these include adopting or subscribing to ethical theories, including humanist, feminist, and social ethics, adhering to ethical principles, and cultivating virtues. The Code of Ethics for Nurses reflects all of these approaches. The words "ethical" and "moral" are used throughout the Code of Ethics. "Ethical" is used to refer to reasons for decisions about how one ought to act, using the above mentioned approaches. In general, the word "moral" overlaps with "ethical" but is more aligned with personal belief and cultural values. Statements that describe activities and attributes of nurses in this Code of Ethics are to be understood as normative or prescriptive statements expressing expectations of ethical behavior.

The Code of Ethics for Nurses uses the term *patient* to refer to recipients of nursing care. The derivation of this word refers to "one who suffers," reflecting a universal aspect of human existence. Nonetheless, it is recognized that nurses also provide services to those seeking health as well as those responding to illness, to students and to staff, in health care facilities as well as in communities. Similarly, the term *practice* refers to the actions of the nurse in whatever role the nurse fulfills, including direct patient care provider, educator, administrator, researcher, policy developer, or other. Thus, the values and obligations expressed in this Code of Ethics apply to nurses in all roles and settings.

The Code of Ethics for Nurses is a dynamic document. As nursing and its social context change, changes to the Code of Ethics are also necessary. The Code of Ethics consists of two components: the provisions and the accompanying interpretive statements. There are nine provisions. The first three describe the most fundamental values and commitments of the nurse; the next three address boundaries of duty and loyalty, and the last three address aspects of duties beyond individual patient encounters. For each provision, there are interpretive statements that provide greater specificity for practice and are responsive to the contemporary context of nursing. Consequently, the interpretive statements are subject to more frequent revision than are the provisions. Additional ethical guidance and detail can be found in ANA or constituent member association position statements that address clinical, research, administrative, educational, or public policy issues.

The Code of Ethics for Nurses with Interpretive Statements provides a framework for nurses to use in ethical analysis and decision-making. The Code of Ethics establishes the ethical standard for the profession. It is not negotiable in any setting nor is it subject to revision or amendment except by formal process of the House of Delegates of the ANA. The Code of Ethics for Nurses is a reflection of the proud ethical heritage of nursing, a guide for nurses now and in the future.

AMERICAN OCCUPATIONAL THERAPY ASSOCIATION

Code of Ethics

Preamble

The American Occupational Therapy Association's Code of Ethics is a public statement of the common set of values and principles used to promote and maintain high standards of behavior in occupational therapy. The American Occupational Therapy Association and its members are committed to furthering the ability of individuals, groups, and systems to function within their total environment. To this end, occupational therapy personnel (including all staff and personnel who work and assist in providing occupational therapy services, (e.g., aides, orderlies, secretaries, technicians) have a responsibility to provide services to recipients in any stage of health and illness who are individuals, research participants, institutions and businesses, other professionals and colleagues, students, and to the general public.

The *Occupational Therapy Code of Ethics* is a set of principles that applies to occupational therapy personnel at all levels. These principles to which occupational therapists and occupational therapy assistants aspire are part of a lifelong effort to act in an ethical manner. The various roles of practitioner (occupational therapist and occupational therapy assistant), educator, fieldwork educator, clinical supervisor, manager, administrator, consultant, fieldwork coordinator, faculty program director, researcher/scholar, private practice owner, entrepreneur, and student are assumed.

Any action in violation of the spirit and purpose of this Code shall be considered unethical. To ensure compliance with the Code, the Commission on Standards and Ethics (SEC) establishes and maintains the enforcement procedures. Acceptance of membership in the American Occupational Therapy Association commits members to adherence to the Code of Ethics and its enforcement procedures. The Code of Ethics, Core Values and Attitudes of Occupational Therapy Practice (AOTA, 1993), and the Guidelines to the Occupational Therapy Code of Ethics (AOTA, 1998) are aspirational documents designed to be used together to guide occupational therapy personnel.

Principle 1. Occupational therapy personnel shall demonstrate a concern for the well-being of the recipients of their services. (beneficence)

Principle 2. Occupational therapy personnel shall take reasonable precautions to avoid imposing or inflicting harm upon the recipient of services or to his or her property. (nonmaleficence)

Principle 3. Occupational therapy personnel shall respect the recipient and/or their surrogate(s) as well as the recipient's rights. (autonomy, privacy, confidentiality)

Principle 4. Occupational therapy personnel shall achieve and continually maintain high standards of competence. (duties)

Principle 5. Occupational therapy personnel shall comply with laws and Association policies guiding the profession of occupational therapy. (justice)

Principle 6. Occupational therapy personnel shall provide accurate information about occupational therapy services. (veracity)

Principle 7. Occupational therapy personnel shall treat colleagues and other professionals with fairness, discretion, and integrity. (fidelity)

References

American Occupational Therapy Association. (1993). Core values and attitudes of occupational therapy practice. *American Journal of Occupational Therapy, 47,* 1085–1086.

American Occupational Therapy Association. (1998). Guidelines to the occupational therapy code of ethics. *American Journal of Occupational Therapy, 52,* 881–884.

Authors

The Commission on Standards and Ethics (SEC):

Barbara L. Kornblau, JD, OTR, FAOTA, Chairperson
Melba Arnold, MS, OTR/L
Nancy Nashiro, PhD, OTR, FAOTA
Diane Hill, COTA/L, AP
Deborah Y. Slater, MS, OTR/L

John Morris, PhD

Linda Withers, CNHA, FACHCA

Penny Kyler, MA, OTR/L, FAOTA, Staff Liaison

April 2000

Adopted by the Representative Assembly 2000M15

Note: This document replaces the 1994 document, *Occupational Therapy Code of Ethics* (*American Journal of Occupational Therapy, 48,* 1037–1038).

Prepared 4/7/2000

© 2000 by the American Occupational Therapy Association, Inc.

AMERICAN PHARMACISTS ASSOCIATION
Code of Ethics

Preamble

Pharmacists are health professionals who assist individuals in making the best use of medications. This Code, prepared and supported by pharmacists, is intended to state publicly the principles that form the fundamental basis of the roles and responsibilities of pharmacists. These principles, based on moral obligations and virtues, are established to guide pharmacists in relationships with patients, health professionals, and society.

I. A pharmacist respects the covenantal relationship between the patient and pharmacist. Considering the patient-pharmacist relationship as a covenant means that a pharmacist has moral obligations in response to the gift of trust received from society. In return for this gift, a pharmacist promises to help individuals achieve optimum benefit from their medications, to be committed to their welfare, and to maintain their trust.

II. A pharmacist promotes the good of every patient in a caring, compassionate, and confidential manner. A pharmacist places concern for the well-being of the patient at

Adopted by the membership of the American Pharmacists Association October 27, 1994 (then the American Pharmaceutical Association).

the center of professional practice. In doing so, a pharmacist considers needs stated by the patient as well as those defined by health science. A pharmacist is dedicated to protecting the dignity of the patient. With a caring attitude and a compassionate spirit, a pharmacist focuses on serving the patient in a private and confidential manner.

III. A pharmacist respects the autonomy and dignity of each patient. A pharmacist promotes the right of self-determination and recognizes individual self-worth by encouraging patients to participate in decisions about their health. A pharmacist communicates with patients in terms that are understandable. In all cases, a pharmacist respects personal and cultural differences among patients.

IV. A pharmacist acts with honesty and integrity in professional relationships. A pharmacist has a duty to tell the truth and to act with conviction of conscience. A pharmacist avoids discriminatory practices, behavior or work conditions that impair professional judgment, and actions that compromise dedication to the best interests of patients.

V. A pharmacist maintains professional competence. A pharmacist has a duty to maintain knowledge and abilities as new medications, devices, and technologies become available and as health information advances.

VI. A pharmacist respects the values and abilities of colleagues and other health professionals. When appropriate, a pharmacist asks for the consultation of colleagues or other health professionals or refers the patient. A pharmacist acknowledges that colleagues and other health professionals may differ in the beliefs and values they apply to the care of the patient.

VII. A pharmacist serves individual, community, and societal needs. The primary obligation of a pharmacist is to individual patients. However, the obligations of a pharmacist may at times extend beyond the individual to the community and society. In these situations, the pharmacist recognizes the responsibilities that accompany these obligations and acts accordingly.

VIII. A pharmacist seeks justice in the distribution of health resources. When health resources are allocated, a pharmacist is fair and equitable, balancing the needs of patients and society.

AMERICAN PHYSICAL THERAPY ASSOCIATION

Code of Ethics

Preamble

This Code of Ethics of the American Physical Therapy Association sets forth principles for the ethical practice of physical therapy. All physical therapists are responsible for maintaining and promoting ethical practice. To this end, the physical therapist shall act in the best interest of the patient/client. This Code of Ethics shall be binding on all physical therapists.

PRINCIPLE 1. A physical therapist shall respect the rights and dignity of all individuals and shall provide compassionate care.

PRINCIPLE 2. A physical therapist shall act in a trustworthy manner towards patients/clients, and in all other aspects of physical therapy practice.

PRINCIPLE 3. A physical therapist shall comply with laws and regulations governing physical therapy and shall strive to effect changes that benefit patients/clients.

PRINCIPLE 4. A physical therapist shall exercise sound professional judgment.

PRINCIPLE 5. A physical therapist shall achieve and maintain professional competence.

PRINCIPLE 6. A physical therapist shall maintain and promote high standards for physical therapy practice, education and research.

PRINCIPLE 7. A physical therapist shall seek only such remuneration as is deserved and reasonable for physical therapy services.

PRINCIPLE 8. A physical therapist shall provide and make available accurate and relevant information to patients/clients about their care and to the public about physical therapy services.

PRINCIPLE 9. A physical therapist shall protect the public and the profession from unethical, incompetent, and illegal acts.

PRINCIPLE 10. A physical therapist shall endeavor to address the health needs of society.

PRINCIPLE 11. A physical therapist shall respect the rights, knowledge, and skills of colleagues and other health care professionals.

AMERICAN SOCIETY FOR CLINICAL LABORATORY SCIENCE
Code of Ethics

Preamble

The Code of Ethics of the American Society for Clinical Laboratory Science (ASCLS) sets forth the principles and standards by which clinical laboratory professionals practice their profession.

I. Duty to the Patient

Clinical laboratory professionals are accountable for the quality and integrity of the laboratory services they provide. This obligation includes maintaining individual competence in judgement and performance and striving to safeguard the patient from incompetent or illegal practice by others.

Clinical laboratory professionals maintain high standards of practice. They exercise sound judgment in establishing, performing and evaluating laboratory testing.

Clinical laboratory professionals maintain strict confidentiality of patient information and test results. They safeguard the dignity and privacy of patients and provide accurate information to other health care professionals about the services they provide.

II. Duty to Colleagues and the Profession

Clinical laboratory professionals uphold and maintain the dignity and respect of our profession and strive to maintain a reputation of honesty, integrity and reliability. They contribute to the advancement of the profession by improving the body of knowledge, adopting scientific advances that benefit the patient, maintaining high standards of practice and education, and seeking fair socioeconomic working conditions for members of the profession.

Clinical laboratory professionals actively strive to establish cooperative and respectful working relationships with other health care professionals with the primary objective of ensuring a high standard of care for the patients they serve.

III. Duty to Society

As practitioners of an autonomous profession, clinical laboratory professionals have the responsibility to contribute from their sphere of professional competence to the general well being of the community.

Clinical laboratory professionals comply with relevant laws and regulations pertaining to the practice of clinical laboratory science and actively seek, within the dictates of their consciences,

---

(by permission of the American Society for Clinical Laboratory Science)

to change those which do not meet the high standards of care and practice to which the profession is committed.

Pledge to the Profession

As a clinical laboratory professional, I strive to:

- Maintain and promote standards of excellence in performing and advancing the art and science of my profession
- Preserve the dignity and privacy of others
- Uphold and maintain the dignity and respect of our profession
- Seek to establish cooperative and respectful working relationships with other health professionals
- Contribute to the general well being of the community.

I will actively demonstrate my commitment to these responsibilities throughout my professional life.

AMERICAN SOCIETY OF RADIOLOGIC TECHNOLOGISTS
Code of Ethics

Preamble

Ethical professional conduct is expected of every member of the American Society of Radiologic Technologists and every individual registered by the American Registry of Radiologic Technologists. As a guide, the ASRT [American Society of Radiologic Technologists] and the ARRT [American Registry of Radiologic Technologists] have issued a code of ethics for their members and registrants. By following the principles embodied in this code, radiologic technologists will protect the integrity of the profession and enhance the delivery of patient care.

Adherence to the code of ethics is only one component of each radiologic technologist's obligation to advance the values and standards of their profession. Technologists also should take advantage of activities that provide opportunities for personal growth while enhancing their competence as caregivers. These activities may include participating in research projects, volunteering in the community, sharing knowledge with colleagues through professional meetings and conferences, serving as an advocate for the profession on legislative issues and participating in other professional development activities.

By exhibiting high standards of ethics and pursuing professional development opportunities, radiologic technologists will demonstrate their commitment to quality patient care.

Code of Ethics

- The radiologic technologist conducts himself or herself in a professional manner, responds to patient needs and supports colleagues and associates in providing quality patient care.

- The radiologic technologist acts to advance the principal objective of the profession to provide services to humanity with full respect for the dignity of mankind.

- The radiologic technologist delivers patient care and service unrestricted by concerns of personal attributes or the nature of the disease or illness, and without discrimination on the basis of sex, race, creed, religion or socio-economic status.

- The radiologic technologist practices technology founded upon theoretical knowledge and concepts, uses equipment and accessories consistent with the purpose for which they were designed and employs procedures and techniques appropriately.

- The radiologic technologist assesses situations; exercises care, discretion and judgment; assumes responsibility for professional decisions; and acts in the best interest of the patient.

- The radiologic technologist acts as an agent through observation and communication to obtain pertinent information for the physician to aid in the diagnosis and treatment of the patient and recognizes that interpretation and diagnosis are outside the scope of practice for the profession.

- The radiologic technologist uses equipment and accessories, employs techniques and procedures, performs services in accordance with an accepted standard of practice and demonstrates expertise in minimizing radiation exposure to the patient, self and other members of the health care team.

- The radiologic technologist practices ethical conduct appropriate to the profession and protects the patient's right to quality radiologic technology care.

- The radiologic technologist respects confidences entrusted in the course of professional practice, respects the patient's right to privacy and reveals confidential information only as required by law or to protect the welfare of the individual or the community.

The radiologic technologist continually strives to improve knowledge and skills by participating in continuing education and professional activities, sharing knowledge with colleagues and investigating new aspects of professional practice.

Glossary

Act utilitarianism: The doctrine that skips any reference to principles and rules and judges the right action be the one that brings the greatest happiness to the greatest number.

Active euthanasia: Actively assisting the process of death.

Acupuncture: A standard treatment modality for traditional Chinese medicine in which needles are inserted into the skin to assist the energy flow throughout the body.

Ad litem: A guardian ad litem is a person given the power and duty to act on behalf of another, for example, a legally incapacitated person, for purposes of a lawsuit.

Advanced directives: Documents that relate your wishes in regard to treatment options or in regard to who should make the decisions for you should you lose the ability to relate these matters yourself.

AIDS: Acquired immunodeficiency syndrome; generally accepted as a collection of specific, life-threatening, opportunistic infections that result from an underlying immune deficiency.

Agape: An ethical theory based on the principle of love for humanity, general goodwill. From the Greek *agape*, altruistic love.

Allele: A variant form of a given gene, which may determine a trait such as having type O or type A blood.

Altruism: Concern for the welfare of others; selflessness.

Amoral: To be without morals; neither moral nor immoral.

Authentic decision: A decision in keeping with the individual's past choices and known preferences.

Autonomous: Independent, self-governing, self-determining.

Autonomy: Personal self-determination; the right of patients to participate in and decide questions involving their care.

Beneficence: The principle that imposes on the practitioner a duty to seek the good for patients under all circumstances.

Benevolent deception: The view that one can lie to a patient for his own good. It is the mechanism most often used when paternalism is advanced over patient autonomy.

Best-interest standard: A proxy decision-making standard in which the guardian is directed to make the decision in the best interest of the individual; often used in cases in which the individual was never in a position to make an autonomous decision.

Biological life: Life that separates the living from the nonliving (e.g., that separates plants from rocks). Life in this sense is not uniquely human but is that which we share with all other living things.

Born Alive Infant Protection Act: This law states that infants born alive, at any stage of development, and regardless of circumstances of birth are persons and entitled to equal protection under the law.

Categorical imperative: The statement formulated by Immanuel Kant that one is obligated to act on that principle that is binding for all people, in all situations, at all times.

Classism: The doctrine that holds that one particular social class of persons is superior to another.

Clear and convincing evidence standard: Following the Nancy Cruzan case, the courts have asked for clear and convincing evidence of the individual's wishes in regard to continuing or ceasing life support. This has created a new emphasis on the need of advanced directives.

Code of ethics: A document usually created by a profession that provides guidelines for the ethical behavior of its membership. These documents are often seen as meeting the self-regulating criteria for a profession.

Cognitive sapient state: A condition in which the individual has the ability to reason.

Competency: Having the ability to make sound, authentic judgments for oneself. Usually this means that the patient is able to understand the nature of the condition, the options available, and the risks involved in the potential options.

Conceptus (single-celled zygote): The union of spermatozoon and an ovum at conception.

Confidentiality: The principle that binds the practitioner to hold in strict confidence those things learned about a patient in the course of medical practice.

Consequence-oriented system (teleological perspective): An ethical system holding that the right action is one that maximizes some good. The right thing to do in the end is based on what is the good thing to do. One cannot know what is right without an examination of the consequences.

Contractarian theory: A theory of morality that grounds all claims to rights in the principle of justice founded on collective choice.

Correlative obligations: In matters of rights, when one person has a right, others have obligations to either refrain from hindrance or provide the required goods and services associated with the right. As an example, an individual's right to autonomy creates the correlative obligation of disclosure (informed consent).

Culture shock: A high-stress situation in which one finds oneself in another culture in which former behavior patterns are ineffective and one fails to understand the basic cues of social intercourse.

Disparagement: To belittle, or criticize the skill, knowledge, or qualifications of another professional.

Distributive justice: Refers to just distribution in society, structured by various moral, legal, and cultural rules and principles.

Divine command ethics: The ethical theory that something can be known to be right and good when it is in compliance with God's will and wrong or bad when God condemns it.

Dominant gene: A gene that needs to be present in only one parent in order to have a fifty-fifty chance of affecting each child.

Do-not-resuscitate order (DNR): Those orders issued when a determination is made that the level of life that could be sustained following a resuscitative effort would be such that it would not be in the patient's best interest to perform resuscitation.

Double effect: A doctrine first stated by St. Thomas Aquinas that is commonly used to determine whether an action is morally defensible when the action has more than one consequence, usually both favorable and ill.

Duty-oriented system (deontological perspective): An ethical system that holds that the right action is one that is based on ethical principles known to be right, independent of consequences or whether they serve good ends.

Egalitarianism: A system of allocation that seeks to provide all things equally.

Egoist: One devoted to his own self-interest and advancement.

Embryo: Between two and three weeks into pregnancy and until the eighth week, the identification of the zygote as implanted into the uterine wall.

EMTALA: The Emergency Medical Treatment and Labor Act, which requires that certain emergency room services be provided upon request prior to transfer to other facilities.

Equal consideration of interest: The rule that the interests of all individuals must be considered equally. This rule, if adopted, reduces the harm and scapegoating possible in otherwise hedonistic ethical systems such as utilitarianism.

Ethical dilemma: Any situation that forces us to choose in a way that involves breaking some ethical norm or contradicting some ethical value.

Ethics: Critical reflections about morality and the rational analysis of it. In some sense, *ethics* is a generic term for the study of how we make judgments regarding right and wrong.

Ethnocentric: Belief in the superiority of one's own ethnic group's customs and traditions and a preference for it when considering other traditions.

Etiquette: Any special code of behavior or courtesies.

Eugenics: The study of methods for controlling the characteristics of future human populations through selective breeding.

Euthanasia: Bringing about the death of a person who is suffering from an incurable disease or condition actively, as by administering a lethal drug, or passively, by allowing the person to die by withholding treatment.

Fetus: The unborn offspring of a viviparous animal after it has attained the particular form of the species.

Fiduciary relationship: A special relationship of loyalty and responsibility formed between the patient and practitioner. The practitioner will act with scrupulous good faith and candor. The patient has the right to believe that the practitioner will maintain a higher level of accountability in regard to health care than that expected from most other relationships.

Filial piety: Pertaining to or befitting a son or daughter; respect for parents. In cultures influenced by Confucianism, this was perhaps the highest duty. One example often given is the parent who allows his child to starve so that food is available for the grandparents.

Formal justice: The ethical concern of formal justice is that the criteria are applied equally to all similar cases. Formal justice does not tell us whether the criteria are relevant or ethically valid, only that they are equally applied.

Futile care: Care that has no efficacy or potential for benefit.

Gaming the system: A generic term used for a series of activities designed to get around the system (e.g., adjusting a diagnosis so as to receive the highest potential for payment).

Gatekeeping: A whole series of activities needed to protect the profession from those who would misuse the appropriate functions of that specialty (e.g., the requirement that one professional report the misconduct of another). The term is also used commonly in managed care situations to describe the monitoring system used to ensure compliance with the particular plans or guidelines.

Gene therapy: The treatment of genetic diseases by the administration of genes to correct an absent or defective gene.

Genetic carriers: A person who carries a defective gene that, when combined in reproduction with a similar one from another person, may yield a genetic defect. A carrier does not exhibit symptoms of the disease.

Genetic disease: A disease affected by an individual's genes.

Genetic predisposition: A genetically determined susceptibility to certain health problems. It does not cause the disease itself but, in combination with behavioral and environmental factors, can increase a person's chances of getting a certain disease.

Genome: The complete genetic makeup of a species. The complete set of genes in the chromosomes of each cell of a particular organism.

Harm principle: When the practitioner can foresee a danger to an individual who is outside the patient-provider relationship, potentially caused by the patient, the harm principle provides the rationale for breaching confidentiality to warn the vulnerable individual.

Health Insurance Portability and Accountability Act (HIPAA): Legislation enacted in 1996 to encourage the use of electronic transmission of health information (to assist in cost containment) to provide new safeguards for protecting the security and confidentiality of the information.

Hedonism: The doctrine that holds that the chief good of humans lies in the pursuit of pleasure and the avoidance of personal pain.

Heterozygous: Children inherit one allele from each parent. When the child has one, say, for sickle cell anemia, and one that is normal, we say the child is heterozygous.

High-risk behaviors: A series of behaviors associated with the spread of AIDS infections.

Holistic: Emphasizing the importance of the whole and the interdependence of the parts.

Homozygous: When a child possesses two identical alleles (one from each parent) for a variant gene, the child is homozygous.

Hospice movement: The development of centers for providing palliative care for the terminally ill that focus on the process of relieving pain and suffering.

Impaired colleague: A colleague who can no longer function appropriately within the specialty. This may be due to illness or the use of substances such as alcohol or drugs.

Imperfect obligations: Claims that do not create obligations. An example is the duty to be compassionate or charitable. While we can sense these as obligations, their time and place of performance are left to autonomous choice.

Informed consent: In order for patients to be truly autonomous, they must understand the nature of the condition, the treatment options, and the risks involved. This information forms the basis for informed consent.

Institutional review boards: Review boards that examine the protocol design for research to ensure that the research conforms to appropriate standards for humans.

Involuntary euthanasia: Bringing about the death of someone suffering from terminal illness or intractable pain without the request or consent of the individual.

Joint venturing: In common usage, the situation in which a health professional has an investment interest in a health care facility.

Justice: The basic principle that deals with fairness, just deserts, and entitlements in the distribution of goods and services.

Legal requirements: Requirements proper or sufficient to be recognized by the law; justiciable in the courts.

Legal rights: A power, privilege, or immunity guaranteed under a constitution, statutes, or decisional laws.

Libertarianism: A system of allocation that is generally based on the free market exchange of goods and services.

Material justice: The ethical concern of material justice is that the criteria used in allocation be relevant and ethically valid.

Material risk: A risk or hazard of sufficient significance as to be included within the informed disclosure by the physician. The decision of material risk is made on the basis of whether the information would be significant enough to influence the patient's decision.

Mean: The middle point, the moderate position, the position between extremes.

Medicaid: Title XIX of the Social Security Act, which authorizes federal matching funds to assist the states in providing health care for certain low-income groups.

Medical utility: The allocation of scarce resources to those with the best prognosis.

Medicide: Suggested by Dr. Kevorkian, creation of a new medical specialty with the function of terminating life.

Melting pot: The concept that immigrants come to the United States and they and their culture are mixed in and assimilated into the American culture. *E pluribus unum* (from many, one) is an expression of the concept.

Mercy killing: Active euthanasia, in which the intent is to ease the dying process or end intractable pain.

Monogenic: A disease caused by a single gene.

Moral: Of or concerned with the judgment principles of right and wrong in relation to human actions and character.

Moral duty: An act or course of action that is required by one on the basis of moral position.

Moral option: The power or right to choose among several alternatives on the basis of a moral question.

Morality: The doctrine of moral duties; quality of an action in regard to right and wrong.

Moxibustion: A treatment modality in traditional Chinese medicine in which an herb is burned at select points on the skin so that the energy flow through the body can be enhanced.

Natural rights: Rights that grow out of the nature of man and are necessary to fulfill the ends to which nature calls him, as distinguished from those that are created by law and depend upon civilized society.

Nihilism: A doctrine that all values are meaningless and that nothing is knowable; a rejection of all previous theories of morality.

Nonmaleficence: The principle that imposes the duty to avoid or refrain from harming the patient. The practitioner who cannot bring about good for the patient is bound by duty to at least avoid harm.

Ordinary and extraordinary care: A differentiation used to determine what level of care is ordinary and therefore required, and to differentiate this from that level of care that might be considered extraordinary and therefore optional due to high costs, low effectiveness, or other criteria.

Original position: An imagined state in which individuals make choices under a veil of ignorance, as to the natural attributes and social status of the individuals involved. In this situation, no one making the choice would know what place he would play in the society; he could be a prince or a pauper. Under these conditions, all choices are made so that even the individual who is in the most disadvantaged position would be willing to accept the decision.

Palliative care: Care designed to provide relief from pain and suffering rather than cure.

Parens patria: Originates in English common law, whereby the king had the authority to act as guardian for persons with legal disabilities. In the United States, the parens patria function belongs to the states.

Passive euthanasia: Ceasing therapies that prolong life so that death can occur.

Paternalism: The belief that one should, on the basis of doing good for the patient, limit the patients' personal autonomy. In the best sense, it is a conflict between the basic principles of autonomy and beneficence.

Patient advocate: One who investigates and mediates patients' problems and complaints in relation to the health care services.

Patient-centered standard: A standard holding that the information needed is that required by the individual to make a rational judgment. This would be a very subjective stand, given that some patients may not meet the criteria of a hypothetical reasonable person.

Patient Self-Determination Act of 1990 (PSDA): Mandates that all health care providers receiving federal reimbursements for services provide information to each patient and offer the option of initiating an advanced directive.

Perfect obligations: Claims that justify and create correlative obligations. The right to informed consent is a perfect obligation in that it creates the correlative obligations of providing appropriate information.

Persistent vegetative state (PVS): A state characterized by a permanent eyes-open level of unconsciousness.

Person: A living entity with moral standing, legal rights, and duties (not necessarily equivalent to human).

Personhood: The individual state in which one is accepted as having the criterion of humanity; an entity possessing moral standing, with legal rights and duties.

Placebos: Substances thought to be biologically inert that are given to patients so as to make them believe that they are getting medication. Although useful as a research practice, the clinical use of placebos creates problems in the areas of patient autonomy and the duty of truth telling.

Polygenic: A disease caused by a combination of genes.

Principle of double effect: A doctrine, first stated by St. Thomas Aquinas, that is commonly used to determine whether an action is morally defensible when it has more than one consequence, usually both favorable and ill.

Principle of utility: The principle that holds that the right action is the one leading to satisfaction of those desires that the individual prefers to have satisfied.

Professional autonomy: Once a patient–health care professional relationship is established, the practitioner has a duty to provide care but is not obliged to perform services that he or she finds morally repugnant. Health care providers may, under such circumstances, withdraw from their obligations to provide services.

Professional code of ethics: A document usually created by the profession that provides guidelines for the ethical behavior of its membership. These documents are often seen as meeting the self-regulating criteria by which professions are defined.

Professional community standard: A standard stating that the amount of care or amount of disclosure provided should be judged appropriate if it is equal to that provided by other practitioners in the local community.

Quickening: The point at which the mother feels the fetus move.

Reasonable patient standard: A standard that holds that the physician must provide enough information to the patient so that a hypothetical reasonable person could understand and make autonomous decisions.

Recessive gene: A gene that must be present in both parents for a child to inherit it. On average, when both parents are carriers, the child will have a one-in-four chance of being free of the gene altogether.

Recipient rights: Rights that provide an interest or title in an object or property; a just and legal claim to hold, use, or enjoy it, or to convey or donate it, as one may please. This form of right is often called a positive right, which provides a claim to goods or services.

Recombinant DNA: The practice of altering DNA by splicing parts of one into another.

Red-tagged: A term used to indicate a do-not-resuscitate order.

Regenerative medicine: A term used to describe advancements in medicine based on the opportunities to regenerate tissues. The term is often used in connection with discussions of stem cells and cloning as possible avenues for medical advancement.

Relativism: The doctrine that truth is not an absolute but is relative to the individual or group that holds the belief.

Right: A justified claim that demands respect.

Right to privacy: The right to be left alone; the right of a person to be free from unwarranted publicity.

Role fidelity: Each specialty in health care has a prescribed role of practice. Role fidelity is the faithful practice of the duties contained in the particular practice. Role fidelity forms the basis for the ethical system known as virtue ethics.

Rule utilitarianism: The doctrine that certain rules have been found to have a high utility, that is, have brought about the greatest happiness for the greatest number. The rule utilitarian justifies actions by appealing to universal rules such as "Thou shalt not steal," which are justified by the principle of utility.

Safe harbor rules: Rules that allow a questionable practice such as self-referral to continue due to the special circumstances of a particular case whereby the practice serves the patient's interests.

Safe sex: A series of practices designed to be used in sexual contact that does not spread sexually transmitted diseases. The most important aspect of these practices is the use of condoms.

Scope of practice: The tasks that are included within the practice of a specialty. Often the scope of practice is set forth in the legal regulations that allow the practice within a state. Scope of practice is an important consideration in the determination of questions regarding role fidelity.

Self-referral: A process in which a patient or the patient's family is introduced to additional health resources in the community in which the referring practitioner has a financial interest.

Social utility: The allocation of scarce resources to those who are most useful or valued by the society.

Speciesism: Discrimination based solely on one's membership in a species.

Standard precautions: Techniques adopted by health care providers that provide a barrier for acquiring AIDS. These are protective measures against contamination by blood or body secretions.

Stem cells: Immature cells that function as blank slates capable of becoming any cell of the body.

Substituted-judgment standard: A proxy decision-making standard whereby the guardian is directed to make the decision compatible with the previous wishes of the individual.

Therapeutic privilege: The right of the health care practitioner to provide care for patients without informed consent. Generally, these are rare cases in circumstances that involve emergency care, incompetent patients, or in which sound medical judgment dictates that the truth would be a greater harm to the patient than the overcoming of his or her personal autonomy.

Third-party payers: Agencies such as insurance companies or governmental programs that are called on to pay for health care services.

Triage: A system that divides the patient cases into categories so that care can be allocated effectively.

Utilitarianism: The doctrine that utility is the sole standard of moral conduct; the doctrine of the greatest happiness for the greatest number.

Utilization review: A review of the appropriateness of care and the various types of patient care provided within an institution. It is usually designed to ensure appropriate and cost-effective care.

Value: A principle, personal standard, or quality considered worthwhile or desirable.

Value cohort: A group of individuals who experience a particular set of historical events and are values programmed or shaped by the events as a group. For example, those who experienced the great depression of the 1930s often share the same values toward thrift and poverty.

Veracity: Truth telling. The practice of health care is best served in a relationship of trust in which practitioner and patient are bound to the truth.

Viability: The stage at which the fetus can live independent of the mother's body.

Virtue ethics (aretaic): Virtue-based ethical systems are often called *aretaic ethics*. From the Greek word *arête*, which is translated as virtue or excellence.

Voluntary euthanasia: Actively assisting the process of death for someone who has requested assistance in the dying process.

Worldview: An individual's set of subjective values derived from his or her religious background, cultural heritage, and personal experiences.

Xenografting: The use of tissues from another species for human transplants.

Xenophobic: Undue fear or contempt for strangers or foreigners.

Zygote (multicelled zygote): Comes into being in first twenty-four hours with the splitting of the conceptus and continues until the zygote becomes implanted into the uterine wall.

Index